RECENT DEVELOPMENTS IN
ALCOHOLISM
VOLUME 13
ALCOHOL AND VIOLENCE

RECENT
DEVELOPMENTS IN

Edited by

MARC GALANTER

New York University School of Medicine
New York, New York

Associate Editors

HENRI BEGLEITER, RICHARD DEITRICH,
RICHARD FULLER, DONALD GALLANT,
DONALD GOODWIN, EDWARD GOTTHEIL,
ALFONSO PAREDES, MARCUS ROTHSCHILD,
and DAVID VAN THIEL

Assistant Editor
DEIRDE WINCZEWSKI

An Official Publication of the American Society of Addiction Medicine
and the Research Society on Alcoholism.
This series was founded by the National Council on Alcoholism.

ALCOHOLISM

VOLUME 13
ALCOHOL AND VIOLENCE

Epidemiology
Neurobiology
Psychology
Family Issues

PLENUM PRESS • NEW YORK AND LONDON

The Library of Congress has catalogued this work as follows:

Recent developments in alcoholism: an official publication of the American Medical Society on
Alcoholism, and the Research Society on Alcoholism, and the National Council on Alcoholism—Vol.
1——New York: Plenum Press, c1983–
   v.: ill.; 25 cm.
   Cataloging in publication.
   Editor: Marc Galanter.
   ISSN 0738-422X = Recent developments in alcoholism.

   1. Alcoholism—Periodicals. I. Galanter, Marc. II. American Medical Society on Alcoholism. III.
Research Society on Alcohol (U.S.) IV. National Council on Alcoholism. [DNLM:
1. Alcoholism—periodicals. W1 RE106AH(P)]

HV5001.R4	616.86'1'05—dc19	83-643791
Library of Congress	[8311]	AACR 2 MARC-S

ISBN 0-306-45358-4

© 1997 Plenum Press, New York
A Division of Plenum Publishing Corporation
233 Spring Street, New York, N. Y. 10013

http://www.plenum.com

10 9 8 7 6 5 4 3 2 1

Contributors

Nancy Asdigian, Family Research Laboratory, University of New Hampshire, Durham, New Hampshire 03824

Ronet Bachman, Department of Sociology, University of Delaware, Newark, Delaware 19716

D. Caroline Blanchard, Bekesy Laboratory of Neurobiology, Department of Anatomy and Reproductive Biology, University of Hawaii at Manoa, Honolulu, Hawaii 96822

Robert J. Blanchard, Department of Psychology, Bekesy Laboratory of Neurobiology, University of Hawaii at Manoa, Honolulu, Hawaii 96822

Jenia Bober Booth, Laboratory for the Study of Addictions and UCLA Drug Abuse Research Center, West Los Angeles Veterans Administration, Los Angeles, California 90073

Brad J. Bushman, Department of Psychology, Iowa State University, Ames, Iowa 50011-3180

Cheryl J. Cherpitel, Alcohol Research Group, Western Consortium for Public Health, Berkeley, California 94709

Mark A. Cohen, Owen Graduate School of Management, and Vanderbilt Institute for Public Policy Studies, Vanderbilt University, Nashville, Tennessee 37212

James J. Collins, Health and Social Policy Division, Research Triangle Institute, Research Triangle Park, North Carolina 27709-2194

Joseph F. DeBold, Department of Psychology, Tufts University, Medford, Massachusetts 02155

Richard A. Deitrich, Department of Pharmacology, Alcohol Research Center, University of Colorado Health Sciences Center, Denver, Colorado 80262

M. Elena Denison, Laboratory for the Study of Addictions and UCLA Drug Abuse Research Center, West Los Angeles Veterans Administration, Los Angeles, California 90073

James H. Derzon, Vanderbilt Institute for Public Policy Studies, Vanderbilt University, Nashville, Tennessee 37212

William R. Downs, Center for the Study of Adolescence, University of Northern Iowa, Cedar Falls, Iowa 50614

Annemoon M. M. van Erp, Department of Psychology, Tufts University, Medford, Massachusetts 02155

Richard K. Fuller, Division of Clinical and Prevention Research, National Institute on Alcohol Abuse and Alcoholism, Bethesda, Maryland 20892-7003

Edward Gottheil, Department of Psychiatry and Human Behavior, Thomas Jefferson University, Philadelphia, Pennsylvania 19107

Ellen F. Gottheil, Department of Psychiatry and Behavioral Sciences, University of Washington Medical School, Seattle, Washington 98195

J. Andy Henrie, Department of Chemistry, University of Hawaii at Manoa, Honolulu, Hawaii 96822

J. Dee Higley, Laboratory of Clinical Studies, Primate Unit, National Institute on Alcohol Abuse and Alcoholism, Poolesville, Maryland 20837

Glenda Kaufman Kantor, Family Research Laboratory, University of New Hampshire, Durham, New Hampshire 03824

Larry A. Kroutil, Health and Social Policy Division, Research Triangle Institute, Research Triangle Park, North Carolina 27709-2194

W. Vernon Lee, Penn Recovery Systems, Philadelphia, Pennsylvania 19104-1953

Markku Linnoila, Laboratory of Clinical Studies, Division of Intramural Clinical and Biological Research, National Institute on Alcohol Abuse and Alcoholism, Bethesda, Maryland 20892-1256

Mark W. Lipsey, Vanderbilt Institute for Public Policy Studies, Vanderbilt University, Nashville, Tennessee 37212

Eugene Maguin, Research Institute on Addictions, Buffalo, New York 14203

Susan Ehrlich Martin, Prevention Research Branch, Division of Clinical and Prevention Research, National Institute on Alcohol Abuse and Alcoholism, Rockville, Maryland 20892-7003

Klaus A. Miczek, Departments of Psychology, Psychiatry, and Pharmacology, Tufts University, Medford, Massachusetts, 02155

Brenda A. Miller, Research Institute on Addictions, Buffalo, New York 14203

Marlee Moore-Gurrera, Health and Social Policy Division, Research Triangle Institute, Research Triangle Park, North Carolina 27709-2194

Alfonso Paredes, Laboratory for the Study of Addictions and UCLA Drug Abuse Research Center, West Los Angeles Veterans Administration, Los Angeles, California 90073

Judith Roizen, Institute of Population Studies, University of Exeter, Exeter EX4 6DT, England

E. Joyce Roland, Health and Social Policy Division, Research Triangle Institute, Research Triangle Park, North Carolina 27709-2194

Walter Tornatzky, Department of Psychology, Tufts University, Medford, Massachusetts 02155

Matti Virkkunen, Department of Psychiatry, Helsinki University Central Hospital, Helsinki 00180, Finland

Stephen P. Weinstein, Department of Psychiatry and Human Behavior, Thomas Jefferson University, Philadelphia, Pennsylvania 19107

Helene Raskin White, Center for Alcohol Studies, Rutgers University, Piscataway, New Jersey 08855-0969

David B. Wilson, Vanderbilt Institute for Public Policy Studies, Vanderbilt University, Nashville, Tennessee 37212

Errol Yudko, Department of Psychology, University of Hawaii at Manoa, Honolulu, Hawaii 96822

Preface

From the President of the Research Society on Alcoholism

On behalf of the Research Society on Alcoholism, I am pleased to introduce this thirteenth volume of *Recent Developments in Alcoholism* about alcohol and violence. Current concepts are presented in well-organized sections that focus on epidemiology, neurobiology, psychology, and family issues. It is becoming increasingly clear that age, gender, socioeconomic circumstances, and genetics affect aggressive behavior and vulnerability to alcoholism. This volume contains up-to-date discussions of these issues. Indeed, the information presented here will help all alcohol researchers to identify biological and social factors that contribute to the comorbidity of alcoholism and aggression. The editors and associate editors should be congratulated for bringing together such important information. This volume will be a valuable resource for investigators and therapists alike.

Ivan Diamond M.D., Ph.D.
President, Research Society on Alcoholism

From the President of the American Society of Addiction Medicine

The American Society of Addiction Medicine is honored to continue its cosponsorship with the Research Society on Alcoholism of *Recent Developments in Alcoholism*. The topic of alcohol and violence is a particularly timely one, given the growing number of studies that are examining the relationship between the two. These studies are consistent with the hypothesis that alcohol can increase aggression and contribute to both domestic and criminal violence. Intoxicating blood levels of alcohol have been found to be especially prevalent in those injured in fights and assaults. Despite this growing body of evidence, there still is a great deal to be learned about what causes alcoholics to become aggressive and violent. Additional resesarch is also needed relative to self-directed violence and suicide in relation to alcohol. This volume on alcohol and violence ranges from epidemiology and neurobiology to psychology and family issues and will make an important addition to the body of knowledge relative to this complex phenomenon.

David E. Smith, M.D.
President, American Society of Addiction Medicine

Contents

I. Epidemiology

Richard K. Fuller, Section Editor

Overview
Richard K. Fuller

Chapter 1

Epidemiological Issues in Alcohol-Related Violence
Judith Roizen

Chapter 2

The Relationship of Alcohol to Injury in Assault Cases
Susan Ehrlich Martin and Ronet Bachman

Chapter 3

Alcohol and Spouse Abuse: Ethnic Differences
Glenda Kaufman Kantor

Chapter 4

**Longitudinal Perspective on Alcohol Use and Aggression
during Adolescence**
   Helene Raskin White

Chapter 5

Alcohol and Violence-Related Injuries in the Emergency Room
   Cheryl J. Cherpitel

II. Neurobiology

Richard A. Deitrich, Section Editor

Overview
Richard A. Deitrich

Chapter 8

Serotonin in Early-Onset Alcoholism
   Matti Virkkunen and Markku Linnoila

Chapter 9

**A Nonhuman Primate Model of Excessive Alcohol Intake:
Personality and Neurobiological Parallels of Type I-
and Type II-Like Alcoholism**
   J. Dee Higley and Markku Linnoila

III. Psychology

Alfonso Paredes, Section Editor

Overview
Alfonso Paredes

Chapter 10

Effects of Alcohol on Human Aggression:
Validity of Proposed Explanations
Brad J. Bushman

Chapter 11

**Is There a Causal Relationship between Alcohol Use and Violence?
A Synthesis of Evidence**
  *Mark W. Lipsey, David B. Wilson, Mark A. Cohen,
  and James H. Derzon*

Chapter 12

Alcohol and Cocaine Interactions and Aggressive Behaviors
  M. Elena Denison, Alfonso Paredes, and Jenia Bober Booth

IV. Family Issues

Edward Gottheil and Ellen F. Gottheil, Section Editors

Overview
Edward Gottheil and Ellen F. Gottheil

Chapter 13

When Women Are under the Influence: Does Drinking or Drug Use by Women Provoke Beatings by Men?
Glenda Kaufman Kantor and Nancy Asdigian

Chapter 16

Issues in the Linkage of Alcohol and Domestic Violence Services
James J. Collins, Larry A. Kroutil, E. Joyce Roland,
and Marlee Moore-Gurrera

I

Epidemiology

Richard K. Fuller, Section Editor

Overview

Richard K. Fuller

It is both appropriate and timely that this volume of *Recent Developments in Alcoholism* is devoted to alcohol and violence, since violence is regarded by many as the most important problem facing our society today. Daily, we hear or read stories of domestic violence, child abuse, homicides, and gang violence; and the public perception is that alcohol often has an important role in these events. Epidemiological studies of perpetrators and victims of interpersonal violence indicate that alcohol has often been consumed shortly prior to the violent act. However, drinking is a common social activity for most adult Americans, particularly young males who are those most likely to commit a violent act; and "therefore it is to be expected that drinking will often occur proximate to violence."[1] A key question is whether alcohol use is coincidental to aggression or whether it plays a causal role in aggression. The consistency of the relationship between alcohol and aggression across many studies suggests that it is a real association and not spurious. Despite many studies, our understanding of the precise role of alcohol in aggression and violence is in its infancy.

At this point in time, it appears that alcohol is one of several factors leading to violence.[1] The other types of factors contributing to aggression appear to be biochemical, genetic, psychological, and environmental in nature. Other sections of this volume discuss these factors. Another key question is how does the mix of all these factors increase aggression in some individuals but not in others?[2]

The public health model may be useful in answering this question. The premise of the public health model is that alcohol-related problems arise from an interaction of individual (host) variables, alcohol (agent), and environmen-

Richard K. Fuller • Division of Clinical and Prevention Research, National Institute on Alcohol Abuse and Alcoholism, Bethesda, Maryland 20892-7003.

Recent Developments in Alcoholism, Volume 13: Alcoholism and Violence, edited by Marc Galanter. Plenum Press, New York, 1997

tal factors. Host variables include traits and life experiences that influence the individual's vulnerability to the effects of alcohol. Alcohol (the agent) varies by type, pattern of drinking, and availability. Environmental factors include interpersonal interactions, social milieus, cultural norms surrounding both the use of alcohol and aggressive behavior, and factors regulating a person's exposure to alcohol. Epidemiology is one of the disciplines that generates knowledge for the public health model.

In Chapter 1, Dr. Roizen discusses that epidemiological studies of alcohol and violence can be divided into two categories: event-based studies and general population studies. Event-based studies are based on samples of perpetrators or victims of the violent event. In her discussion of event-based studies, Dr. Roizen focuses on the role of alcohol in one type of violent act, i.e., rape. An example of a general population study is the one described in Chapter 2, by Drs. Martin and Bachman. General population studies use samples drawn from a community, county, state, region, or country to determine the prevalence of alcohol-related violent behavior. Dr. Roizen's discussion indicates that both of these types of studies have limitations.

While alcohol is frequently consumed prior to acts of violence, the lack of a comparison group in some event-based studies makes the interpretation of the results difficult, if not meaningless. Another methodological problem for event-based studies is the selection of an appropriate control group. Is the person who lives next door an appropriate "control" for a habitual child molester?[3]

Other methodological criticisms of event-based studies include use of samples of convenience, which results in sample selection bias, and subjects in these studies may not be representative of all violent offenders, victims, or their drinking patterns. Furthermore, since these studies are cross-sectional, they do not allow causal inferences about the relationship between alcohol and aggression.

As Roizen points out in Chapter 1, population surveys also have limitations. Population samples, even good ones, may miss the small segment of the population given to violence. A limitation to both types of studies is that those interviewed may have selective recall or be reluctant to admit to deviant acts. Dr. Roizen selects one population study to discuss in detail. She selected the study done in Thunder Bay, Ontario, by Kai Pernanen because of its methodological rigor.

Another limitation of epidemiological studies is that if there are a number of variables related to aggression, the strength of the role of alcohol in the web of causation leading to aggressive behavior is not testable unless those other variables are also measured.

Like Dr. Roizen, the authors of the other chapters in Section I also discuss the limitations of the studies described in their chapters. While these limitations should lead to caution in drawing causal inferences, there is much valuable information provided by the epidemiological studies reviewed in the chapters in this section. They show that alcohol is prevalent in violent acts and they further our understanding of alcohol's role in aggression and violence by focusing on specific issues.

Kai Pernanen, who has made a life-long study of alcohol and violence, has called for data on the role of alcohol in the escalation of aggressive behavior, e.g., from verbal threats to physical violence.[4] In Chapter 2, Drs. Martin and Bachman test several hypotheses posited by Pernanen[4] by examining the role of alcohol in the escalation of hostile interactions. They review the literature and use the National Crime Victimization Survey (NCVS) to provide new information on the escalation from threat to assault without injury to assault causing injury. The NCVS is a large, nationally representative sample of the US population 12 years and older and obtains information on crimes including incidents not reported to the police.

In Chapter 3, Dr. Kaufman Kantor evaluates ethnic differences in the role of alcohol in spouse abuse. She examines the interplay among ethnicity, structural factors (e.g., poverty), and cultural factors (e.g., "machismo drinking" in Hispanic culture).

Dr. Raskin White, in Chapter 4, discusses the relationship of alcohol-related violence and ethnicity among adolescents. There have been few studies of alcohol and violence in youth per se. Dr. Raskin White reviews several models for explaining the role of alcohol in violent acts committed by adolescents and arrives at some surprising conclusions.

In Chapter 5, the final chapter of this section, Dr. Cherpitel examines the role of alcohol and drinking patterns in violent and nonviolent admissions to emergency departments. She reviews studies that used probability samples of all injured patients representative of those served by these facilities.

Studies such as those presented in the section contribute to our understanding of the role of alcohol in aggression and violence. This epidemiologic knowledge, when integrated with the knowledge derived from other disciplines, can provide the basis for designing prevention strategies to reduce the violence that is related to alcohol use.

References

1. Collins JJ, Messerschmidt MA: Epidemiology of alcohol-related violence. *Alcohol Health Res World* 17:93–100, 1993.
2. Gordis E: Alcohol, aggression, and injury. *Alcohol Health Res World* 17:91, 1993.
3. Roizen J: Issues in the epidemiology of alcohol and violence, in Martin SE (ed): *Alcohol and Interpersonal Violence: Fostering Multidisciplinary Perspectives* (DHHS NIH Publication No. 93-3496). Washington, DC, US Government Printing Office, 1993, pp 3–36.
4. Pernanen K: *Alcohol in Human Violence.* New York, Guilford Press, 1991.

Epidemiological Issues in Alcohol-Related Violence

Judith Roizen

Abstract. Epidemiological research on alcohol and violence exhibits a number of methodological limitations. This is the case whether it is event based (i.e., based on samples of victims and/or perpetrators of violence) or based on samples of the general population. The chapter identifies some of the limitations that confront researchers, policymakers, and other end-users of the research. The methodological issues are illustrated by exploring one type of violent event—rape—and one general population study—Kai Pernanen's research on alcohol-related violence in a Canadian community. It is argued that epidemiological research would benefit from further qualitative research on the natural history of violent events.

1. Defining the Problem

1.1. Introduction: The Six Dilemmas

In this chapter and the longer work from which it is drawn,[1] I review a number of studies on alcohol and violence that come under the umbrella of epidemiological research. I take a very broad view of what is meant by "epidemiological," often looking at small populations and at analyses rarely carried out by an epidemiologist or with the rigor of epidemiological research at its best. The work reviewed here is among the best empirical research on alcohol and violence from North America. These are studies of different populations that contribute to our knowledge of the distribution and correlates of alcohol-related violence. The chapter focuses on alcohol use in violent events rather

Judith Roizen • Institute of Population Studies, University of Exeter, Exeter EX4 6DT, England.

Recent Developments in Alcoholism, Volume 13: Alcoholism and Violence, edited by Marc Galanter. Plenum Press, New York, 1997

than the chronic alcohol problems of those who are violent or the relationship between alcohol use and abuse and criminal careers. Table I shows the range in percentages of alcohol-present cases in studies based on violent events and, for comparative purposes, other untoward and serious events. The width of the ranges in the proportion of alcohol-present cases in different studies is the result of a number of factors. These include variable definitions of alcohol use and the violent behavior itself, inconsistent attention to alcohol in the event, and small sample sizes. The fact that there are few definitive studies in this area and that studies are of uneven quality means that a close look at each study reviewed is needed rather than the more usual concise review of many studies.

Readers seeking to draw conclusions about alcohol and violence from epidemiological research will find themselves caught in a number of dilemmas. First, despite decades of research on these problems and although alcohol use often precedes violence, we still know little about alcohol's role in violent behavior. Much of the evidence on which judgment will depend comes from data collected for entirely other purposes, such as data collected in police reports or emergency room intake forms. Yet, purposive research is expensive and there is very little theoretically guided empirical work to build on. Even after many decades of research on alcohol and violence, Pernanen[2] has asserted,

> For the time being, we still need a much firmer empirical foothold, in order to assess the validity of the relationship between alcohol use and violence in potentially less biased samples of violence episodes and of actors in these episodes than those available in official documents. We need information on the potential role of alcohol in the choice of different types of violent acts and in escalations in seriousness of aggression and physical violence, as well as in the use of indiscriminate aggression in partial or total obliviousness to the nature of the victim, the setting, and the general social context.

In relation to a social problem as important as alcohol and child abuse, Leonard and Jacob have concluded,[3]

> A final difficulty worth noting is simply the paucity of literature attempting to examine this issue. Few studies have been conducted and most of these have methodological problems. . . . Additionally, these few child abuse studies are frequently concerned with only one or two specific forms of child abuse, thus rendering comparisons between studies or conclusions regarding one specific form of abuse difficult to make.

We know that an alcohol presence in violent events does not necessarily mean that alcohol affected the behavior of any of the participants. And more than half of violent crimes and other incidents of violence do not involve alcohol use by the victim or the offender. Further, as is the case in much epidemiological research, the precise mechanism for a relationship between the independent and dependent variables is not known, and there is no gen-

Table I. Summary of Studies Reporting Alcohol Presence[a] at the Time of the Event (in percent)

	Number of studies	Range
Casualty		
Accidents (nontraffic)		
Fatal		
Aviation	15	0.7–44
Drowning	14	12–80
Fire/burns	19	9–83
Falls	8	17–70
Work	1	15
Other accidents	7	9–45
Coroners' studies	13	14–64
Nonfatal		
Fire/burns	7	12–62
Falls	3	13–25
Work	2	1–16
Other accidents	5	21–83
Emergency room/trauma studies	3	23–63
Traffic accidents		
Fatal		
Drivers	33	32–64
Passengers	8	16–49
Pedestrians	26	21–83
Motorcycle	8	25–63
Drivers		
Single vehicle	19	41–72
Multivehicle	15	18–51
Responsible		
All fatal accidents	6	45–75
Multivehicle accidents	3	31–44
Nonresponsible	3	7–12
Nonfatal		
Drivers	6	3–25
Crime		
Arrested populations		
Homicide offenders	13	28–86
Assault offenders	3	24–37
Robbery offenders	3	7–72
Sex offenders	18	13–60
Homicide victims	29	14–87
Assault victims	5	25–60
Robbery victims	2	12–16
Sex victims	5	6–40
Prison populations		
Offenders	17	14–100
Suicide		
Attempters	6	30–70
Completers	13	18–66

continued

Table I. Continued

	Number of studies	Range
Casualty		
Accidents (nontraffic)		
Fatal		
Family abuse		
Marital violence (men's drinking)	6	6–57
Marital violence (women's drinking)	2	10–27
Child abusers/neglecters	1	13
Child molesters	6	32–54

*a*Studies use measures such as BACs, police reports of driving, witness reports, self reports.

eral agreement about which alcohol effects might be operating. More is written about the possible contributions alcohol might make to violent and criminal behavior than is written from research that attempts to establish whether there is an empirical relationship and what that relationship might be. Alcohol's presence is often considered presumptive of a causal relationship.

The second dilemma that we face is the lack of cumulation in work on alcohol and violence generally and in important specific areas such as alcohol and rape or family violence. Research is scattered among disciplines, journals, and countries. If one could characterize an area of research as very "preparadigmatic,"[4] this would be it. The task in reviewing this work is to try to glean findings from work that springs from little or no common base. The process of gleaning results from disparate studies of uneven quality means that there cannot be the usual overview. We can learn something from these studies only by taking a pointillist view, observing small parts in relation to the whole.

The third dilemma that we confront in relation to research in this area is that social research in the last two decades or so has become increasingly complex. Looking for multiple causes of attitudes and behavior and using multivariate methods for examining these potential causes have become part of the stock-in-trade of the social scientist. Behavior was ever this complex, but it is now recognized that we are no longer looking for a single or direct cause of complex behavior. Good research of the last 15 years acknowledges this in design and analysis, but the consequences are rarely explored. First, the messiness involved in interpreting multivariate findings means that there will be no simple or single consequence for policymakers. Correlatively, this raises the question of how research on social problems should be divided among administrative agencies and research groups.

For example, over the last two decades, as those looking at alcohol problems were slowly coming to grips with the multivariate causes of untoward behavior, drugs became more frequently implicated in many of the behaviors that we were seeking to understand. In Collins' 1981 book[5] on alcohol and crime, drugs other than alcohol played a small part in our analyses. Drug use is now present in violent behavior, especially criminal behavior, to a degree that makes it questionable whether it is sensible to look at alcohol and violence apart from other drugs. The work of the Drug Use Forecasting group shows that 59% of arrestees for violent crimes had been using drugs, often in conjunction with alcohol, in the days prior to the offense. A good case can be made that it is not just criminal violence that shows this drug presence but much other violent behavior as well. R. Room (personal communication, 1993), however, has argued against including drugs routinely in research on alcohol and crime on the grounds that the "alcohol will get lost" due to the often greater attention to drug problems where both are under investigation. Perhaps this need for the separation of in-depth investigation of alcohol and drug problems in part reflects the fact that administrative control over research and policy on alcohol and drugs is divided among different agencies with differing agendas. But it is also symptomatic of the increasing difficulty we have in handling multivariate explanations of social problems.

The fourth dilemma, related to the third, arises because we live in a multivariate world in which our improved methods of social analysis have capabilities beyond what the data will usually support. In part this is because it is generally easier to develop new analytic methodologies than to find new ways of measuring behavior. It is, in part, linked to the allocation of prestige in disciplines. As Stinchcombe has argued,[6]

> the higher the prestige of a piece of sociological work, the less people [who are analyzed in it] are sweaty, laughing, ugly or pretty, dull at parties, or have warts on their noses. . . . If we range theories from the prolix fashion of Herbert Blumer—who knows how people will define the situation and consequently what they will do—to the lean and spare rational actors models that allow us to use maximization mathematical methods to specify at least one feature of the behavior exactly (e.g., what the net profit will be), it is the theories that are most divorced from blood, sweat and tears that have highest prestige.

It is a conclusion of many who write on alcohol and violence (e.g., Pernanen,[2] Collins,[7] Roizen[8]) that we need to know a great deal more about what actually happens in violent situations: Who does what to whom and for what reasons. This means systematic, in part, qualitative, studies to find out how people actually act in situations that result in violence. There is often little prestige in this and nothing exotic in looking at the natural history of events that affect the people next door.

The fifth dilemma is that the police, courts, and medical professionals need to make judgments about alcohol's role in violence at a time when we actually know relatively little about it. Murphy et al.,[9] examining the relationship between substance abuse and child abuse on behalf of the agencies concerned with child protection in Boston, frustratedly argued,

> Orme and Rimmer's 1981 review[10] of the research on alcoholism and child abuse concluded that the studies done up until that time had failed to provide the empirical data necessary to support the association between

alcoholism and child abuse. . . . Although from a scientific point of view it is important to maintain this methodological skepticism, it is equally important to note that from a practical point of view, courts, protective workers, and clinicians are called upon to make decisions about the welfare of children even when definitive evidence about the impact of factors like substance abuse is not available. It is important to keep in mind that the majority of the previous studies as well as prevailing legal and clinical opinion agree that untreated, serious substance abuse plays a clear role in increased levels of risk for child mistreatment.

They go on to assert, despite the limited empirical evidence, that

Substance abuse has been so clearly and consistently associated with child mistreatment that the Boston Juvenile Court, like other family courts, now accepts serious, untreated substance abuse as *prima facie evidence of parental inability to adequately care for a child.* [emphasis added]

However, these families often have many other problems apart from their history of substance abuse.

The last dilemma is that although some may argue that the contribution of alcohol to violent behavior is "less than meets the eye,"[7] the problem of explaining the very great proportion of violent acts of all kinds that have alcohol and intoxicated actors present remains (see Parker[11]). Presently, we can explain neither to what degree alcohol is effectively involved in these events nor why an alcohol presence is so prevalent.

The epidemiological research on alcohol and violence is large, diverse, and poorly integrated. This chapter uses two approaches in assessing the role of alcohol in violent behavior from an epidemiological perspective. Studies of a single category of violent behavior—rape—are discussed using different research windows based on different study populations. The same exercise can be carried out in relation to other violent behaviors.[1] Another approach is to review in detail a single epidemiological study of alcohol and violence, in this case, Pernanen's *Alcohol in Human Violence,*[2] in order to illustrate many of the key issues in epidemiological research that will need to be addressed in the next decade.

Any review of research on alcohol and violence must make a choice between a broad overview of many studies and a detailed look at a few. The importance of detailed analysis can be illustrated by an example of a review paper that discusses studies reviewed in this chapter. Antonia Abbey,[12] in a review article, "Acquaintance Rape and Alcohol Consumption on College Campuses: How are they Linked," uses two studies to establish that there is a link between these two behaviors. (These studies, Koss and Dinero[13] and Muehlenhard and Linton,[14] are reviewed in the second section of this chapter.) Abbey's review devotes only 14 lines to the actual evidence for the association. Three lines are devoted to Koss and Dinero.[13] They read, "Alcohol use at the time of the attack was one of the four strongest predictors of the likelihood of a college woman's being raped." But this 1989 article used typical alcohol use of women as the alcohol measure, not alcohol use at the time of event, and it proved to be a fairly weak predictor. Alcohol use by men is found to be a risk factor in Koss and Dinero.[13] They measured alcohol use at the time of the event on the part of men, but this factor is buried in myriad other risk factors and is undefined. The remaining 11 lines are devoted to Muehlenhard and Linton's[14] study of 635 psychology students on a college campus. On this thread of evidence, alcohol begins to be perceived as a cause of acquaintance rape.

1.2. Definitions of Violence

Violent behavior, as well as drinking behavior, covers an enormous number of different acts. Looking at only a single type of violent act, such as assault, a number of physically and socially different acts are implicated: the threat of assault, assault with a deadly weapon, assault accompanied by physical injury. The same objective act may be characterized as directed against a spouse, a child, or in war. Violent acts can also be typologized by how they are subjectively perceived. Perhaps the single most important typology of violent acts is achieved by dividing those that are legal from those that are not. These may be the same objective acts with the same physical and emotional consequences for the victim but may never come to the attention of the police or welfare agencies.

Pernanen[15] acknowledged the difficulty in aggregating all violent acts in his 1976 review of alcohol and aggression. By separating instrumental crimes, such as crimes for gain, from others, he sought some explanatory simplicity:

> I will almost exclusively deal with noninstrumental and interindividual crimes of violence. The emphasis will be on homicide partly because it is an easily definable category of crime and thus there is the least possible definitional variation between cultures and jurisdictions. Homicides are definitely interindividual. A proportion of homicides are, however, instrumental for various reasons and one criterion is not optimally fulfilled.

"Assaults," he argued, "are probably the most noninstrumental category of violent crimes." He noted, however, "If robbery, rape and arson were included [in an analysis] just because they are classified as violent crimes for nonscientific purposes, the explanatory accounting would have been extremely complex and more often misleading than not"

In the last decade, proportionately more homicides are instrumental, especially those with some drug involvement, and therefore even they involve an extension of the explanatory framework. In his recent empirical work, Pernanen[2] defined violence operationally by specific acts of physical violence, measured at three behavioral levels: actual physical harm, threats of violence, and witnessing violence. To be counted as an act of violence, "the assailant must clearly have shown the intention to hurt, or shown that he/she gave higher priority to reaching some other instrumental goal than to avoid hurting the respondent."

The focus of most research on alcohol and violence, especially criminal violence, has been on noninstrumental, expressive acts of violence because it is the (often unstated) belief of investigators that these are more likely to be related to alcohol use. This is changing with the development of a body of work on nonviolent criminal offending that contributes to our understanding of alcohol and violence by illustrating the many nonviolent behaviors that show a considerable alcohol presence (see, for example, Cordilia,[16] Petersilia et al.,[17] Ladouceur and Temple[18]). Other dimensions of violence that should be but rarely are used in assessing the relationship of alcohol and violence include the intensity of violent acts, duration in time, the rate of violent episodes in a time period, and the physical consequences of a single violent act.

1.3. Measurement of Alcohol Use and Alcohol Problems

Just as there are a number of types of violent acts and ways of measuring them, there are a large number of ways of measuring alcohol use. These include blood or urine alcohol levels, self-reports of quantity and frequency of drinking, drinking problems, types of beverages, congener contents of these beverages, observer reports of drinking, speed of drinking, and alcoholism. There is, in addition, variation in the cultural climate, temporally and geographically, in which drinking occurs and the alcohol-specific norms that will affect drinking behavior.

There is a wide range of effects attributed to alcohol. These include effects on coordination, eye movements, cognition, and judgment. There are also "expectancy" effects: behavior may change when someone thinks they have been drinking or when they think others have. Within the literature there is considerable debate over the importance of pharmacological and cultural effects, a debate that sometimes borders on the ideological.

In analyzing alcohol and violent events, we are typically concerned with distinguishing the acute effects of alcohol from the chronic or long-term effects. Thus, we separate out the use of alcohol in the event from the alcohol problems of those involved in the event. In addition, we consider separately those who are defined by their alcohol use and problems, that is, alcoholics.

Much of the research on alcohol, crime, and other violence in the last 15 years is far better than that which was reviewed in the wide-ranging review of alcohol, casualties, and crime carried out by Aarens et al.,[19] in 1977. The epidemiological research on drinking patterns and problems is working its way into the literature. Nonetheless, there remain many methodological problems connected with the measurement of drinking. A blood alcohol measurement must be taken on a person within a few hours after drinking has occurred. Self-reports of alcohol use may involve some element of deviance disavowal. Police may ignore women's drinking because they do not expect them to be drinking heavily. Not all members of a sample will have an alcohol measure taken, leading to possible biases in the alcohol-present subsample.

The time order of these behaviors is not always clear: violent behavior may cause drinking, both by the victim and the offender. (These methodological problems and other aspects of the measurement of drinking behavior and a discussion of alcohol effects can be found in Aarens *et al.*,[19] Greenberg,[20] and Roizen.[1])

The complexity of the relationship between alcohol and violence, even from an epidemiological perspective, is captured by Pernanen.[21] In this exercise, he proposes that we consider all possible measurements of alcohol as a set and then consider all violent acts as a set:

> Formally, all possible relationships between the elements of the sets would be represented by the Cartesian product of those sets: {alcohol use × {violent acts}. In addition, [there will be] some interactive combination of elements in the alcohol use variables . . . contemplating this way of representation may make us more sensitive to the indeterminateness of much of the discussion in this area.

(I have substituted "violent acts" for "crime" in this quotation.) We are, then, engaged in the examination and evaluation of the research on some hundreds of possible empirical relationships.

2. An Overview of Methodological Problems in Research on Alcohol and Violence

Methodological and conceptual problems that arise in the definition and measurement of violence and alcohol have been briefly discussed in the previous sections. This section outlines some of the other important methodological problems and constraints. (There are a number of comprehensive methodological critiques of research on crime and alcohol, including Pernanen,[15] Greenberg,[20] and Roizen and Schneberk.[22]) This chapter focuses on event-based studies and studies of the general population, each of which has different methodological problems.

2.1. Event-Based Research

By event-based research we mean samples of people to whom a serious event has occurred (e.g., victims of rape or assault) or samples of people who have initiated such an event (e.g., rapists or assaulters). For our purposes, we are looking at the amount of alcohol consumed before these events or the frequencies and kinds of alcohol problems these people have.

Perhaps the single most important methodological failing in event-based studies is the lack of, or an inappropriate, comparison group. Thus, in evaluating the alcohol problems of a sample of battered women, it is essential to know the level of alcohol problems in a sample of women comparable on other variables. Since it is often the case that event-based samples do not have comparison groups, distributions of alcohol problems in a general population sample are sometimes used. However, the cases in the events sample may differ on many other characteristics, making a general population sample inappropriate. Where comparison groups do exist, they are often convenient to the researcher rather than appropriate. Emergency room (ER) studies of trauma, for example, will use other types of ER patients. When the purpose of the research is to measure drinking problems, it may be questionable to include in a comparison group women in labor, victims of heart attack, and those suffering from surgical problems, all of whom are relatively unlikely to have been drinking.

Elsewhere, Aarens et al.[19] have argued that attempts to find comparison groups for events that involve intentional behavior, as most violent acts do fully or in part, are difficult if not impossible. A comparison group must be based on ceteris paribus criteria. It is questionable whether these criteria can be established for someone who has murdered his wife or shot someone in a robbery. Is the person who lives next door a reasonable "control" for someone who habitually assaults children? Assessing and controlling for the degree of intentionality in violent behavior is a problem that needs to be addressed in any study of violent behavior.

A second problem with event-based samples is that they are a highly selective subgroup of all cases of the occurrence of the event, with perhaps the single exception of homicide victims, most of whom are eventually discovered. Women who are victims of domestic violence may only come to public notice because they have nowhere else to go. This is more likely to be the case for poor women than those who are wealthy. Severely battered women may come to an ER, while others only slightly less injured nurse themselves at home. Prison offenders will have been through the highly selective processes of the courts, including plea bargaining and diversion.

Event samples typically include the "worst cases." Only a small proportion of rape victims, for example, ever report their rape. These reported cases are the ones that gain public attention in some way. Often these worst cases have multiple social, economic, and personal problems and many live on the fringes of society. For this reason much of the possible variation in important explanatory variables is attenuated. Disproportionate numbers in these samples are poor, ill, use drugs, and are poorly educated. (See, as a dramatic example of these multiple problems, the review of Barnard et al.[23] in a later section.)

Last, much of the data collected on events comes from intake and evaluation forms that are meant for other purposes, such as police reports, ER intake, and initial interviews with women seeking shelter. They are not purposefully drawn questionnaires. Correlatively, often the data analysis is in the hands of someone who is "interested in the problem" but is not skillful in the analysis of the often complicated data.

The methodology of the study of events is underdeveloped and a significant contribution to the study of alcohol and violence (or indeed other serious events) would be made by further work in this area. Pernanen's recent work is a good beginning.

2.2. Studies of the General Population

We are here concerned only with those methodological constraints on general population surveys that are relevant to studying substance abuse and violence or other untoward events. The single most important constraint is that in most social surveys, even large ones, there will be too few cases of serious events such as violent behaviors or victimizations to justify the costs of including the relevant questions. This problem becomes even more acute when it is a *relationship* that is under investigation, such as the relationship between alcohol and violence. Related to this is the fact that neither drinking patterns and problems nor violent behavior are randomly distributed in the population. Looking at the joint relationship may involve a biased subset of relevant cases.

General population samples, even very good ones, miss large numbers of people; indeed, this is true even of censuses. These missing individuals are likely to be (or so we may think) those who have many of the problems in which we are interested. Thus, thinking in terms of Venn diagrams, we may have a large overlap between event samples and the general population; alternatively, we may have little or no overlap. That is, it is possible that a general population survey may miss altogether those most given to serious violence, although the work of Straus and Gelles[24] suggests that this is not always the case. If extreme cases of the dependent variable, such as criminal behavior, are undersampled in the general population survey, suspected risk factors may appear to be relatively weak when in fact they are of considerable importance (see, for example, Greenfield and Weisner[25]). One of the important and unaddressed questions in the research on the epidemiology of violence is the degree to which there is a continuum of violent behaviors or whether there is a sharp disjunction, with extreme acts of violence being qualitatively different from other violence.

In this chapter I am looking in part at the epidemiology of "events" described in general population surveys—events that may occur to a relatively few people—in contrast to attitudes toward violence, which might characterize the whole of a sample. Thus, a fourth problem, which is in part described by Pernanen,[2] can be stated as follows: Although the sample of "events" from a general population survey is less selective than in event-based samples, even these are not random samples of events. There is selective recall and, as argued above, the events that find their way into a general population sample may well be a biased sample of all events. The fact that in many cases the (retrospective) period from which these events are drawn extends back in time many years creates a problem of its own. The types of violent events in recent years may be of a different nature to those that occurred 20 years ago. Patterns of violence and its modes of expression change. Thus, the distribution of types of recent events may differ from those that occurred to people some time ago but are still the most recent event they experienced. Furthermore, without other types of events (e.g., weddings, birthday parties) than violent events for comparison, it is impossible to say with any certainty what the effects an independent variable such as alcohol may have. A factor that must be accounted for in both event-based and general population surveys on problems of the type under investigation here is the reluctance of some people to admit to acts that are deviant and that consequently they may seek to disavow or reinterpret.

3. Evidence on Alcohol and Rape

3.1. Event-Based Research on Alcohol and Rape

Research drawn from data on arrested populations largely explores the immediate situational characteristics of criminal events rather than long-term personal, social, or economic problems of offenders or victims. The principal foci of this research are violent "index" crimes according to the Uniform Crime Report; that is, crimes against persons, such as robbery, rape, assault, and homicide. The most well-considered event-based research on these specific crimes follows the basic design of the initial work of Wolfgang[26] on homicide. This design has been used in several subsequent studies of homicide, and at least one study modeled after Wolfgang is found among those of rape, robbery, and assault. In these studies the focus is on the characteristics of the case as a whole rather than the characteristics of victims *or* offenders. The data sets include a wide range of variables: ethnicity of victims and offenders, alcohol use of victims and offenders, previous criminal record of offenders, temporal patterns, spatial patterns, degree of violence, method, motive, and various observations concerning victim–offender relationships. Alcohol use is included as a single variable in these studies but is often only covaried with some of these other variables. These studies have influenced more recent victims studies, which continue to be an important source of data on alcohol and violence.

The quality of these studies depends, in large part, on the quality of the police records. Some of the studies reviewed here have been reviewed elsewhere by Roizen and Schneberk[22] and Roizen[27]: Only the better studies are discussed here, with an emphasis on the United States. The ranges of alcohol estimates in these studies are shown in Table I. Looking only at the better studies has the effect of narrowing the range of estimated alcohol presence in criminal events. It also allows us to dispose of studies that fail to meet even minimum scientific standards.

Forcible rape is defined in the Uniform Crime Report[28] as "the carnal knowledge of a female forcibly and against her will" and has been redefined to include males in some states. Assaults or attempts to commit rape by force or threat of force are also included; however, statutory rape (without force) and other sex offenses are excluded. In 1975, the rate of rapes was 51 per 100,000 women in the United States; in 1988, it was 73 per 100,000. This varied from 83 in large cities to 36 in rural areas. In 1988, 52% of the known rapes were cleared. Forty-three percent of rape arrestees were under the age of 25; 53% were white and 46% black. Rape is perhaps the most underreported index crime, although report rates have grown as support for victims has increased and attention has been brought to the problem (see US Dept. of Justice, Law Enforcement Assistance Administration,[29] and Bureau of Justice Statistics,[30] for government estimates of victimization and underreporting). Arrest leads to a conviction in only a small proportion of cases. Dietz[31] estimated that only 16% of reported rapes led to a conviction, and nearly a quarter of these were for lesser offenses (see also Clark and Lewis[32]). Thus, offenders found in captured populations probably differ from the universe of rapists.

There is a wide range of alcohol involvement reported in studies of rape as shown in Table II. The Selling[33] study is noteworthy because it gives a self-reported alcohol measure, which is unusual in samples of arrestees (see also Visher[34] for self-reported alcohol use by arrestees for all violent crimes). The level of reported alcohol use by offenders in these studies more closely approximates the estimates of self-reported alcohol use prior to the most recent

Table II. Empirical Studies: Rape Offenders and Victims

Author, date, location	Sample	Percent alcohol offender	Percent alcohol victim	Alcohol measure
Selling (1940) Detroit MI[33]	100 cases male sex offenders	43	—	Combination self-reports and police reports
Shupe (1954) Columbus OH[58]	42 apprehended rapists	50	—	Urine alcohol content
President's Commission on Crime (1966) Washington[59]	151 cases of rape 200 offenders 151 victims	13	6	Police reports alcohol presence
Amir (1971)[35] Philadelphia	646 cases of rape 1292 offenders 646 victims	24	31	Police reports alcohol presence
Tardif (1966) Montreal[60]	112 cases of rape 67 offenders 112 victims	31	16	Police reports alcohol presence
Johnson (1978) Winnipeg[36]	217 "founded" cases of rape	37	36	Police reports alcohol presence

offense from sex offenders in prison than the estimates of use based on police reports.

Estimates of alcohol use prior to criminal events vary considerably among studies apparently similar in design for several reasons. These include differences between studies in the number of cases (small numbers leading to chance variation), quality of data, or ecological differences. Both the Washington, DC, and Philadelphia studies (Table II) use a study design modeled on the 1958 Wolfgang[26] research on homicide. A closer look at these studies can illustrate the difficulty the analyst has in trying to reconcile disparate findings. The difference in estimates of alcohol involvement is considerable, although both use police reports (see Table II). Both studies were carried out in large metropolitan areas with populations comparable on most major demographic characteristics except ethnicity. In the years in which these studies were carried out, 61% of the population of Washington, DC, was nonwhite (largely black), while blacks made up only 18% of the population of Philadelphia. There are known differences in alcohol use by ethnic group. Amir[35] reported that 42% of white rape arrestees had been drinking prior to the alleged crime, contrasted with 24% of black rape arrestees, an ethnic difference supported by other research. This ethnic difference in reported drinking prior to the crime could in part explain the difference in measured alcohol presence between these two studies. However, the data from Washington and Philadelphia show similar ethnic distributions of arrestees, although there are different ethnic distributions in the population. Thus, this substantial difference in ethnic distributions in the two communities in this case does not explain the difference in alcohol presence. However, differences in demographic characteristics of samples are potentially important to explanations of differences between studies in reported alcohol involvement; these are rarely fully analyzed in relation to the alcohol variables.

Other possible explanations for the variation in alcohol presence in these studies include differences in the level of attention paid to drinking that occurs prior to criminal events in the different cities, in the availability of alcohol in neighborhoods where crimes are likely to occur, or, as Johnson *et al.*[36] argued, they may be the result of a "real difference" in the use of alcohol in different geographic areas. Whatever the explanation, these two studies underscore the difficulty in obtaining consistent estimates of alcohol involvement in criminal events even when research designs are similar and studies are restricted to one type of criminal event.

The Amir[35] study has gathered the most complete data on alcohol presence in rape events, although the study is not primarily focused on alcohol use and some of the quantitative analysis is relatively poor. At the time the Amir research was carried out, its value lay in the fact that it expanded the focus of the investigation of criminal behavior beyond the offender to the event and its situational and social context. This detailed analysis of 646 rape events shows, for example, that over 40% of rapes involve multiple offenders; in half of the rapes the victim and offender were acquainted and in 20% they were neighbors. Half of the offenders had a criminal record, but few had previous records of sexual offenses. The place of initial "meeting" of offender and victim is frequently (41%) and somewhat surprisingly in one of their homes. However, 42% occur "on the street." Only 11% of rapes occur near a bar.

These data also show a strong association between alcohol use and type of interpersonal victim–offender relationship. Alcohol use was twice as likely to be found in rapes involving strangers (in 44% of the rape events alcohol had been used) compared with rapes involving primary relations (21% of cases involved alcohol). It is particularly noteworthy that when only the victim had been drinking, the victim and offender were strangers in 77% of the cases. Thus, drinking in rape, as in other crimes, may play any one of a number of different roles: It may be present but have no effect; it may enhance chances of victimization when the parties are strangers; it can be present in the offender alone and exert an effect only on the offender, such as misreading social cues in relation to prevailing norms; or it may begin an evening gathering of a group of men that ends in drunkenness and rape.

Several other alcohol-specific findings are noteworthy from this study. When rape involved a pair of men compared with a single man or a group of men, the offenders were considerably more likely to have been drinking. A number of studies of drinking and crime show excess force in alcohol-present situations. Although the number of cases in which alcohol is present in the offender only is small, all of them involved excess force against the victim. Sexual humiliation was also more likely when alcohol was present. Alcohol was present in 40% of the rapes committed on the weekend and 28% of those committed during the week. Of those cases where alcohol was present in the victim only, 40% occurred on a single day of the week, Saturday.

The Amir research shows that two thirds of the alcohol-present rapes involved drinking by both victim and offender. For some investigators this raises the question of whether or not the behavior of the victim may contribute to her victimization. "Victim precipitation," or the victim's own role in influencing the course of the rape, is a socially sensitive issue. Progress has been made in relation to the problem of blaming the victim by police, the courts, and the general public in the two decades since Amir's work. Amir's analysis is not sensitive to these issues. However, keeping this in mind, Amir's work contains some alcohol relationships that deserve further investigation. Amir[35] defined victim precipitation as

> rape in a particular situation [in which] the behavior of the victim is interpreted by the offender either as a direct invitation for sexual relations or as a sign that she will be available for sexual contact if he will persist in demanding it. Excluded are the situations where no interaction was established between the offender and the victim, and when the offense was a sudden event which befell the victim.

Approximately one in five rapes was considered to be victim precipitated. Victim-precipitated rape was more likely than other rape to involve a white victim and/or a white victim and white offender pair. In the majority of cases the offender and victim were at least acquaintances. Fifty-three percent of victim-precipitated rapes involved alcohol compared with 29% of nonvictim-precipitated rapes. In 35% of victim-precipitated rapes both the victim and the offender had been drinking; in 18% only the victim had been drinking. The proportion of victims-only drinking in victim-precipitated rape was more than twice that in nonvictim-precipitated rape. However, the degree to which a victim's drinking may evoke a presumption, on the part of the police or others, of blame for her involvement in the rape event has been the subject of relatively little research (see, however, Richardson and Campbell[37]).

The finding that 60% of the victim-precipitated rapes involved sexual humiliation, in contrast to 18% of other rapes, is a startling one. Amir[35] argued that this is very likely due to misread signals on the part of the offender:

> [S]ubjecting the victim to forced sexual intercourse means that the imputation of sexual availability was a false interpretation on the offender's part. He may still hold to his views and try to prove them by subjecting her to sexual humiliation, other than forced intercourse, or he may humiliate her as a revenge just because of the failure of his imputation.

Drinking may contribute to the misreading of signals on the part of both the victim and the offender.

Although "victim precipitated" is the wrong term for describing these rapes, they are rapes in which the victim may have increased her vulnerability by her own behavior. Drinking or some types of pub or bar behavior may be factors that increase a woman's vulnerability. Deming et al.,[38] in their study of fatal sexual assaults, report a positive blood alcohol content (BAC) for 40% of the victims; of these, half were intoxicated. These investigators suggested that the victims may have contributed to their deaths by their behavior and judgment, including the inability to escape.

The research of Johnson et al.[36] on alcohol and rape in Winnipeg shows a much higher proportion of alcohol-present cases in their series, although the study design is similar. In their series, 74% of victims or offenders were drinking prior to the event. This difference may be geographic or more likely the result of increased attention to reporting alcohol use since the Amir research. Again, in the majority of alcohol-present cases, both the offender and the victim had been drinking. This study shows a significant difference in the use of physical force in alcohol-present compared with alcohol-absent rapes. Rapes in which both the victim and offender had been drinking involved substantial force in 37% of the cases; this is contrasted with 18% of the cases in which no alcohol had been used. Looking at all alcohol-present cases, 85% involved the use of some force contrasted with 68% of cases in which no alcohol had been used. However, the highest level of force as measured in their index of force was rarely (in 5% of the cases) but equally used in both alcohol-present and alcohol-absent cases.

Few sexual assaults end in homicide. Those that do end in death frequently show injuries and perversion. Deming *et al.*[38] reported on 41 female cases of proven fatal sexual assault over a 10-year period in Dade County, Florida, nearly half of whom were physically traumatized and injured. Thirty percent of the victims were black, in a county in which nonwhite residents averaged 16% of the population over the period covered. Of the 37 victims tested, 40% tested positive for alcohol use. More than half of those tested had a BAC of 0.10 or higher. Only two of the victims were known to be prostitutes. The role of alcohol in sexual assault with serious injury or resulting in homicide is one that needs further investigation, especially in light of new evidence that a substantial proportion (estimated to be between a quarter and a third) of sexual offenders are reconvicted of a sexual or violent offense,[39] and the fact that these events are impulsive/explosive events that may involve a drinking victim.

3.2. Studies of Prison Offenders

Research based on prison offenders offers a second window on the relationship between alcohol and violence. Estimates of alcohol involvement in criminal events based on the self-reports of convicted offenders show a different pattern of relationships between criminal behavior and alcohol use than that based on samples of arrestees. While the prison data support the view that a substantial proportion of violent offenders were drinking or drunk at the time of the crime, these data show considerable alcohol presence in other crimes as well. A detailed reanalysis of data from an early national survey of prison offenders[22] showed that although drinking at the time of the crime varied by type of crime and was greater for violent interpersonal crime than for property crime, these differences were not large. Among those who had been drinking, "drunkenness" at the time of the crime was no less common for property than for crimes against the person, despite the greater skill assumed to be required for property crimes.

This pattern of relationships of drinking and type of crime from prison studies is in marked contrast to the pattern found in arrested populations. The arrest data show a strong relationship between seriousness of the crime and alcohol presence in the offender and similarly significant differences in alcohol presence in personal violent crime compared with property crime. Research of similar design based on arrest record data shows 7% of robberies,[40] 34% of rapes,[41] 24% of assaults,[42] and 55% of homicides[26] involved a drinking offender. Comparable proportions based on the US Department of Justice[43] prison offender sample are 39%, 57%, 61%, and 53%, respectively. The prison data also reveal that a large proportion of burglaries (47%) and car thefts (46%) are committed after drinking. The national survey of prison inmates carried out in 1979 largely supports the data from the earlier national survey. However, the 1979 survey,[43] based on personal interviews with 12,000 inmates, including women, gives a more detailed picture of the drinking habits of prisoners than the earlier national survey. Violent offenders and property offenders were about equally likely to have been drinking prior to their current offense (50% and 46%, respectively). Of those who were drinking, 60% of violent offenders and 68% of property offenders reported drinking very heavily. As well, the proportions who reported being very heavy drinkers in the year prior to the offense for which they were incarcerated were also approximately equal. Thirty-five percent of violent offender and 40% of property offenders reported being very heavy drinkers.

Ladouceur and Temple,[18] using these data, compared the drinking behavior of rapists and other prison offenders. Their analysis shows that rapists are no more likely to drink heavily before the offense for which they are incarcerated than are those convicted of assault or burglary, and that they are about as likely to report feeling drunk as those committing burglary. Ladouceur and Temple[18] noted, "This study finds no differences for heavy alcohol use or for level of drunkenness between offenders who committed violent and nonviolent, or sexual or nonsexual crimes." Further, their results show that both rapists and other offenders are likely to drink less heavily at the time of the offense than on a typical drinking occasion in the past year. While almost 90% of rapists drank moderately to heavily in the year prior to incarceration, only 60% drank prior to the offense. The fact that there are no significant differences in drinking behavior by offense group suggests that criminal *behavior* may not be seriously influenced by drinking in the event, but rather that criminal offenders generally are very heavy drinkers and if there is any contribution made by alcohol, it is in this way. Ladouceur and Temple[18] concluded,

> Because drinking during the past year is not typically associated with the commission of a crime, we conclude that drinking at the time of offense is likely to reflect a typical drinking pattern, or in some other way is unrelated to the commission of the crime. If there was a causal link between alcohol use and crime, such that heavy drinking increased the probability of committing the crime, then we would expect offenders to drink more heavily at the time of offense than on typical drinking occasions.

The work of Barnard and colleagues[23] suggests that future research on alcohol and rape, based on samples of prison offenders, should differentiate offenders with a long history of drinking problems from others. These investigators came to conclusions that are similar to those of Ladouceur and Temple in relation to the failure of acute alcohol effects to explain rape or other criminal behavior. Although it has a small number of cases, the Barnard *et al.*[23] study is important for its attention to the multiple social and psychological problems most offenders have. These investigators reviewed the psychiatric evaluations prepared for the Florida courts of 88 offenders charged with rape. Of the 88, 60 were classified as nonalcoholic, although others met some of the investigators' criteria for alcoholism. Both groups of offenders had experienced problems in their parental families either through divorce or death. Nearly half of the offenders had a parent die or the parents divorce by the time the offender reached age 18. Both groups had school problems and low levels of educational attainment. The alcoholic group began drinking considerably earlier than the nonalcoholic group: at about 14 for alcoholics and over 16 for nonalcoholics. Of those called for military service, 69% of alcoholics and 44% of nonalcoholics were either rejected at entrance or received a dishonorable discharge. Work histories show frequent impulsive changes or firings. While 82% of the alcoholics had been married at some time, only 27% were married at the time of the offense. Comparable percentages for nonalcoholics are 53% and 25%, respectively. The groups differ significantly in criminal histories. While 36% and 45% of the alcoholics had been convicted of assault or other violent charges, respectively, this was the case for only 18% and 13% of nonalcoholics. About half of both groups had previously used drugs. The two groups differ significantly in their relationship to their victims. Thirty-two percent of the alcoholics raped a relative and 41% an acquaintance. This was the case for 11% and 28% of the nonalcoholics. In both groups, substantial proportions of offenders had medical and psychiatric problems.

In relation to the alleged offense, nearly 60% of the alcoholics reported drinking heavily at the time of the incident compared with 30% of the nonalcoholics. Seventeen offenders reported blackouts due to alcohol and could not describe the context of the offense at all. Barnard et al.[23] concluded that

> For both the alcoholic and non-alcoholic prisoners, long-standing and multifaceted histories of disturbed behavior were recorded. It appears therefore that alcohol abuse is but one part of the picture, with sociopathy and other forms of interpersonal disturbance contributing to the criminal act. . . . The alcoholics stand out as more severely disturbed than the nonalcoholics in the amount and pattern of deviant behavior. . . . [T]he data suggest that such immediate effects of alcohol [as are seen] are not sufficient to account for the observed cases of rape which arise out of long-standing patterns of deviance.

Collins and Schlenger[44] carried out a multivariate analysis of the relationship of acute and chronic alcohol effects (i.e., the effects of long-term alcohol use rather than the immediate effects, whether pharmacologically or culturally defined) in a sample of those recently admitted to North Carolina prisons. They found that chronic effects were not significantly associated with either incarceration for a violent offense or with committing a violent offense in the year prior to incarceration. Age, race, marital status, education, and criminal career variables were included in the logistic regression models. These investigators concluded that "it is the proximal effect of alcohol use, rather than characteristics associated with being alcoholic, that is associated with increased likelihood of violence."

Can the conclusion from these different studies be reconciled? Does alcohol contribute to violent criminal behavior? Is the evidence in? The answer is that it is not. What is clear is that broad categories of offense do not adequately distinguish the actual behavior involved. Even specific event types (e.g., "rape" as compared to "violent crime") may mask significant variation in alcohol use in different types of rape events. That is, sadistic rape or date rape or incest (as compared to other types of rape or sexual offense) may well be caused by different alcohol effects and characterized by different levels of drinking, insofar as alcohol is a determinant of rape at all. Research on criminal behavior and alcohol and drug effects, therefore, must be more theoretically driven and these theoretical investigations must control for the other social, economic, mental health, and other health problems of the offender. The theory that alcohol use is only a marker for an intercorrelated set of other problems must be considered in any investigation.

Groth and Birnbaum's[45] extensive empirical work on rape suggests directions for further theoretically based empirical research on drinking and rape. Based on interviews with a sample of 500 sexual offenders, Groth and Birnbaum outline three patterns:

1. Anger rape: "Sexuality becomes a means of expressing and discharging feelings of pent-up anger and rage. The assault is characterized by physical brutality."
2. Power rape: "In these assaults, it is not the offender's desire to harm his victim but to possess her sexually. Sexuality becomes a means of compensating for underlying feelings of inadequacy and serves to express issues of master, strength, control . . ."
3. Sadistic rape: "Both sexuality and aggression become fused. . . . There is a sexual transformation of anger and power so that aggression itself becomes eroticized."

We would expect alcohol to play a different role in these types of rape. For example, in anger rape, alcohol may enhance assaultive feelings. In power rape, alcohol may be used for "Dutch courage" or, as some cases suggest, as a way of trying to suppress sexual responses. Sadistic rape fits a pattern of alcohol-related violence that involves sexual humiliation and excess violence. Rada,[46] for example, has suggested that in some offenders alcohol has a direct, triggering effect on both violent sexual fantasies and behavior. The fact that many rapists report that they cannot have intercourse in the rape situation may also be an alcohol effect, one that leads to angry and sadistic responses.

Unfortunately, Groth and Birnbaum[45] paid little attention to alcohol in their work, arguing that

> The use of alcohol, in and of itself, is insufficient to account for the offense. Although some offenders were to some extent intoxicated at the time they committed their assaults, these same men were more often not sexually assaultive when intoxicated. Our data suggest that alcohol may at most serve as a releasor only when an individual has already reached a frame of mind in which he is prone to rape.

However, they also argued

> that alcohol may contribute to the releasing of rape impulses or assaultive

tendencies in some offenders . . . may impair such cognitive functions as reasoning and judgment . . . may be a necessary component in a process that evolves into an assault. . . . in other cases, alcohol abuse and sexual abuse may constitute two parallel but independent symptoms of personality dysfunction.

3.3. Rape in the General Population

A third window on the relationship between alcohol and rape comes from general population victimization surveys. Official surveys such as the national crime survey[30] and parallel surveys in other countries estimate the overall level of victimization and the degree of underreporting of crimes such as rape. They give little or no attention, however, to risk factors such as alcohol. Pernanen's important recent work on alcohol and violence in a general population sample does not treat sexual offenses separately. The best source of data on alcohol and rape based on a sample of the general population is the work of Koss and her colleagues,[47,48] although this work is limited to college students. The most recent research is based on a national sample of college and university undergraduates and includes 6159 men and women in 32 higher education institutions. Twenty-seven percent of women reported a sexually coercive experience since the age of 14 that met the legal definition of rape, including rape attempts. Fifteen percent of women reported having been raped and 12% reported attempts. Eight percent of men reported perpetrating an act that met the legal definition of rape. Five percent admitted rape and 3% admitted attempts. The difference in these percentages between men and women suggest either that women's sexually coercive experiences were with men outside the higher education system, for example, with a family member, or that there are considerable differences in women's and men's perceptions of how coercive these sexual events were. There is, of course, no reason to believe that all men will admit in a questionnaire to having committed a violent act such as rape, even if they believe in the anonymity of their responses.

Eight percent of women reported having had unwanted sexual intercourse because "a man had given you alcohol or drugs." (Unwanted sex as a result of the woman's own drinking and perceived loss of control was not included.) A man's giving unwanted intoxicants was considerably less important, however, than being "overwhelmed by a man's continual arguments and pressure," which 25% of women reported.

Although the fact that women's drinking patterns are found to be a risk factor for rape and alcohol use had predictive power in the discriminant analyses used, the relationship between alcohol and rape is not a particularly strong one.[13] Using measures of typical drug use (i.e., frequency of drinking, frequency of drunkenness, and usual numbers of drinks per drinking occasion), the raw means of the drinking index, which is unreported but has a range of 3–15, were as follows: nonvictimized, 6.89; sexual contact, 7.38;

sexual coercion, 7.98; attempted rape, 7.82; and rape, 8.01. Four categories of sexual coercion are used in this analysis. Sexual contact includes kissing and fondling under pressure; sexual coercion includes sexual intercourse under pressure but not by use of force.

As these data show, the differences in these scores on the alcohol use index cover a narrow range of drinking behaviors given the scope of the index, with its potential range of scores from 3–15. The investigators noted,

> An inspection of the means on alcohol used indicated that women who had been raped on average received a score that reflected a usual drinking pattern of (a) 1–3 times a month; (b) usually no more than 4 cans of beer (or equivalent in wine or spirits); and (c) getting drunk less than once a month but at least once per year. The score for the group of women who had not been victimized represented the next lower usage level in any one of these three categories.

Since the great majority of college women drink and as many as 12% may be considered heavy drinkers, the level of drinking represented by those women who have been raped is by no means rare (Johnson et al.,[49] Engs and Hanson,[50] Gleason[51]). Drinking patterns vary by area of the country and type of higher education institution, as no doubt do sexual norms and behaviors. These factors need further analysis before drinking can be seen as a risk factor for the sexual victimization of college women.

Women's and men's alcohol use in the event is analyzed in Koss et al.[52] Comparing stranger ($n = 52$) and acquaintance rape ($n = 416$), based on the survey described above, shows substantial alcohol and drug presence in both types of rape. Women had been drinking and/or taking drugs in 68% of the stranger rapes and 55% of the acquaintance rapes. Comparable numbers for the men involved were 76% and 67%, respectively. About 45% of both men and women in both types of rape had used alcohol only; the remaining cases had used alcohol and drugs or drugs only. The use of alcohol and drugs varied by type of acquaintance rape. The proportions of women and men (respectively) using alcohol and/or drugs in the different types of rape events were 65 and 75% in "nonromantic" rapes, 78 and 84% for rapes occurring on casual dates, 45 and 55% on steady dates, and 13 and 42% in rapes involving a spouse or family member. (Men's use of intoxicants is as perceived by the women involved.)

The level of force used by the offender varied by type of rape. Greatest force was used in stranger rapes and those involving family members. The least force was used on casual dates. However, alcohol use was greatest on casual dates for both women and men. Eighty-one percent of the men involved in rape on a casual date had used alcohol, as had 70% of the women. While the work of Koss and her colleagues suggests that alcohol use might be a risk factor for rape, there is no simple positive association between force and alcohol use. Family and spouse rape involved the least alcohol and drug use on the part of the offender, while alcohol and drugs were used by three quarters of stranger rapists. In both types of rape the use of offender force is considerable. Thirty one percent of spouse/family rapes involved choking, beating, or using a weapon (11%). Comparable proportions in stranger rapes were 32% (16% of offenders used a weapon). Unfortunately, the Koss survey does not report the amount of alcohol and drug use nor other characteristics of the rape events, information that would help establish the role of alcohol and drugs, if any, in these rape events. Furthermore, as with all violent acts, there is a great range in the severity of the threat and the outcome. Although the rapes and attempts found in the Koss sample meet the legal definition of rape, they no doubt differ in many characteristics from the rapes found in samples of arrested and convicted rape offenders. Only 23% of the women to whom acquaintance rape happened described themselves as victims of rape; 44% of the victims reported having sex with the offender again.

Muehlenhard and Linton,[14] in a much smaller study of college students at a single university, show a significant relationship between alcohol and drug use and sexual aggression. Comparisons of most recent dates with dates in which unwanted sexual activity occurred showed that significantly more dates in which sexual aggression occurred involved acting or feeling moderately or extremely intoxicated (as a result of alcohol and/or drugs). This was true for both women and men based on the responses of women and men reported separately. The difference in reported intoxication between the two types of dates is considerably greater from women's reports than men's. Women reported heavy use of intoxicants by both themselves and the man involved four times as frequently on dates involving sexual aggression contrasted with the most recent date. Men reported heavy use about twice as frequently. However, this study's definition of sexual aggression is very broad (i.e., including anything from kissing and touching to forced oral sex and sexual intercourse) and occurred to 78% of the women and was perpetrated by 57% of the men.

These studies raise important questions about alcohol and drug use and sexual activity. The degree to which men excuse their own sexual aggression and women explain their sexual activity to themselves and others by using drinking explanations needs further investigation. But considerably more refinement of the alcohol measures, description of the context of the event, and controls for usual drinking and drug taking are needed.

In this review of alcohol and rape we have seen the complexity in assessing the contribution of alcohol to this type of violent behavior. A number of contextual factors are shown to be related to alcohol in the rape event. However, many rapists have multiple social and personal problems that may themselves explain this deviant sexual behavior. Rape offenders, like other violent offenders, are typically heavy drinkers and drug users. Alcohol use in the event may represent no more than everyday use. Extending the study of rape into the student population as Koss and her colleagues have done suggests, however, a rather different set of correlates of rape than we find in the prison offender population.

In the next section we turn to a single study that looks in detail at alcohol's role in violence and is the most important contribution to the epidemiological literature in this area of research in many years.

4. The Recent Work of Pernanen

The recently published work of Kai Pernanen,[2] *Alcohol in Human Violence*, deserves a special place in this chapter for a number of reasons. First, the work is wholly devoted to the problem of alcohol and violence, whereas much of the other work reviewed here has many competing agendas, often raising more questions than giving answers to the question of the relationship between alcohol and violence. Second, and of very considerable importance, is the fact that Pernanen's work is cumulative in relation to the study of alcohol and violence. Unlike many of those who carry out research on alcohol and violence, he is not making an occasional foray into the field. His work is based on his own considerable work in this area of research and a close reading of that of others, including the very large related experimental literature. This sort of cumulative research is rare in contemporary social science where analysts often move from problem to problem as funding or interest compels. Third, the work is of a very high standard. The survey is a classic piece of survey research in an area of research that is extremely patchy with respect to quality.

As Pernanen[2] wrote, "The main strength of these data is that they represent 'real' naturally occurring events of aggression and violence," which can provide much needed descriptive analyses of aggressive episodes and their incidence and prevalence and can serve as models for controlled studies of aggression. As he argued, "Both middle range theories and middle range data have been missing from the study of human aggression." While underscoring the importance of description in the study of violence and the paucity of good data, despite the many studies of alcohol and violence, it is description in the service of providing an explanatory framework for alcohol-related violence that is the strength of this research.

Inevitably, in a tightly argued book-length manuscript, the reviewer must select among the many findings a few that give the flavor of the work and that epitomize its essential contribution. The summarized findings below include some of the important descriptive findings from the survey as well as several that will contribute to explanation and theory in this area of research.

The survey is based on a probability sample (Thunder Bay, Ontario) of 933 men and women aged 20 and over representing a city of 112,500. Of these 933 respondents, 492 had been victims of violence at some time since they were 15 years of age. The most recent incident of violence is the subject of most of the analyses. Violent incidents in the 12 months prior to the survey are also analyzed, but these numbers are smaller. About 10% of the 495 men in the survey had been victims of violence, 10% had been threatened with violence in the previous year, and 39% had witnessed violence. Comparable figures for women are 10%, 6%, and 28%, respectively.

This is a victimization study in the sense that violent incidents are described from the perspective of the victim. The focus of the study, then, is the role of alcohol in violent victimizations, not the role of alcohol in the aggressive and violent behavior of the respondents. A comparison study of violent crimes ($n = 781$) based on police records was carried out at roughly the same time. Only 4% of the violent episodes from the interview survey were recorded by the police in the year of the study, although the police were made aware of 15% of the episodes. This demonstrates the fact that the analysis of cases from police records involves a small and selective subset of all cases of violence, although these probably consist predominantly of the most serious cases.

Although the risk of violent victimization in the 12 months preceding the survey was about equal for men and women, 60% of male and 44% of female respondents reported having been victimized since age 15. There is the problem of the adequacy of recall for the violent incidents that make up the main analysis: 40% of the index incidents, that is, the 492 incidents, occurred during the 3 to 4 years prior to the survey; however, another 40% occurred more than 8 years prior to the survey. Of these incidents, men were disproportionately likely to have had their last victimization in their youth, while women reported more recent incidents. Some of the major findings of this work are outlined below.

4.1. Pervasiveness of Alcohol

In more than half of the index incidents of violence in the community sample and 42% of the violent crimes reported in the police sample, either the victim, the assailant, or both were drinking. In the interview study, 51% of the assailants (note: as perceived by the victims) and 30% of the victims had been drinking; in the violent crime study the comparable percentages were 31% and 26%, respectively. Pernanen[2] concluded:

> We now have some evidence that, at least in a cultural sphere where alcohol is implicated in criminal violence, it is also abundantly present in day-to-day violent confrontations. The relationship between alcohol use and severe aggression, as reflected in studies of police and court records and in emergency room samples of injured persons, does not seem to be mainly an artifact created by biasing selection processes.

Nor, as he rightly concluded, can this relationship be seen as pertaining only to a small group or particular subcultures in the population. The question of the representativeness of event samples is often raised, and this work of Pernanen's gives us an answer based on a general population survey in one community.

4.2. Differential Risk of Alcohol-Involved Violence

Many studies show that both heavy drinking and drinking problems are related to gender and age. The data from Thunder Bay, perhaps not surprisingly, also demonstrate that particular demographic groups in the population have higher risks than others of alcohol-involved violence and that this is in excess of what would be expected merely by the frequency of their drinking. Young men are most at risk, although all young adults are at greater risk than others.

The risk of injury from the index violent incidents (i.e., not those in the year prior to the survey) was surprisingly high. Twenty-six percent of the incidents resulted in a physical injury; 11% involved seeking medical attention. It is an important finding of this work that alcohol-present episodes did not result in any greater rate of injury than those that did not involve alcohol. However, the risk of injury increased with the amount of alcohol consumed by the victim.

4.3. Selected Findings on Alcohol and Violence from Pernanen's Work

The findings reported here are important in their own right in the development of both empirical research and theory in this field; they are also some of the findings that refer to themes from other studies reviewed in this chapter and in the longer paper from which it is drawn. Included is a comparison of drinking during violent episodes contrasted with usual drinking patterns and an examination of differential alcohol involvement in violent episodes involving acquaintances versus strangers, with different gender mixes of victim and assailant, and in different locations.

1. The amount of alcohol consumed by both men and women in their index (i.e., most recent) victimization was considerably higher than the mean levels of consumption during their most recent drinking episodes. This suggests the need for further work on victim precipitation or vulnerability to violence.

2. Alcohol involvement differed according to the gender of the victim and assailant. Total alcohol involvement in episodes of a male victim and assailant was 62%, a female victim and male assailant was 53%, and of a female assailant was 27%. Violent episodes between men not only had higher levels of alcohol involvement but were also more likely to lead to injury.

3. Alcohol involvement differed according to the relationship between the victim and the offender. Total alcohol involvement was greatest in episodes between strangers. Seventy-eight percent of these incidents involved either a drinking victim or assailant. In 36%, both were drinking. More needs to be known about these "stranger" episodes that make up nearly a quarter of violent episodes.

Over half of the violent incidents reported by women involved conflicts with their spouses. Only 12% of the incidents reported by men were reported as family violence. This difference is difficult to explain without more data. It may be the case that men "forget" their incidents of family violence or that men do not see them to be as serious as women do. (As we have seen in the previous section, some men have perceptions of sexual coercion that are quite different from those of women.) Nearly half of the violent episodes between spouses involved drinking by the victim or the assailant. The victim (in most cases the wife) was drinking in only a third of these episodes. Pernanen[2] noted, "The serious nature of alcohol use in some marital violence is probably reflected in the finding that divorced or separated respondents had an alcohol involvement of 69 percent in their most recent subjection to violent acts". He notes that the sample is small ($n = 37$). One fifth of episodes of family violence resulted in an injury.

4. Based on the episodes of violence in the year prior to the survey, Pernanen[2] found no

> clear-cut relationships between the typical drinking frequency of the individual and the three types of experiences of aggression during the preceding year: men who were more frequent drinkers were not more likely to experience acts of violence, threats and witness violence than were other men.

The same relationship was not true for women. Among both men and women, those who drank once or twice a week were considerably more likely to witness violence (and presumably to increase their chances of being participants) than more frequent drinkers. He observed,

> The point that this discontinuous finding should make clear is that, even though a statistical connection between alcohol use and aggressive encounters seems very likely in many jurisdictions and cultural spheres, we should not expect a linear relationship between frequency of drinking and these experiences.

This is an important point, one that has consequences both for choice of analytic methods and choice of alcohol variables used in research on alcohol and violence. There is growing evidence that heavy infrequent or binge drinkers may be disproportionately involved in violent behavior (see, for example, Kantor and Straus[53]). This needs further exploration.

5. The findings on violence that occurred in a tavern are noteworthy. All except one of the assailants had been drinking. The victim had been drinking in about 80% of the cases. The proportion of injuries resulting from these violent encounters was almost twice as great as from incidents that occurred in the respondents' own home. This may reflect the fact that tavern violence reported in the interviews occurred in large part among strangers.

4.4. Contributions of Pernanen's Recent Work to Theoretical Debate

Pernanen[2] considers three "clusters of hypotheses" that are relevant to determining the role of alcohol in violence: these include severity and persistence hypotheses, indiscrimination hypotheses, and elicitation hypotheses. The latter is not dealt with in Pernanen's book but will be in later work; it suggests that when alcohol is added to any situation, the risk of eliciting an aggressive response is greater. The other two hypotheses are briefly reviewed below.

4.5. Alcohol and Severity of Choice of Acts and Outcomes

Tests of seriousness of the choice of violent acts and their consequences in relation to alcohol-involved violence are important in the development of a coherent theory of alcohol-related aggression. Severity hypotheses are relevant both to disinhibition-type theories and to establishing whether a dose–response relationship exists in relation to alcohol and untoward outcomes. The persistence hypothesis is related: that an intoxicated aggressor will persist in violence beyond what would occur in "normal" violence. Wolfgang[26] and his students have called this "excess violence."

Pernanen[2] concludes that "no support has been found for a general severity hypothesis in these data." This is largely based on the failure to find a difference in injury outcome between drinking and nondrinking episodes and the failure to find a difference in rate of injury related to the assailant's drinking. There is limited conditional support for finding a difference in rate of injury when the assailant was judged to be drunk, but the difference is not a large one.

In my view, the evidence is not in on this question. These data are not sufficiently finely drawn to support such a conclusion. The fact that there were both (1) a clear relationship between very heavy drinking on the part of the victim and the risk of injury and (2) an elevated risk when the assailant was judged to be drunk suggest that there may indeed be a relationship between level of drinking and severity. Furthermore, it is in the nature of the sample that it may not capture many very heavy and frequent drinkers. Thus, if there were a relationship between amount of alcohol consumed and the severity of the outcome, this relationship would be attenuated. The two weakest aspects of this research program as a whole are the alcohol variable for assailants' drinking (i.e., the respondent's memory of what the assailant had been drinking) and the length of time between an index incident and the survey.

4.6. Indiscrimination in Acts of Violence and Alcohol

Pernanen defines these hypotheses as follows:

The "indiscrimination" hypotheses state that acts of aggression after drinking will not be as well attuned as acts of sober aggression to the requirements of the situations and the social norms applying to it, such as the restraints (or "inhibitions") related to the location, the types of acts performed, the characteristics of the target of aggression, and so forth. . . . [A]cts performed would be as serious as in other social contexts, regardless of normally attenuating factors.

There is some evidence in this work of "less discrimination" in the use of violence in relation to how well the assailant and the victim know one another. For example, in relation to the gender of the victim, Pernanen concludes that his data contain "rather clear evidence of the continued importance of conditional social-contextual cues and normative factors in the determination of types of aggression and physical violence after drinking." In the alcohol-present episodes, more violent acts such as punching and kicking were used against both male and female victims, but the difference in types of acts between alcohol-present and alcohol-absent is small. Less severe and less indiscriminate violence is generally used against female victims, and this does not change substantially even when alcohol is involved in the incident and when the assailant is drinking.

Pernanen[2] concludes, "It can be said that once aggression occurs in connection with drinking, it has the same general character of a 'guided doing' [using Goffman's term] as in sober conflict." Even in incidents involving both violence and drinking, normative constraints are still operative. This is, of course, consistent with the theories of drunken comportment of MacAndrew and Edgerton[54] and others. However, Pernanen is not yet prepared to declare this debate over. He further argues,

> Nonspecific "indiscrimination" and "excessiveness" may be more characteristic of determination in the initial stage of a conflict, in the processes involving instigating cues and cognitive issues in angry arousal, and in the process by which these instigations produce open conflict.

These are important findings. However, we must question the extent to which such findings are generalizable. Certainly they have relevance to everyday violence, but as Pernanen himself points out, "Samples of violence that occur in specific subcultures with more extreme drinking habits, such as 'skid row' . . . could yield different results altogether." Larger, more urban communities with a greater representation of those who use excessive violence, alcohol, and drugs may yield different results.

Although Pernanen is concerned with motivations and meanings, social surveys such as his, however well carried out, do not allow us to pull out the important scenarios that may give greater insights into alcohol involvement in violence. Looking at "victim–offender" relationship, location, and so forth separately is no substitute for getting into the context of violent events and the "minds" of those involved. The fine work of Tony Parker,[55,56] who has sensitively interviewed a sample of men and women who are or have been imprisoned for murder, is an important contribution. Although these are a small number of "ideal typical" cases and are not meant to be a random sample of such offenders, they give no support to theories that suggest that substance abuse is a major determinant of homicidal behavior. Interviews of this type done with violent offenders who were drinking or drinking heavily at the time of the event would be an important contribution to work on alcohol and violence.

5. The Future of Epidemiological Research on Alcohol and Violence

One section of this chapter concentrated on a single type of violent behavior and another on a single study of violent behavior generally. The longer review from which this chapter is drawn looks in similar detail at other types of violent criminal behavior and at the research on domestic violence using the same "windows" as in this chapter. What can we conclude from this research about the relationship between alcohol and violence?

First, although there is a considerable alcohol presence in both offenders and victims involved in violent events, there is evidence that they have many other social, economic, and mental health problems.[57] Additionally, alcohol use is related to a number of situational variables that describe violent events. These different types of variables are rarely included in the same piece of research. The strength of the alcohol explanation is therefore not tested. In addition, there is some evidence that the co-occurrence of multiple social and health problems may preclude a clear explanation of alcohol's relation to many violent behaviors. This is, in part, a consequence of the multivariate explanations of social behavior, and it is a problem that research and policy-making have not adequately confronted.

Second, typologies of violent events that are theoretically driven are rare in this research. Global divisions of behaviors into such categories as "violent" versus "nonviolent," or even groups of behaviors such as "homicide" or "domestic violence," do not offer enough specificity to establish clearly alcohol's relationships with the behavior in question, although there is often considerable alcohol presence in samples of these behaviors.

Third, empirical studies of alcohol and violence are typically unclear about precisely what effects of alcohol are under investigation. Thus, in the same piece of research the sociobehavioral effects of alcohol as an excuse for untoward behavior are not distinguished from the pharmacological or other effects. There is growing evidence that violence is a rational choice of particular actors. Yet alcohol-involved violence is often viewed as irrational, uncontrollable behavior. But these effects are often not clearly explicated. Often researchers do not even address the question of why alcohol is included in their research. Why, for example, do Koss and her colleagues include alcohol and drugs as risk factors for sexual aggression? What theories of alcohol's effects lie behind the inclusion?

Fourth, the methodology of studying untoward events such as violence is underdeveloped. This is particularly evident in the paucity of work on appropriate comparison groups for violent events. Finding appropriate "controls" is essential if the use of alcohol by persons who are similarly situated in relation to variables of theoretical importance in a given study is to be evaluated.

The past decade has seen changing perceptions of the victim–aggressor relationship. This has been the case especially in relation to spousal violence in which the woman as aggressor has been perceived by some courts, by special interest groups, and by others as having committed justifiable violence because of past victimization. This has also characterized some abusive parent–child relationships that have involved violence, including homicide. The possible contribution of alcohol and/or drugs to these violent outcomes must be assessed not only in relation to the final violent event but to what might have been an aggressive interaction over a long period of time, with the aggression in some cases coming from each party at different times. The victim–offender relationship in these cases is a mutable one. It is essential then that the analyst is clear in denoting who is the victim and who is the aggressor in relation to a specific act, and whether the analysis of the "final" act is the proper unit of analysis. Ideally, a time scale for the interaction should be specified. The Pernanen-type questions (i.e., those used in Pernanen) do not clearly specify each of these. Indeed, the respondent is labeled the "victim," because the study is a "victimization" survey that takes the perspective of the respondent, despite the fact that in an unknown proportion of cases the "victim" may have "started" the conflict. An analysis of the time scale of violent interactions and the use of alcohol over time in these interactions will depend on more qualitative evidence than is typically collected. This need for both quantitative and qualitative evidence analyzed within the same study is a significant challenge for future work.

If epidemiological research on alcohol and violence is to contribute to our understanding of the role of alcohol in violent events and violent lives, each of these four factors needs considerably greater attention in future research. Ironically, this progress may depend on the development of qualitative research on the natural history of violent events rather than epidemiological research itself.

ACKNOWLEDGMENT. An earlier version of this chapter appeared in "Alcohol and Interpersonal Violence: Fostering Multidisciplinary Perspectives," published in 1993 by the National Institutes of Health as NIAAA Research Monograph 24. Preparation of the chapter was supported by the Alcohol Research Group, Berkeley, California, from its NIAAA Center Grant.

References

1. Roizen J: Alcohol and violence: An evaluation of the evidence from epidemiological research. Prepared for the Working Group on Alcohol-related Violence: Fostering Interdisciplinary Perspectives, convened by the National Institute on Alcohol Abuse and Alcoholism, Washington, DC, May 14–15, 1992.
2. Pernanen K: *Alcohol in Human Violence.* New York, Guilford Press, 1991.

3. Leonard KE, Jacob T: Alcohol, alcoholism and family violence, in Van Hasselt V, *et al* (eds): *Handbook of Family Violence*. New York, Plenum Press, 1990, pp 383–406.
4. Kuhn T: *Structure of Scientific Revolutions*. Chicago: University Press, 1970.
5. Collins JJ Jr: Alcohol use and criminal behavior: An empirical, theoretical, and methodological overview, in Collins JJ Jr (ed): *Drinking and Crime: Perspectives on the Relationships between Alcohol Consumption and Criminal Behavior*. New York, Guilford Press, 1981, pp 288–316.
6. Stinchcombe A: The origins of sociology as a discipline. *Acta Sociol* 27:51–61, 1984.
7. Collins JJ Jr: Alcohol and interpersonal violence: Less than meets the eye, in Weiner N, Wolfgang M (eds): *Pathways to Criminal Violence*. Newbury Park, CA, Sage Publications, 1989, pp 49–67.
8. Roizen J: Alcohol and trauma, in Giesbrecht N, Gonzalez R, Grant M, *et al* (eds): *Drinking and Casualties*. London, Routledge, 1989, pp 21–66.
9. Murphy JM, Jellinek M, Quinn D, *et al:* Substance abuse and serious child mistreatment: Prevalence, risk, and outcome in a court sample. *Child Abuse Neglect* 15:197–211, 1991.
10. Orme TC, Rimmer J: Alcoholism and child abuse: A review. *J Stud Alcohol* 42:273–287, 1981.
11. Parker RN: *Bringing "Booze" Back In: The Relationship between Alcohol and Homicide*. Berkeley, CA, Prevention Research Center, 1992.
12. Abbey A: Acquaintance rape and alcohol consumption on college campuses: How are they linked? *J Am College Health* 39:165–169, 1991.
13. Koss MP, Dinero TE: Discriminant analysis of risk factors for sexual victimization among a national sample of college women. *J Consult Clin Psychol* 57:242–250, 1989.
14. Muehlenhard CL, Linton MA: Date rape and sexual aggression in dating situations: Incidence and risk factors. *J Counsel Psychol* 34:186–196, 1987.
15. Pernanen K: Alcohol and crimes of violence, in Kissin B, Begleiter H (eds): *The Biology of Alcoholism: Social Aspects of Alcoholism*. New York, Plenum Press, 1976, pp. 351–444.
16. Cordilia A: Alcohol and property crime: Exploring the causal nexus. *J Stud Alcohol* 46:161–171, 1985.
17. Petersilia J, Greenwood PW, Lavin M: *Criminal Careers of Habitual Felons*. Washington, DC, US Government Printing Office, 1978.
18. Ladouceur P, Temple M: Substance abuse among rapists: A comparison with other serious felons. *Crime Delinquency* 31:269–294, 1985.
19. Aarens M, Cameron T, Roizen J, *et al* (eds): *Alcohol, Casualties and Crime*. Alcohol, Casualties and Crime Project Final Report, Report No. C-18, Social Research Group, University of California, Berkeley, 1977.
20. Greenberg SW: Alcohol and crime: A methodological critique of the literature, in Collins JJ Jr (ed): *Drinking and Crime: Perspectives on the Relationships between Alcohol Consumption and Criminal Behavior*. New York, Guilford Press, 1981, pp 70–109.
21. Pernanen K: Theoretical aspects of the relationship between alcohol use and crime, in Collins JJ Jr (ed): *Drinking and Crime: Perspectives on the Relationships between Alcohol Consumption and Criminal Behavior*. New York, Guilford Press, 1981, pp 1–69.
22. Roizen J, Schneberk D: Alcohol and crime, in Aarens M, *et al* (eds): *Alcohol, Casualties and Crime*. Alcohol, Casualties and Crime Project Final Report No. C-18, Social Research Group, University of California, Berkeley, 1977.
23. Barnard GW, Holzer C, Vera H: A comparison of alcoholics and non-alcoholics charged with rape. *Bull Am Acad Psychiatry Law* 7:432–440, 1979.
24. Straus MA, Gelles RJ: Societal change and change in family violence from 1975–1985. *J Marriage Family* 48:465–479, 1986.
25. Greenfield TK, Weisner C: Drinking problems and self-reported criminal behavior, arrests and convictions: 1990 national alcohol and 1989 county surveys, presented at the American Public Health Association 120th Annual Meeting, Washington, DC, November 8–12, 1992.
26. Wolfgang ME: *Patterns in Criminal Homicide*. Philadelphia, University of Pennsylvania Press, 1958.
27. Roizen J: Estimating alcohol involvement in serious events, in *Alcohol Consumption and Related Problems*. Alcohol and Health Monograph No. 1. DHSS Publication No. (ADM 82-1190), Washington, DC, US Government Printing Office, 1982, pp 179–219.

28. US Department of Justice, Federal Bureau of Investigation: *Crime in the United States: Uniform Crime Reports.* Washington, DC, US Government Printing Office, 1988.
29. US Department of Justice, National Criminal Justice Information and Statistics Service: *Census of State Correctional Facilities 1974 Advance Report.* NPS Special Report, July. Washington, DC, US Government Printing Office, 1975.
30. US Department of Justice, Bureau of Justice Statistics: *Criminal Victimization in the United States, 1982* (publication No. NCJ-92820). Washington, DC, US Government Printing Office, 1984.
31. Dietz PE: Social factors in rapist behavior, in Rada RT (ed): *Clinical Aspects of the Rapist.* New York, Grune & Stratton, 1978.
32. Clark L, Lewis D: *Rape: The Price of Coercive Sexuality.* Toronto, The Women's Press, 1977.
33. Selling LS: The role of alcohol in the commission of sex offenses. *Med Rec* 151:289–291, 1940.
34. Visher C: Reported use of alcohol by DU arrestees. Drugs and Crime 1990 Annual Report: Drug Use Forecasting. Washington, DC, National Institute of Justice, 1990.
35. Amir M: *Patterns in Forcible Rape.* Chicago: University of Chicago Press, 1971.
36. Johnson SD, Gibson L, Linden R: Alcohol and rape in Winnipeg, 1966–1975. *J Stud Alcohol* 39:1887–1894, 1978.
37. Richardson D, Campbell JL: The effect of alcohol on attributions of blame for rape. *Pers Soc Psychol Bull* 8:468–476, 1982.
38. Deming JE, Mittleman RE, Wetli CV: Forensic science aspects of fatal sexual assaults on women. *J Forensic Sci* 28:572–576, 1983.
39. Gibbens T, Soothill K, Way C: Sex offenses against young girls: A long-term record study. *Psychol Med* 11:351–357, 1981.
40. Normandeau A: *Trends and Patterns in Crimes of Robbery.* Ann Arbor, University Microfilms International, 1968.
41. Amir M: Alcohol and forcible rape. *Br J Addict* 62:219–232, 1967.
42. Pittman DJ, Handy W: Patterns in criminal aggravated assault. *J Criminal Law, Criminol Police Sci* 55:462–470, 1964.
43. US Department of Justice, Bureau of Justice Statistics: *Survey of Inmates of State Correctional Facilities, 1979.* (ICSPR 7856) 2nd ICSPR ed. Ann Arbor, International Consortium for Social and Political Research, 1981.
44. Collins JJ Jr, Schlenger WE: Acute and chronic effects of alcohol use and violence. *J Stud Alcohol* 49:516–521, 1989.
45. Groth AM, Birnbaum HJ: *Men Who Rape: The Psychology of the Offender.* New York, Plenum Press, 1979.
46. Rada RT: Alcoholism and forcible rape. *Am J Psychiatry* 132:444–446, 1975.
47. Koss MP, Gidycz CA, Wisniewski N: The scope of rape: Incidence and prevalence of sexual aggression and victimization in a national sample of higher education students. *J Consult Clin Psychol* 55:162–170, 1987.
48. Koss MP, Dinero TE: Predictors of sexual aggression among a national sample of male college students. *Ann NY Acad Sci* 528:133–146, 1988.
49. Johnson LD, O'Malley PM, Bachman JG: *Drug Use, Drinking and Smoking: National Survey Results from High School, College and Young Adult Populations, 1975–1988.* National Institute on Drug Abuse, DHHS Pub. No. (ADM) 86-1638, 1989.
50. Engs R, Hanson D: The drinking patterns and problems of college students. *J Alcohol Drug Educ* 31:65–83, 1983.
51. Gleason N: *Toward a Model for Preventing Alcohol Abuse by College Women: A Relational Perspective.* The Stone Center for Developmental Services and Studies, Wellesley College, 1992.
52. Koss MP, Dinero TE, Seibel C, *et al:* Stranger, acquaintance and date rape: Is there a difference in the victim's experience? *Psychol Women Q* 12:1–24, 1988.
53. Kantor GK, Straus MA: The drunken bum theory of wife beating. *Social Problems* 34:213–231, 1987.
54. MacAndrew C, Edgerton R: *Drunken Deportment: A Social Explanation.* Chicago, Aldine, 1969.
55. Parker T: *Life After Life.* London, Martin Secker and Warburg, 1990.
56. Parker T: *The Violence of Our Lives.* London: HarperCollins, 1995.

57. Abram KM, Teplin LA, McClelland GM: The effects of co-occurring disorders on the relationship between alcoholism and violent crime, in Martin SE (ed): *Alcohol and Interpersonal Violence: Fostering Multidisciplinary Perspectives.* NIH Publication No. 93-3496, Rockville, MD, National Institutes of Health, 1993.
58. Shupe LM: Alcohol and crime: A study of the urine alcohol concentration found in 882 persons arrested during or immediately after the commission of a felony. *J Criminal Law, Criminol Police Sci* 44:661–664, 1954.
59. President's Commission on Crime: *Report on the President's Commission on Crime in the District of Columbia.* Washington, DC, US Government Printing Office, 1966.
60. Tardif G: *La Criminalite de Violence.* MA Thesis, University of Montreal, 1966.

The Relationship of Alcohol to Injury in Assault Cases

Susan Ehrlich Martin and Ronet Bachman

Abstract. Little is known about the precise role of alcohol in the escalation of interactions from threats into physical violence or its contribution to the risk of injury. Experimental studies indicate that intoxicated subjects (allegedly) give markedly higher electric shocks than sober subjects and are less sensitive to their cries of pain. However, few studies in a naturalistic setting have examined whether aggressive acts become more serious and result in higher injury rates when the assailants have been drinking than when they are sober. This chapter reviews the two bodies of research on the effects of alcohol on interpersonal aggression and violence; presents new data on the escalation of threatening interactions to assaults and the likelihood of victim injury given an assault, using data from the National Crime Victimization Survey for the years 1992 and 1993; and suggests future directions for research based on our findings that alcohol's impact on both escalation and injury differed according to the victim–assailant relationship.

In the past three decades, more than 100 studies have confirmed the widespread belief that alcohol frequently has been consumed by offenders and victims prior to violent incidents. These findings have been summarized in several reviews of the literature on alcohol consumption and violence[1-7] and indicate that a majority of homicide and assault cases involve alcohol use. Another body of research, focused on the contribution of alcohol to aggression in a laboratory setting, also has found that alcohol is a potent antecedent of aggressive behavior. Nevertheless, there is surprisingly little empirical data concerning alcohol's precise role in the escalation of hostile interactions or threatening situations into physical violence, particularly assaults that do not

Susan Ehrlich Martin • Prevention Research Branch, Division of Clinical and Prevention Research, National Institute on Alcohol Abuse and Alcoholism, Rockville, Maryland 20892-7003. **Ronet Bachman** • Department of Sociology, University of Delaware, Newark, Delaware 19716.

Recent Developments in Alcoholism, Volume 13: Alcoholism and Violence, edited by Marc Galanter. Plenum Press, New York, 1997

result in homicide. Similarly, knowledge is limited regarding the contribution of alcohol to the risk of injury or injury severity in incidents in which violence occurs. Nor are the mechanisms or mediating factors by which alcohol consumption affects aggression well understood.

This chapter reviews the research literature on the contribution of alcohol to: (1) the escalation from threats to violence in naturalistic settings; (2) the risk of victim injury and injury severity given an assault; and (3) acts of aggression in experimental laboratory settings. It next tests two hypotheses regarding the contribution of alcohol to incident severity and to the perpetrator's lack of discrimination in the use of violence, using a large nationally representative sample of victims of violence from the National Crime Victimization Survey. It concludes with a discussion of explanatory frameworks and future research directions for studying alcohol's contribution to assault.

1. Research on Alcohol in Human Violence

Evidence regarding the role of alcohol in human violence comes primarily from two types of research: correlational studies of naturally occurring alcohol use and violent behavior and laboratory experiments.

1.1. Correlational Studies

Surveys have typically focused on real-life incidents of violence reported by victims or perpetrators and have frequently found associations between violence and drinking or drunkenness. For example, in an update of an earlier study, Roizen[8] reported that in 14 studies of homicide, alcohol was present in between 28 and 86% of the offenders; in eight studies of assaults, it was present in 24 to 72% of the assault offenders. Alcohol also was present in 21 to 50% of the victims or assailants in seven studies of marital violence. Another review of studies of alcohol and violent crime that included five studies with data on assaults, using data primarily from police records, found that between 24 and 82% of assault offenders and between 24 and 40% of assault victims had been drinking prior to the assault.[3]

In addition to data on alcohol prevalence, findings from several studies suggest that alcohol is positively associated with the severity of injuries resulting from violence. One study examined the contribution of alcohol to injury by comparing the frequency of its presence in incidents of specific types of aggression of differing degrees of severity. In all four comparisons, alcohol was more likely to be involved in the act producing the greatest injury.[9] For example, 28% of marital cases of threatening behavior but 49% of marital assaults and 34% of common assaults but 46% of assaults causing injuries involved alcohol.

Surveys of incarcerated offenders also find they frequently used alcohol alone or in combination with other drugs prior to the assault for which they were locked up, including 34% of youth in custody[10] and 54% of jail inmates.[11] While these data are suggestive of an alcohol–violence association, samples of arrested or incarcerated offenders are neither representative of all violent offenders nor of their patterns of alcohol consumption.

Research focused on victims of violence, such as emergency room (ER) studies of injuries using a case-control methodology, also has found alcohol consumption to be associated with violence-related fatal and nonfatal injuries[8,12,13] (for a review of injury studies). For example, one study found that 29% of persons with severe violence-related injuries reported drinking more than 10 drinks in the 12 hr preceding their injury compared with 18% with only minor injuries, suggesting a positive association between the degree of victim's intoxication and the severity of the injury.[14] A Finnish study found that alcohol intoxication increased the likelihood of hospitalization for male assault victims treated in an ER (odds ratio 1.5; $P < 0.06$).[15] A third study reports a higher proportion of coroner cases (47%) that were alcohol-related compared with violence-related ER nonfatal injury cases (19%).[16]

Emergency room studies primarily focus on the presence of alcohol in the blood, breath, or tissues of a victim of violence who receives medical treatment. They rarely ascertain data on the presence of alcohol in the perpetrator of the violence or document the processes of violence escalation. Thus, the contribution of ER studies to understanding of assault severity is limited.

In the past two decades, dozens of new studies have focused specifically on the role of alcohol in violence among intimates. Several reviews have pointed out the methodological shortcomings of such studies and their consistent finding that drinking is associated with intimate-perpetrated domestic violence.[17–20] Often the research has focused on distal influences such as husband's drinking pattern and socioeconomic status. While such an approach can identify high-risk groups, it sheds little light on the underlying processes that lead to marital violence and on the proximal influence of alcohol consumption on the event.[19]

Evidence regarding acute effects of drinking on the escalation of conflicts to violence among intimates and the interactions of alcohol effects with contextual factors in the escalatory processes is quite limited. Estimates of the proportion of violent events among intimates that are associated with alcohol use range from 22[20] to 60%.[21] It is noteworthy, however, that in many of these violent incidents only the assailant (usually the man) is drinking, whereas in violent incidents involving other victim–assailant relationships it is more likely that both the offender and victim have been drinking. For example, police records from one community over a 1-year period found that in reports involving marital abuse, 44% of the assailants but only 14% of the victims had been drinking (compared with 31 and 26% of all of the violent crime incidents).[6] The 1985 National Family Violence Resurvey (NFVR), based on a nationally representative sample of 5159 couples,[20] found that 22% of the husbands and 10% of the wives had been drinking prior to incidents of spousal violence (while overall, 24% of the incidents involved drinking).

Studies of the effect of alcohol on the severity of the spousal violence, usually measured as the extent of injuries, provide inconsistent findings. Fagan and colleagues[22] reported that the severity of spouse abuse was positively associated with alcohol use by the assailant (while there was a weak, negative association with use of other substances). Conversely, an analysis of 262 domestic disturbance calls to which the police responded found that the man's drinking pattern was related to the severity of the victim's injuries but drinking by the offender and victim were unrelated to the injury.[23] Kantor and Straus'[24] reanalysis of NFVR findings found that the husband's drunkenness was associated with higher rates of minor violence but not severe violence against their wives.

This finding, as well as those of more than 100 studies of spouse abuse in the past 15 years, is based on the Conflict Tactics Scale (CTS), which classifies cases of spousal assault as minor or severe in a way that corresponds to the legal distinctions between simple and aggravated assault.[25,26] Thus, the CTS has a scale for physical aggression that is subdivided into minor and severe violence. Minor violence includes pushing, grabbing, and slapping; severe violence includes kicking, punching, hitting with an object, choking, beating up, and using a knife or gun. It also includes threatening with a knife or gun, since such threats meet the legal definition of assault. But threats do not involve actual physical contact or violence, although they constitute nearly a third of all assaultive incidents between intimates and more than half of all assaults in a nationally representative sample of victimization.[27] Kantor and Straus'[24] inclusion of threats in their measure of severe violence, therefore, may be partly responsible for their failure to find drunkenness to be a predictor of serious violence among intimates.

In a uniquely comprehensive study of the role of alcohol in human violence that used multiple methods to study one community, Kai Pernanen[5] conducted interviews with 933 community residents aged 20 and over drawn from a probability sample of the general population in one medium-sized Canadian community (Thunder Bay, Ontario). Of those interviewed, 435 reported experiencing violent victimization and provided details on their most recent experience involving an actual physical assault, including the drinking behavior of both the assailant and victim prior to the assault.

Pernanen explored two hypotheses regarding the role of alcohol in naturally occurring violent events. The "severity" hypothesis argues that the rate and extent of injuries will be more serious when assailants have been drinking than under similar conditions when the assailants are sober. The "indiscrimination" hypothesis states that acts of aggression after drinking are less likely to be tailored to the situation and social norms applying to it than acts of sober aggression. For example, drinking would be expected to loosen restraints on serious violence directed at "restricted" targets such as women and children; if such acts occur after drinking, they are expected to be as serious as sober acts.

Although alcohol was involved in more than half of the 435 incidents examined in detail, Pernanen's data provided no support for a general severity hypothesis. Injury rates were closely related to the age, gender, and relationship of victim and perpetrator, but were not consistently associated with whether the assailant was drinking. For example, men were more likely to be injured when their assailants had been drinking and women were at higher risk when their assailants were sober. Nevertheless, the finding that the injury rate was significantly higher when the assailant was judged to be drunk provides conditional support for the severity hypothesis.

Support for the indiscrimination hypothesis was similarly inconsistent. There was a tendency to greater rather than diminished discrimination by gender of victim when alcohol had been used. Drinking, even drunkenness, did not lead men to abandon the normative restrictions regarding the types of violence deemed permissible when a man is fighting a woman. Drinking, however, did increase likelihood that victimizations by strangers would result in injury.

1.2. Experimental Studies

Experimental research provides the second source of evidence on the role of alcohol in human violence and served as the primary basis for severity and indiscrimination hypotheses. Reviews of the many studies of alcohol-induced aggression under controlled conditions have concluded that alcohol is a potent determinant of aggression.[28-30] Pernanen's severity hypothesis is predicated on studies using variations of the Buss[31] "aggression machine," which measures aggression in the form of the intensity and/or duration of electric shocks (allegedly) administered by subjects to other subjects.[32-36] In general, these studies have found that intoxicated subjects give markedly higher shocks than sober subjects, particularly under conditions of frustration, provocation,[37] or threat.[38]

Similarly, there is experimental support for the indiscrimination hypothesis. For example, following administration of controlled doses of alcohol, researchers have found that subjects showed less sensitivity to cries of pain from a decoy victim[39] and were less sensitive to empirical contingencies in the evaluation of feedback and in the aggression committed.[40] However, experimental findings also have shown that intoxicated subjects are influenced by social pressure from a "bystander" and by social norms.[41-43]

The prevailing explanation for these findings is that alcohol has an impairing effect on information processing. This view was expanded by Steele and Joseph[44] into a broader theory of the affective and interpersonal consequences of "alcohol myopia." However, in the past several years there has been little follow-up research testing measures of information processing or mediating factors such as emotions that may be affected by attentional impairment.[45]

1.3. Limitations of Existing Studies

The limitations of both correlational and experimental studies suggest the need for additional research on the effects of alcohol on the escalation and severity of injury in assaults. The principal problems of laboratory studies are the limitations related to the artificiality of the drinking situation and the difficulty of successfully carrying off variations of the balanced placebo design that include the "expectancy effect" that has been found for direct physical aggression. Other problems include the extent to which pain thresholds vary across trials, the putative analgesic effect of alcohol, and the failure of the commonly used aggression paradigms to study the interactions between people who know each other.[45]

Correlational studies in general and Pernanen's analyses in particular also have a number of limitations. First, most studies do not include incidents of threat only and therefore cannot examine the contribution of alcohol consumption to the risk of an incident escalating from threat to physical attack. Second, small sample size limited Pernanen's ability simultaneously to control for other important contextual characteristics of the incident (e.g., both gender and the victim–assailant relationship) in examining the contribution of alcohol to the risk of injury.

2. The NCVS Study

To ameliorate the shortcomings and to test more refined versions of the severity and indiscrimination hypotheses, we used data from a much larger, nationally representative sample of the US population aged 12 years and over. We focused on the effects of alcohol on assault severity and on discrimination in the use of violence for five types of assault determined by the victim's and offender's gender and the victim–offender relationship. Specifically, analyses were performed separately for men's assaults on male friends and acquaintances and on male strangers and for men's assaults against women who were intimates (i.e., husbands, boyfriends, and former husbands and boyfriends), acquaintances, and strangers. The initial descriptive analysis revealed too few cases of female-perpetrated assaults involving alcohol to include in multivariate analysis.

2.1. Sample

The data used in our analysis come from the Bureau of Justice Statistics-sponsored National Crime Victimization Survey (NCVS) for 1992 and 1993. The NCVS obtains information about crimes, including incidents not reported to the police, from a continuous, nationally representative sample of households in the United States, which is more fully detailed elsewhere.[27] The redesign has added questions that directly ask respondents about attacks that were perpetrated by relatives or other persons known to them, permitting collection of fuller information about intimate violence.[46] Prior to 1992, NCVS estimates of intimate-perpetrated violence against women were much lower than estimates obtained from other national surveys,[47] probably because the NCVS did not directly ask respondents about attacks that were perpetrated by relatives or other offenders known to them. Prompted by criticism of this earlier methodology, a new NCVS screening instrument gradually was implemented into the sample beginning in 1989. By 1992, the entire NCVS sample was using the redesigned survey and the number of victimizations reported to interviewers, particularly assaults perpetrated by intimates, had greatly increased.[48]

In this chapter we focus exclusively on single-offender assaults. The NCVS defines assault as an unlawful physical attack, including attempted or threatened attacks upon a person. The offenses categorized as assaults in our analyses range in severity from minor incidents such as attempted and verbal threats of assault to more severe incidents such as those involving use of weapons and resulting in injury. However, because NCVS classifies victimizations according to a seriousness hierarchy, a number of the more serious incidents may have been excluded from the analysis. For example, an assault also involving theft is classified as a robbery; similarly, rapes and attempted rapes are categorized separately.

2.2. Measures

2.2.1. Dependent Variables: Assault Severity. The severity of assault was operationalized in two ways. The first dependent variable we examine indicates whether or not the assault actually culminated in a physical attack by the offender. To operationalize this variable victims were asked, "Did the offender hit you, knock you down, or actually attack you in any way?" In the multivariate analyses, the variable was coded 1 if the answer was yes and 0 if only a threat of assault was involved.

The second dependent variable indicated whether victims sustained any injuries. In the multivariate analysis, this variable was coded 1 if the victim was injured and 0 if no injuries had been sustained. In the bivariate analysis displayed in Tables II–IV, however, we treated these variables as three values of a single assault variable, namely, threat only, assault without injury, and assault with injury. We would have liked to have determined the extent to which alcohol increased the severity of injuries sustained, adding a "severe injury" category. However, because the distribution of assaults resulting in injury from this sample primarily consisted of minor injuries such as bruises and scratches, there was not enough variation in injury severity to investigate the extent to which alcohol increased the seriousness of an injury.

2.2.2. Independent Variables. A number of independent variables were used in the analyses, including alcohol use, location of occurrence, victim–assailant relationship, and demographic controls including victim's gender, age, and marital status. The determination of assailant's alcohol use was based solely on victim perceptions. Victims were asked, "Was the offender drinking or on drugs?" If the reply was affirmative, they were next asked, "Which was it, drinking, drugs, or both?" If victims said the offender had been drinking, this variable was coded 1. If the assailant was not perceived to be under the influence of any substance, this variable was coded 0. To make the comparison categories as pure as possible, all assailants perceived to be under the influence of drugs other than alcohol or perceived to be under the influence of both substances were excluded from the analysis.

The location of the occurrence was dichotomized as occurring in a public place (coded 1) or at or near a private residence (including the home of the victim, a friend, or neighbor; coded 0). Age of victim was a continuous variable ranging from 12 to 84 years. Marital status was coded 1 if married, 0 for single, separated, divorced, or widowed.

2.3. Analytic Procedures

The effects of alcohol on assault severity were examined for five different types of assault, determined by the victim's and assailant's gender and the victim–assailant relationship. Specifically, analyses were performed separately for male-on-male assaults involving friends and acquaintances and those involving strangers. Male assaults against females were examined separately for intimates, acquaintances, and strangers. Intimate was defined as all husbands or ex-husbands, and boyfriends or ex-boyfriends. Nonintimate relatives were excluded from the analyses.

We first conducted bivariate analyses predicting the assault severity measure using assailant's alcohol use only. For relationships found to be significant at the bivariate level, we performed multivariate logistic regression analysis to control for other factors that may affect assault severity.

2.4. Findings

The descriptive characteristics of the victim sample and the victimization category are displayed in Table I. This table indicates that most "assault" incidents (58%) involved threats rather than actual physical attacks. Men were more likely than women to be victims of assaultive incidents, but female victims were more likely than male victims actually to be both physically attacked and injured.

Escalation from threat to attack also was closely related to the victim's age; the younger the victim, the greater the likelihood of an actual physical assault. Most attacks occurred in public places, but those that occurred in private places were more likely to result in an attack and injury to the victim.

Table I. Characteristics of Victim Sample by Percent in Victimization Category

	Threat	Assault without injury	Assault with injury
Total (*N* = 5592)	58%	19%	23%
Gender of victim			
Male (*N* = 3234)	60	20	20
Female (*N* = 2358)	55	18	27
Age of victim			
12–18 (*N* = 1587)	46	25	29
19–29 (*N* = 1679)	56	19	25
30–45 (*N* = 1732)	65	16	19
46 and up (*N* = 594)	69	14	17
Location of incident			
Public (*N* = 3973)	61	19	20
Private (*N* = 1619)	49	20	31
Victim–assailant relationship			
Intimate (*N* = 613)	32	22	46
Acquaintance (*N* = 1650)	55	22	23
Stranger (*N* = 1321)	68	19	13
Assailant's perceived alcohol use			
Not drinking (*N* = 2064)	58	20	22
Had been drinking (*N* = 941)	50	23	27

Most assaults involved people who know each other, and the closer the relationship between victim and assailant, the greater the likelihood of escalation to attack.

Table I also indicates that most assailants were not perceived to have been drinking prior to the assault incident. Nevertheless, the consumption of alcohol increased the chance that an incident would result in physical violence and victim injury, providing preliminary support for the severity hypothesis.

In Table II, we explore the joint percentage distributions of the assault severity measures by assailant's alcohol use and present the results of the Chi square analysis. The upper portion of the table presents male-on-male assaults by victim–assailant relationship. For assaults involving friends or acquaintances, both measures of assault severity appear to be unaffected by the perpetrator's alcohol use. Similar percentages of assaults culminate in actual attacks in the presence and absence of alcohol; likewise, the proportion of male victims that sustained injuries was unchanged by whether the assailant had been drinking.

In contrast to the findings for acquaintance assaults, alcohol did affect the severity of male-on-male assaults involving strangers. Men who had been drinking were significantly more likely to physically attack another man during an assault incident (39%) than men who had not been drinking (26%). The assailant's use alcohol did not, however, increase the likelihood that the assault would result in injury to the victim.

Assaults involving male perpetrators and female victims are presented in the lower portion of Table II. For two of the three relationships, assault severity escalated if the man was perceived to have been drinking. Both the percentage of women actually assaulted and the percentage of women who were injured increased if a male intimate or stranger had been drinking; a male acquaintance's drinking did not affect the incident. The only relationship to attain statistical significance, however, was the increased likelihood of injury for women assaulted by intimates who had been drinking (54%) in contrast to nondrinking intimates (43%).

We next examine whether the use of alcohol by the assailant increases the probability of an assault escalating to a physical attack even after controlling for other important contextual characteristics of the assault. Table III displays the results for the logistic regression analysis predicting a physical attack (coded 1) versus a threat only (coded 0) for male-on-male assaults involving strangers. This table indicates that men's encounters with male strangers were significantly more likely to escalate from threat to physical attack when the assailant had been drinking compared to incidents in which he had not. In

Table II. Contribution of Alcohol to Assault Victimizations by Victim and Assailant Gender and Relationship

	Assailant perceived as using alcohol	Assailant not perceived as using alcohol
Male assailant/male victim		
Acquaintance assaults		
Threat	50%	50%
Assault without injury	26	27
Assault with injury	24	23
Stranger assaults		
Threat	61[a]	74[a]
Assault without injury	24	14
Assault with injury	15	12
Male assailant/female victim		
Intimate assaults		
Threat	26	34
Assault without injury	20	23
Assault with injury	54[a]	43[a]
Acquaintance assaults		
Threat	64	64
Assault without injury	19	14
Assault with injury	17	22
Stranger assaults		
Threat	64	74
Assault without injury	22	16
Assault with injury	14	10

[a]Indicates Chi-square between assailants perceived to be using and not to be using alcohol was significant at $P < 0.05$ level.

Table III. Logistic Regression of Male Physical Attack on Male Strangers Controlling for Other Contextual Characteristics

	B	S.E.	Sig.	Exp (B)
Assailant drinking	.6300	.1538	.0001	1.877
Incident in public place	−.2221	.2591	.3914	.800
Victim's age	−.0300	.0069	.0001	.970
Model Chi-square = 38.55; $P < 0.0001$

fact, the odds of an assault resulting in a physical attack were almost twice as great for assailants who have been drinking (Exp(B) = 1.877) compared to those not under the influence of alcohol.

In addition to the assailant's use of alcohol, the victim's age was also significant in predicting assault severity in male-on-male assaults involving strangers. Assaults involving younger victims were significantly more likely to result in physical attacks than assaults involving older victims. Whether the assault occurred in a public place, however, did not affect the likelihood of a male-on-male stranger incident escalating into a physical assault.

Table IV presents the results of the logistic regression model predicting the probability that female victims sustained injuries from the assault (coded 1) versus assaults that did not result in injury (coded 0) by male assailants who were intimates, while simultaneously controlling for location and victim's age and marital status. The results of this logistic regression model indicate that alcohol use by the perpetrator was significant in predicting assault severity (i.e., victim injury), even after controlling for location, marital status, and victim's age. The odds of a woman sustaining an injury in an assault by an intimate partner who had been drinking increased by a factor of 1.49 compared to women attacked by a nondrinking partner. In addition, injury was significantly more likely when the assault occurred in a private home. Age and marital status did not affect assault severity for male-on-female assaults involving intimates.

Table IV. Logistic Regression of Male Assailants' Injury of Intimate Female Victims, Controlling for Other Contextual Characteristics

	B	S.E.	Sig.	Exp (B)
Assailant drinking	.4023	.1820	.0271	1.495
Incident in public place	−.4725	.2421	.0509	.623
Victim's age	−.0068	.0083	.4095	.993
Married	.2162	.2437	.3750	1.241

Model Chi-square = 11.42; $P < 0.0222$

2.5. Discussion

Based on data from the NCVS, we have found that the effects of drinking by the assailant on the escalation and outcome of assaultive behavior varies according to the assault context. Specifically, alcohol's contribution to the escalation of an incident from a threat to a physical attack and to injuries sustained by the assault victim varies with the gender of the victim and the victim–assailant relationship.

In male-on-male acquaintance assaults, alcohol has no effect either on the likelihood of a threat escalating to an attack or on it resulting in injury. Similarly, alcohol has no effect on either outcome in male-on-female acquaintance attacks, although a smaller proportion of these incidents (36%) than male-on-male incidents (50%) result in actual attacks regardless of alcohol involvement.

The pattern of escalation from threat to assault with and without victim injury is similar in male-on-male and male-on-female stranger assaults, although alcohol's effect on the escalation only achieves statistical significance in the male-on-male incidents. Multivariate analysis indicates that even after controlling for other variables, alcohol increases the likelihood that a threat will escalate to an attack in male-on-male incidents but does not increase the probability of injury to the victim.

Assailant alcohol use also affected the outcome of male-on-female assaults between intimates. While alcohol use by the assailant did not increase the likelihood that an intimate partner would escalate his threat to physical violence, drinking by the perpetrator did increase the likelihood that the female victim would sustain an injury even after controlling for her marital status and age and the location of the incident. It should also be noted that male assaults on intimate female partners were more likely to result in actual attacks and in victim injury compared to any other victim–offender relationship regardless of alcohol use by the offender.

Our findings differ somewhat from those obtained by Pernanen. After controlling simultaneously for victim–perpetrator relationship and gender, we found that men's drinking increases the already-elevated probability of injury to an intimate female partner. This suggests that violent acts are less limited and tailored to the situation and relationship in the presence of alcohol.

The extremely high rate of injury to female intimates from male partner violence (46% of all such assaults irrespective of alcohol involvement and 54% of the assaults when the man had been drinking) in contrast to the injury rates in all other victim–perpetrator categories needs some explanation. Our findings are consistent with other studies that have found that alcohol abuse is a relatively strong and consistent correlate of partner aggression.[18–20,49] Going beyond measures of the prevalence of alcohol in intimate violence, however, we have found that alcohol also significantly increases the likelihood of injury in such incidents. It is unclear, however, the extent to which psychological, situational, and pharmacological factors contribute to women's alcohol-related injury by an intimate.

An alternative interpretation of this finding, however, may be related to the NCVS data. Although the redesign has increased the rate at which victimizations by intimates are reported, women may still use a different threshold for reporting violence by an intimate than they use in similar incidents involving acquaintances and strangers. Threats by nonintimate men may be viewed as more unusual, more memorable, and thus more likely to be reported in a survey, whereas spousal threats may rarely be regarded as "criminal" or worth reporting in a survey except when they culminate in an attack or injury.

Several other limitations of the NCVS data supported here should be noted. The alcohol-related information contains only the victim's report of the perpetrator's drinking and indicates only the apparent presence of alcohol. There is no information on the victim's use of alcohol, which is a serious limitation given the frequency with which the victim has been found to have been drinking in assault and spousal assault cases.[3,6,7,20] Furthermore, data are lacking on the amount consumed by the perpetrator. Moreover, the presence of alcohol does not necessarily indicate that it had a casual role. The NCVS data also lack information on many cognitive influences (e.g., provocation) and cultural expectancies (e.g., the belief that violence toward a spouse is acceptable under certain circumstances) that appear to mediate alcohol-related behavior.

Despite these limitations, our findings provide the first examination of the contribution of alcohol to the escalation of violence and its contribution to victim injury based on a nationally representative sample of naturally occurring episodes of violence. They suggest that drinking by a male assailant does increase the likelihood that he will actually physically attack the victim in an interpersonal confrontation, particularly when the other is a female intimate.

3. Future Research Directions

The limited prior research coupled with the findings from the NCVS presented here suggest the need for expanded research focusing on the contribution of alcohol consumption to the escalation of interactions from threats to actual attacks and the severity of injury given a physical attack. Such research should bridge the theoretical gap between the naturalistic perspective that rests on the view that alcohol's pharmacological effects disinhibit the drinker and the sociocultural perspective that treats drunken behavior as purely determined by social norms.[6,44] This requires developing and testing multivariate models that explore the linkages among interpersonal relationships, situational factors, and social processes as well as blood alcohol concentration levels, individual motivation, and orientation to the situation.

Because violence typically represents a low base-rate phenomenon, promising directions for such research include an expanded community-wide approach using a larger sample than Pernanen's, drawn from a US city with a heterogeneous population and high violent crime rate, to explore the wide range of violent incidents. Alternative strategies for exploring incident escalation and assault severity include secondary analyses of existing data, direct observation of natural episodes of intoxicated behavior, and experimental research using pairs of friends and intimates to explore the social, situational, and individual factors that affect behavior while intoxicated.

Additional secondary analyses of the NCVS might focus on exploring the relationship of the presence of alcohol to the nature of various threats, factors that affect the seriousness of an injury, including the presence of a weapon and of other persons, and the specific types of assaultive acts directed at different types of victims. The size and complexity of the NCVS data set allow for development of more complex models and multivariate analyses to examining the conditional and interactive factors that, together with alcohol ingestion, explain the escalation from threat to violence and victim injury in some assaultive incidents. The addition of alcohol-related questions to the NCVS would greatly enhance its value for exploring the escalation of violent events. Other data sets, particularly the 1985 National Family Violence Resurvey,[20] also may lend themselves to further analyses of the role of alcohol in incidents that do and do not actually result in violence of various types.

Specific questions related to alcohol's role in assaults include the conditions under which social rules related to gender apply. Does alcohol affect the types of violent acts men use against women and men? The application of general norms that restrict violence against women in dating situations and interactions with intimates and spouses? Why was there no alcohol effect on men's violent encounters with friends and acquaintances? Under what conditions does inhibition of conflict increase or decrease? In summary, many questions remain regarding the impact of alcohol consumption on the processes of escalation and discrimination in violent interactions.

ACKNOWLEDGMENT. An earlier version of this chapter was presented at the annual meeting of the American Sociological Association, Washington, DC, August 19, 1995.

References

1. Collins JJ: Alcohol and interpersonal violence: Less than meets the eye, in NA Weiner and ME Wolfgang (eds): *Pathways to Criminal Violence*. Newbury Park, CA, Sage Publications, 1989, pp 49–67.
2. Collins JJ, Messerschmidt P: Epidemiology of alcohol-related violence. *Alcohol Health Res World* 17:93–101, 1993.
3. Murdoch DD, Pihl RO, Ross D: Alcohol and crimes of violence: Present issues. *Int J Addict* 25:1065–1081, 1990.
4. Pernanen K: Alcohol and crimes of violence, in Kissin B, Begleiter H (eds): *The Biology of Alcoholism: Social Aspects of Alcoholism*. New York, Plenum Press, 1976, pp 351–444.

5. Pernanen K: Theoretical aspects of the relationship between alcohol use and crime, in Collins JJ (ed): *Drinking and Crime: Perspectives on the Relationships between Alcohol Consumption and Criminal Behavior*. New York, Guilford Press, 1981, pp 1–69.
6. Pernanen K: *Alcohol in Human Violence*. Guilford, New York, 1991.
7. Roizen J: Issues in the epidemiology of alcohol and violence, in SE Martin (ed): *Alcohol and Interpersonal Violence: Fostering Multidisciplinary Perspectives*. (NIAAA Research Monograph No. 24). NIH Pub. No. 93-3496. Rockville, MD, DHHS, 1993, pp 3–36.
8. Roizen J: Estimating alcohol involvement in serious events, in alcohol consumption and related problems. *Alcohol and Health* (Monograph No. 1) DHHS Publication No. 1 ADM 82-1190. Washington, DC, US Government Printing Office, 1982, pp 179–219.
9. Gerson LW, Preston D: Alcohol consumption and the incidence of violent crime. *J Stud Alcohol* 40:307–312, 1979.
10. Beck AJ, Kline SA, Greenfeld LA: *Survey of Youth in Custody, 1987*. Washington, DC, Bureau of Justice Statistics, 1988.
11. Beck, AJ: *Profile of Jail Inmates, 1989*. Washington, DC, Bureau Justice Statistics, 1991.
12. Cherpitel C: What emergency room studies reveal about alcohol involvement in violence-related injuries. *Alcohol Health Res World* 17:162–166, 1993.
13. Roizen J: Alcohol and trauma, in Giesbrecht N, Gonzales R, Grant M, *et al* (eds): *Drinking and Casualties*. London, Routledge, 1989, pp 21–66.
14. Shepherd J, Irish M, Scully C, Leslie I: Alcohol intoxication and severity of injury in victims of assault. *Br Med J* 296:1299, 1988.
15. Honkanen R, Smith GS: Impact of acute alcohol intoxication on the severity of injury: A cause-specific analysis of non-fatal trauma. *Injury* 21:353–357, 1990.
16. Cherpitel C: Alcohol and casualties: A comparison of emergency room and coroner data. Paper presented at the Research Society on Alcoholism annual meeting, June 18–24, 1993, San Antonio, TX.
17. Hamilton CJ, Collins JJ: The role of alcohol in wife beating and child abuse: A review of the literature, in Collins JJ (ed): *Drinking and Crime*. New York, Guilford Press, 1981, pp 253–287.
18. Hotaling GT, Sugarman DB: An analysis of risk markers in husband to wife violence: The current state of knowledge. *Violence Victims* 1:101–124, 1986.
19. Leonard KE, Jacob T: Alcohol, alcoholism, and family violence, in Van Hasselt VB, Morrison FL, Bellack AS, Herson M (eds): *Handbook of Family Violence*. New York, Plenum Press, 1988, pp 383–406.
20. Kantor GK, Straus MA: The "drunken bum" theory of wife beating. *Social Problems* 34:213–231, 1987.
21. Roberts AR: Psychosocial characteristics of batterers: A study of 234 men charged with domestic violence offenses. *J Family Violence* 2:81–93, 1987.
22. Fagan JA, Stewart DK, Hansen KV: Violent men or violent husbands? Background factors and situational correlates, in Finkelhor D, Gelles RJ, Hotaling GT, Straus MA (eds): *The Dark Side of Families: Current Family Violence Research*. Beverly Hills, CA, Sage Publications, 1983, pp 49–67.
23. Berk RA, Berk SF, Loseke DR, Rauma D: Mutual combat and other family violence myths, in Finkelhor D, Gelles RJ, Hotaling GT, Straus MA (eds): *The Dark Side of Families: Current Family Violence Research*. Beverly Hills, CA, Sage Publications, 1983, pp 197–212.
24. Kantor GK, Straus MA: Substance abuse as a precipitant of wife abuse victimizations. *Am J Drug Alcohol Abuse* 15:173–189, 1989.
25. Straus MA: Measuring intrafamily conflict and violence: The conflict tactics scale. Durham, University of New Hampshire, *Family Research Laboratory*, 1979.
26. Straus MA: The conflict tactics scale and its critics: An evaluation and new data on validity and reliability, in Straus MA, Gelles RJ (eds) *Physical Violence in American Families: Risk Factors and Adaptations to Violence in 8,145 Families*. New Brunswick, NJ, Transaction Books, 1990, pp 49–73.
27. Bureau of Justice Statistics: *Criminal Victimization in the United States, 1992*. Washington, DC, Bureau of Justice Statistics, 1993.

28. Bushman BJ, Cooper HM: The effects of alcohol on human aggression: An integrative review. *Psychol Bull* 107:341–354, 1990.

29. Gustafson R: What do experimental paradigms tell us about alcohol-related aggressive responding? *J Stud Alcohol* (Suppl 11):20–29, 1993.

30. Steele CM, Southwick L: Alcohol and social behavior I: The psychology of drunken excess. *J Personality Social Psychol* 48:18–34, 1985.

31. Buss A: *The Psychology of Aggression.* New York, Wiley, 1961.

32. Gustafson R: Threat as a determinant of alcohol-related aggression. *Psychol Rep* 58:287–297, 1986.

33. Gustafson R: Alcohol, aggression and the validity of experimental paradigms in women. *Psychol Rep* 59:51–56, 1986.

34. Lang AR, Goeckner DJ, Adesso VJ, Marlatt GA: Effects of alcohol on aggression in male social drinkers. *J Abnormal Psychol* 84:508–518, 1975.

35. Pihl RO, Smith M, Farrell B: Alcohol and aggression in men: A comparison of brewed and distilled beverages. *J Stud Alcohol* 45:278–282, 1984.

36. Taylor SP, Schmutte GT, Leonard KE: Physical aggression as a function of alcohol and frustration. *Bull Psychonom Soc* 9:217–218, 1977.

37. Taylor SP, Leonard KE: Alcohol and human physical aggression, in Green RG, Donnerstein EI (eds): *Aggression: Theoretical and Empirical Reviews,* vol 2. San Diego, CA, Academic Press, 1983, pp 77–101.

38. Gantner A, Taylor SP: Human physical aggression as a function of alcohol and threat of harm. *Aggressive Behavior* 18:29–36, 1992.

39. Schmutte GT, Taylor SP: Physical aggression as a function of alcohol and pain feedback. *J Social Psychol* 10:235–244, 1980.

40. Zeichner A, Pihl RO: The effects of alcohol and instigator intent on human aggression. *J Stud Alcohol* 41:265–276, 1980.

41. Jeavons CM, Taylor SP: The control of alcohol-related aggression: Redirecting the inebriate's attention to socially appropriate conduct. *Aggressive Behavior* 11:93–101, 1985.

42. Taylor SP, Gammon CB: Aggressive behavior of intoxicated subjects: The effect of third-party intervention. *J Stud Alcohol* 37:917–930, 1976.

43. Taylor SP, Sears JD: The effects of alcohol and persuasive social pressure on human physical aggression. *Aggressive Behavior* 14:237–243, 1988.

44. Steele CM, Josephs RA: Alcohol myopia: Its prized and dangerous effects. *Am Psychol* 45:921–933, 1990.

45. Lang AR: Alcohol-related violence: Psychological perspectives, in SE Martin (ed): *Alcohol and Interpersonal Violence: Fostering Multidisciplinary Perspectives.* (NIAAA Research Monograph No. 24). Rockville, MD, US Department of Health and Human Services, 1993, pp 121–147.

46. Bachman R, Taylor BM: The measurement of family violence and rape by the redesigned national crime victimization survey. *Justice Q* 11:499–512, 1994.

47. Straus MA, Gelles RJ (ed): *Physical Violence in American Families: Risk Factors and Adaptations to Violence in 8,145 Families.* New Brunswick, NJ, Transaction Books, 1990.

48. Bachman R, Saltzman L: *Violence against Women: Estimates from the Redesigned Survey* (NCJ #154848). Washington, DC, Bureau of Justice Statistics, 1995.

49. Leonard KE: Drinking patterns and intoxication in marital violence: Review, critique and future directions for research, in S Martin (ed): *Alcohol and Interpersonal Violence: Fostering Multidisciplinary Perspectives* (NIAAA Research Monograph No. 24). NIH Pub. No. 93-3496. Rockville, MD, DHHS, 1993, pp 253–280.

3

Alcohol and Spouse Abuse
Ethnic Differences

Glenda Kaufman Kantor

Abstract. This chapter examines theoretical and empirical evidence on the interplay between ethnicity, structural and cultural factors, and alcohol-related assaults against wives and considers whether there is a differential vulnerability to such assaults among varying ethnic groups. Our review demonstrated that structural factors emerged as dominant in their influence on alcohol-related wife assaults in varying ethnic groups. The empirical evidence, though limited, showed that the linkages between drinking and wife beating are not just a problem of poor ethnic minorities. Heavy drinking per se is associated similarly in Hispanic-American and Anglo-American families. However, we also identified differences among Hispanic subgroups, as well as cultural variations in drinking patterns that differentially affected wife assaults. Although data on alcohol–wife assault relationships among African Americans are extremely limited, the available evidence indicates little or no effect of drinking by African-American men on wife assaults, after taking other socioeconomic variables into account. Empirical evidence did not support the saliency of particular cultural beliefs favoring violence toward women as intrinsic to any one ethnic group. The major cultural differences in alcohol-related cognitions are consistent with the greater legitimation of alcohol-related misbehavior and the acceptance of "machismo" drinking by Hispanic Americans compared to Anglo-Americans.

1. Introduction

There is strong empirical grounding for both the existence of linkages between poverty and violent intrafamily crimes, such as wife abuse,[1–3] and the greater prevalence of alcohol-related problems among the impoverished.[4] There is also a considerable body of research, often divorced from socio-economic considerations, that establishes a correlation between excessive

Glenda Kaufman Kantor • Family Research Laboratory, University of New Hampshire, Durham, New Hampshire 03824.

Recent Developments in Alcoholism, Volume 13: Alcoholism and Violence, edited by Marc Galanter. Plenum Press, New York, 1997.

drinking and violent interpersonal crimes.[5] In particular, alcohol has emerged as a consistent predictor of wife assaults in a wide range of studies. A previous study,[6] which did consider socioeconomic factors along with alcohol consumption patterns, found evidence that binge-drinking patterns by blue-collar men, in combination with the approval of violence, were associated with higher wife abuse rates. The study findings supported the need for a comprehensive theoretical framework integrating factors at the individual, structural, and cultural levels. However, research on alcohol-related wife assaults is rarely situated in the context of ethnicity or culture. This chapter examines evidence on the interplay between ethnicity, structural and cultural factors, and alcohol-related assaults against wives and considers whether there is a differential vulnerability to such assaults among varying ethnic groups.

Violence is often an adaptation to stress produced by structural inequalities. If adequate resources are not available, violence may be used by men against wives to maintain their dominant status in the family.[2] Several studies have shown that the stress associated with unemployment or income disparity between husband and wife leads to an increase in marital violence.[2,7] Furthermore, the relationship between socioeconomic stress and family assaults may be mediated by substance abuse. Drug and/or alcohol use may become a method for reducing the stress caused by changes in family interaction.

The susceptibility of minority families to alcohol-related assaults is a plausible assumption because poverty, unemployment, substandard housing, and segregation have characterized the minority experience in the United States.[1] For example, in 1991, the median income for Hispanic families was only 65% of that earned by non-Hispanic families. Over a quarter of Hispanic families lived below the poverty line in 1991 compared to 10% of non-Hispanic families. African Americans also tend to be considerably more impoverished than white Americans.[8]

Despite the fact that Hispanic and African-American families constitute a disproportionate percentage of impoverished families, and that lower socioeconomic status is associated with higher rates of family violence,[2] evidence for the cultural patterning of family violence is limited.[9] There are few studies of family violence using ethnicity rather than class as their central focus. Research examining the linkages between alcohol and wife assaults within differing ethnic groups is even more uncommon. The intent of this current review is not to perpetuate stereotypes that dysfunctional family patterns and family crimes are lower-class phenomena but to consider the available evidence on structural and cultural areas that may have major implications for those concerned with alcohol–aggression relationships and those concerned with preventing violence against women.

Specifically, the questions considered in this chapter are: (1) Do Hispanic and African-American husbands who drink heavily have a higher probability of wife beating than Anglo-American husbands who drink heavily? (2) Does taking into account the effects of other variables such as poverty, acculturation, and gender role attitudes alter the relationship between ethnicity, drinking, and wife beating? (3) Are such linkages between drinking and wife beating found primarily among poor ethnic minorities?

2. Drinking and Violence in Ethnic Groups

Alcohol has been associated with a number of social ills, and over half of all violent crimes are believed to be alcohol related.[10] A substantial literature establishes distinctive cultural drinking patterns and the greater prevalence of alcohol problems, including alcohol-related violence, in certain subgroups of the population.[11-17] Problem drinking has been identified more often among ethnic groups such as the Irish (both in America and in Ireland)[18] and among African-American and Hispanic-American men. While studies specifically designed to examine the presence of alcohol-related aggression in different cultures are uncommon, studies that do so find that aggressive behavior is not a constant in heavy drinking cultures[19] and that alcohol-related aggression is more common in the Southern United States, among youth, and also in some Hispanic subgroups.[20] Additionally, Levinson's[9] cross-cultural analysis of family violence in 90 small-scale and peasant societies found that wife beating occurred in conjunction with the husband's drunkenness in only 9% of societies. In approximately 6% of societies, the husband's intoxication was inconsistently linked to wife beating.

2.1. Problem Drinking in African-American Men

A review of the literature on the extent of drinking among African-American men[21] suggests that the differences between African Americans' and white Americans' drinking are actually small or that African Americans drink less than whites. At the same time, analyses of American drinking patterns have identified greater alcohol problems for African Americans[15,17,22,23] compared to white Americans. The seeming inconsistencies of these findings suggest that while abstention and moderate drinking values prevail among African Americans, there may also be a segment of African-American society where drinking is associated with negative consequences. According to Herd's[17] historical analysis of African-American drinking patterns, the effects of racial oppression and subsequent African-American migration to urban areas, along with the targeting of African Americans first by the illicit alcohol market and then by the legal alcohol industry, sowed the seeds of a heavy-drinking culture.

Excessive drinking and other forms of substance abuse in largely African-American and poor urban areas are often linked to violent crimes.[24] The mechanisms postulated for this association suggest that subcultural values promoting heavy drinking, the accessibility of liquor stores and taverns in poor African-American communities, and the social stresses of poverty leading to escapist drinking are major influences. Anger and frustration at racist forces, unemployment, and feelings of powerlessness may lead to drinking, family disorganization, and violence among some African Americans.[24,25]

2.2. Wife Abuse in African-American Families

Wife-abuse studies of shelter populations most often examine race as a background variable and reach inconsistent conclusions about the relevance of race to wife-abuse situations.[26,27] Studies specifically designed to examine wife abuse in African-American families[28,29] conclude that race effects are not significant when class factors are controlled. However, Lockhart[28] also finds that violence rates are higher for African-American middle-class women compared to white middle-class women. Lockhart[30] explains violent conflict resolution strategies among the African-American middle class as a function of lower-socioeconomic developmental experiences and the stresses resulting from the tenuousness of newly acquired middle-class roles.

One reason for the inconsistent findings of the studies cited above may be the methodological limitations in using clinical or convenience samples to establish ethnic variations or prevalence rates. Prevalence rates of wife abuse are best estimated in large national probability samples.[31] Results from two national surveys (the 1975 and 1985 National Family Violence Surveys)[2,32,33] indicate that wife abuse rates are significantly greater in African-American families compared to white American families even when occupational class factors are controlled. However, few studies using large probability samples have examined the possibility that excessive drinking or variables other than socioeconomic factors contribute to the higher rates of wife assaults by African-American men.

2.3. Moderators of Alcohol-Related Wife Assaults in African-American Families

Failure to specify the complex array of causal and moderating factors implicated in wife assaults by varying ethnic groups is undoubtedly related to the gaps in research. Indeed, Asbury's[34] discussion of African-American women in violent relationships takes wife-abuse researchers to task for failing to mention the race of abused women. Her review of the wife-abuse literature adopts an "afrocentric perspective" (i.e., a worldview that is framed by African-American historical traditions and experiences of slavery, oppression, poverty, and discrimination) in identifying themes relevant to black women's victimizations by spouses. Her themes, derived largely from Roy's[35] list of triggers to wife abuse, emphasize economic difficulties, alcohol use, traditional sex-role socialization, and African-American women's family allegiances as contributors to assaults on black American women. Using a sociological perspective, Asbury[34] also suggests that greater anomie* among black American men unable to achieve societal goals may result in violence toward women and others. Although this is a promising theoretical framework for examining wife assaults among African-American families, no empirical data are provided.

Even research on anomie and violence is limited. In fact, researchers have failed to identify significant linkages between anomie and violence, as well as for anomie and excessive drinking.[37] However, the lack of statistically significant associations may be more a function of the level of abstractness present in the concept of "anomie" and difficulties in operationalization rather than the absence of any relationship between alcohol, anomie, and violence. Such data also do not address the effects of anomie on the occurrence of violence in intimate partnerships.

Most experts on wife assaults concur that these are complex phenomena rooted in both social structural and family processes. There is, for example, speculation that traditional sex roles contribute to assaults on African-American women. Historically, African-American families have been stereotyped as matriarchal and wife dominated. However, other data on marital satisfaction and family role structure suggest that wife-dominant African-American couples are as satisfied with their marriages as their egalitarian counterparts.[38] Additionally, research comparing the gender roles of African-American and white American men has yielded inconsistent results. Generalizations from the body of research on African-American family structure and family violence regarding predictors or moderators of spousal assaults are not easily made because so few studies have been done. There is clearly a need to empirically examine the complex interrelationships between alcohol, socioeconomic status, family structure, marital quality, and marital violence.

2.4. Problem Drinking in Hispanic-American Men

There is also evidence that high rates of alcohol consumption and problem drinking exist among Hispanic men to a greater extent than for other ethnic groups.[13,15] However, with the exception of Caetano's[39] survey, which did examine a representative sample of Americans, most studies of Hispanic-American drinking patterns have had limited generalizability because of the low numbers of Hispanics sampled or sampling limited to specific subgroups or geographical areas.[40–42]

There are several reasons why we would expect to find greater alcohol problems in Hispanic Americans compared to other groups such as their lack of economic and educational resources, lesser access to external social sup-

---

* According to Merton's[36] theory of deviance, anomie leads to deviance when there are disparities between culturally prescribed goals and socially structured avenues to achieve those goals.

ports such as human services,[43,44] and potentially greater social isolation. Using the suppositions of a social stress perspective,[45] the numerous daily life stresses associated with poverty or isolation could increase the likelihood of using alcohol as a coping mechanism. Another explanation is that cultural influences increase the risk of problem drinking.

2.5. "Machismo" Drinking and Wife Assaults

An ethic supporting heavy drinking by Hispanic men, i.e., "machismo drinking," as an indicator of their masculinity, is often assumed to be at the heart of Hispanic drinking problems, but it is also rejected as an inaccurate and pejorative stereotype.[40,46–48] In fact, Kaufman Kantor, Aldarondo, and Jasinski[49] argue that the machismo ethic is actually one where "real" men consume substantial quantities of alcohol *without* demonstrating ill effects and without interference with their work and family roles. In other words, there are both positive and negative aspects of the machismo concept, such that the ethic of machismo drinking supports alcohol tolerance but purportedly without negative consequences to others.

Few studies provide information on how wife assaults and intoxication might be associated in Hispanic families. Despite our assertions about the complexity of the machismo concept, the broader stereotype of alcohol machismo, e.g., the conjunction of heavy drinking and assertion of manliness through physical force, does suggest a possible mechanism. Some support for the stereotype is provided by ethnographic accounts of native Hispanic cultures. One such account[50] describes a practice among the Tzeltal of Mexico where wife beating following the husband's drinking has been formalized to such an extent that it is incorporated into the marriage ceremony. Levinson[50] reports that "the beatings are routinely expected and accepted by Tzeltal wives who excuse their husbands as crazy" (p. 50). Another ethnographic study in Puerto Rico[51] identifies a practice known as "Social Fridays," where men stay away from home all weekend and drink to intoxication. However, no research has examined this pattern in the mainland. If this were so, it suggests a potential source of marital conflict and, at worst, a greater risk of marital assaults, since binge drinking patterns have been linked to wife abuse.[6,52] However, drinking patterns and attitudes approving of drunkenness or violence may also differ depending on the degree to which acculturation has occurred[53–55] or social status has changed.

2.6. Ethnic Comparisons of Wife Abuse

Until recently, few studies examined the occurrence of marital violence in Hispanic-American families. Studies examining differences by race in shelter populations of battered women find no differences between white, African-American, and Hispanic women in the frequency and severity of abuse, but Hispanic women appear to have endured abuse longer before entering shelters.[56–58] Hispanic-American women are said to have a higher "tolerance" compared to Anglo-American women for minor physical abuse such as slapping and for verbal abuse.[58] Hispanic women are also more likely to have larger families and might remain in relationships longer because of their children.[56,58] Although these findings are consistent with some discussions of Hispanic family structure,[59] there are also methodological limitations in generalizing conclusions from studies using clinical samples to the Hispanic population at large.

2.7. Wife Assault Patterns among Hispanic Americans

Straus and Smith's[3] analysis of national data concludes that Hispanic-American husbands assault their wives at a rate more than double that of white American husbands. Although family assaults seem inconsistent with descriptions of Hispanic families as cohesive and close-knit,[60] characterizations of Hispanic families as male dominant,[59,61] along with high levels of poverty and unemployment, are consonant with typical predictors of wife abuse. Authoritarian role structures assigning dominance to the husband and dictating obedience by the wife are said to persist at least as an ideology of Mexican-American, Puerto Rican, and Cuban cultures, if not in practice.[59,62–65] Despite theoretical evidence to support contentions of wife abuse among Hispanics, there is, in fact, little empirical evidence on wife beating in Hispanic families. However, high rates of intrafamily homicides in Hispanic families suggest the possibility of severe spousal violence,[66] and this is supported by reports based on the 1985 National Family Violence Survey[3,67] and the 1992 National Alcohol and Family Violence Survey.[68]

2.8. Drinking and Wife Assaults in Multiethnic Groups

A previous analysis of ethnicity and drinking,[67] using the 1985 National Family Violence Survey, examined the incidence of drinking problems and wife abuse by Hispanic, African-American, and white American husbands. The findings reveled greater prevalence of wife assaults and binge-drinking problems among ethnic minorities (i.e., African-American and Hispanic-American men). Hispanic-American men were approximately three times as likely as white American men and almost four times as likely as African-American men to engage in high-volume binge drinking. This study also found that Hispanic-American women with binge-drinking husbands were more than ten times as likely to be assaulted than were Hispanic-American wives of low-moderate drinkers. The findings also revealed that African-American women were at high risk of assault if their husbands were excessive daily drinkers. Additionally, a multivariate analysis was conducted to examine the joint effects of poverty, drinking, and ethnicity on wife abuse probabilities. The results of the multivariate analysis comparing white and African-American husbands showed that although overall violence rates by minority husbands were generally higher than those of white Americans, the effects of race among African-American respondents dominated those of alcohol in predicting wife assaults even when socioeconomic status was controlled.

In contrast to the findings for African-American husbands, the highest rates of violence by Hispanic-American husbands occurred for those at poverty level with high-volume binge-drinking patterns. The multivariate analysis comparing Hispanic and white American husbands also showed that drinking was the only significant predictor of wife abuse when socioeconomic status and ethnicity were controlled. However, there are also important limits to generalizing the findings of this study regarding Hispanic Americans because subgroup differences between Hispanics and acculturation levels of Hispanic Americans were not measured in this earlier (1985) national study.

2.9. Moderators of Alcohol-Related Wife Assaults in Hispanic-American Families: Acculturation

Acculturation needs to be considered as a potential moderator of differential risks for wife assaults between Hispanic-American subgroups. Acculturation is a process by which an immigrant group takes on the norms and behavior patterns of the host society and modifies customs, habits, language, lifestyle, and values over time.[69,70]

2.9.1. Acculturation and Mental Health. Some have suggested that a number of psychological disorders (e.g., alcoholism, depression, psychosomatic symptoms) are more prevalent among highly acculturated Mexican Americans compared to native born (Mexican born) Mexican Americans.[71–73] This is believed to be caused by prolonged stresses associated with adaptation, such as alienation from Mexican culture, or the experience of discrimination or deprivation relative to Anglo-American society. However, the evidence for detrimental effects of acculturation is not unequivocal. For example, Griffith and Villavicencio[74] found that high acculturation is correlated with social support, extended kin network, and lower incidence of psychological distress in Mexican American families. They also attribute this relationship to the higher socioeconomic status of more acculturated Mexican Americans.

2.9.2. Acculturation and Alcohol. Studies that have examined acculturational influences on alcohol consumption yield mixed results on the direction of the effects, though the majority suggest that drinking increases with acculturation.[72,75,76] For example, Caetano and Medina Mora's[75] study comparing men of Mexican descent in their native country with Mexican Americans in the United States suggests that Mexican-American men drink more frequently in the United States. There is also evidence that escapist drinking patterns characterize lesser acculturated Mexican Americans.[77] Gordon's[55] study of Dominican men demonstrates a shift from macho drinking, i.e., heavy drinking and drunken fighting, to a more conservative lifestyle in the

United States. Yet another study by Gordon[78] finds that Guatemalan men maintain their practices of macho drinking. A more careful examination of these studies suggests that factors other than acculturation, such as altered family structure, work arrangements, socioeconomic status, and drinking opportunities, are responsible for either the maintenance or the severance of drinking behavior patterns. The divergent views on acculturation effects are most likely due to the lack of uniform measures that tap different dimensions of the construct or the failure to control for the confounding effects of socioeconomic status.

2.9.3. Acculturation and Wife Abuse. One would expect that factors likely to modify the linkages between alcohol and wife assaults such as family roles, norms approving violence, and attitudes about drinking and drinking behaviors may be influenced by the level of individual acculturation. However, few studies of Hispanic family violence have specifically measured acculturation. Torres,[79] for example, describes the degree of acculturation for the subject population of battered women in shelters but does not use acculturation as a variable in her empirical analysis. Additionally, a major limitation of previous studies examining the linkages between Hispanic alcohol abuse and wife abuse[67] or studies examining the incidence of intrafamily violence among Hispanic and white families[3] is their inability to adequately measure the concept of Hispanic ethnicity. The validity of categorizing diverse members of society under one classification is questionable. This approach fails to detect the actual subgroup members at risk. One could plausibly assume considerable heterogeneity within and between Hispanic subgroups regarding family roles, attitudes toward alcohol use, and beliefs about the legitimacy of violence. It is not at all clear that Hispanicity is a coherent construct or even that certain subgroups, (e.g., Puerto Ricans, Mexicans, Dominicans) share a unique cultural experience or consistent set of beliefs about issues that may affect the risks of family violence.

Studies that have empirically examined the role of acculturation in wife assaults[68,80] indicate that wife abuse rates are higher among US-born Hispanics. Sorenson and Telles's[80] analysis of Epidemiological Catchment Area data on the prevalence of wife abuse in Los Angeles indicates that Mexicans born in the United States have the highest life-time prevalence of wife assaults compared to Anglos and Mexican-born Hispanics. Thus, using country of birth as an alternative measure for acculturation indicates that acculturation may actually increase the likelihood of wife abuse.

The 1992 National Alcohol and Family Violence Survey (NAFVS)[68] provides a primary source of data on the prevalence and incidence of Hispanic and Anglo-American spousal violence. The research design of this study included face-to-face, bilingual (Spanish–English) interviews with a national probability sample of 1970 persons, including an oversample of approximately 800 Hispanic persons. The study included specific measures of acculturation and perceived ethnicity, among others. The population examined included sufficient numbers of Hispanics representing the three major sub-groups in the United States (Mexicans, Puerto Ricans, and Cubans) to allow for subgroup analyses.

2.10. The 1992 National Alcohol and Family Violence Survey

Using the NAFVS, we examined the relationship between sociocultural status and the incidence of marital violence in Hispanic-American and Anglo-American families.[68] Findings from this study revealed that the highest rates of wife assaults were found among more acculturated Mexican Americans and Puerto Ricans. We also replicated the Sorenson and Telles findings that country of birth (US born) is significantly associated with wife assaults. At the same time, we did not find significant effects of our acculturation *measure* (reflecting language preference and Spanish–English utilization) on wife as-saults when other cultural and socioeconomic indicators were held constant. This suggests that acculturation is confounded with these other measures. Another plausible explanation is that the acculturation measure used in this study, though widely validated, was conceptually limited in its linguistic focus.

The major findings of this study did support the importance of a socio-cultural approach to understanding wife abuse. Similar to the findings of the 1985 National Family Violence Survey,[3,67] this study found that Hispanic Americans, taken as a single ethnic group, do not differ significantly from Anglo Americans in their odds of wife assaults when cultural norms regard-ing violence approval, age, and economic stressors are held constant. Second, our findings provided evidence for not regarding Hispanic Americans as a homogeneous group. Rather, considerable heterogeneity was apparent be-tween ethnic subgroups relative to their extent of acculturation, country of birth, impoverishment, and their acceptance of wife abuse as normative. We found that cultural norms sanctioning wife assaults, while significantly asso-ciated with actual husband-to-wife violence, are not uniquely Hispanic cultur-al values. Our results show that the presence of these norms within any ethnic subculture, regardless of socioeconomic status, is a risk factor for wife abuse. A third important finding of this study, amplifying the discovery of Sorenson and Telles,[80] was that being born in the United States increases the risk of wife assaults by Mexican- and Puerto Rican-American husbands.

One possible and important inference from our study of sociocultural status and our finding of a significant association between country of birth and wife assaults is that family strengths derived from intact cultural values may provide buffers against stresses that might otherwise lead to conflict and violence. This suggests the importance of building and preserving family strengths and kin networks in the prevention of intrafamily violence among Hispanic families. At the same time, nonegalitarian family power structures, which exist in some Hispanic-American families, and problem drinking, which is also higher in Hispanic-American families relative to other groups, can each affect levels of verbal and physical conflict between husbands.

One important limitation to both studies emphasizing acculturation effects on wife assault, discussed above, is that neither of these studies provide information on *how* acculturation or being born in the United States might have such deleterious effects. There is a need to empirically examine the relationship of other dimensions of acculturation to wife assaults such as feelings of cultural marginality[77] and perceptions of social distance and discrimination from the dominant Anglo majority.[81] This is particularly important because studies arguing for a culture of violence interpretation, i.e., more normative acceptance of violence by certain subgroups, rarely specifically test alternative explanations such as acculturation stress or discriminatory effects. Additionally, neither of these studies took alcohol's role in wife beating into account.

2.10.1. Alcohol-Related Wife Assaults in Minority Families. A second analysis of the 1992 National Alcohol Family Violence Survey data[49] evaluated the association between alcohol consumption and wife assaults among the three largest Hispanic subgroups in the United States and among Anglo-American families.

2.10.2. Violence-Related Behaviors. Because variations in violence rates may also be influenced by ethnicity, we first considered the overall incidence rates by ethnic groupings. The results of this second analysis support the findings discussed above. As shown in Fig. 1, the highest rates of assaults on wives occur in Puerto Rican-American families. Rates of wife beating in Puerto Rican-American families are more than double those reported in Anglo families. Assault rates in Mexican-American families are almost equally as high. It can also be seen that rates of wife assaults by less acculturated Mexican husbands living in the United States are virtually the same as those of Anglo-American husbands. However, as shown in Fig. 1, husband-to-wife assaults are rarely reported by Cuban-American families.

2.10.3. Average Drinking Patterns and Marital Assaults. Figure 2 examines the association between husband's average alcohol consumption patterns dichotomized into nonheavy (abstinent through low-volume binge) and heavy (high daily and high-volume binge) drinking patterns and wife assaults. The results based on an analysis of variance show significant main effects of ethnicity and drinking. Consistent with the results of our previous research,[6,82] it is evident that heavy-drinking husbands engage in considerably more wife abuse. The highest proportion of alcohol-associated wife assaults are again found in Puerto Rican families. Heavy-drinking Puerto Rican husbands are five times more likely to hit their wives than their nondrinking counterparts. Virtually the same proportions of wife assaults are reported by

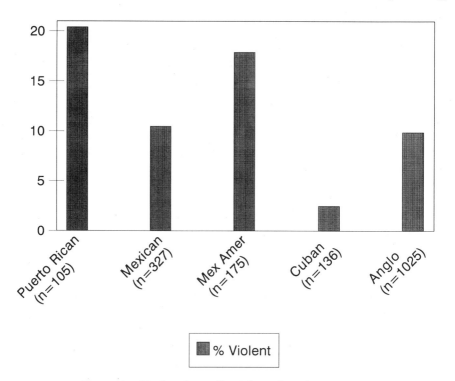

Figure 1.   Husband-to-wife violence by ethnic group.

Anglo- and Mexican-American heavy-drinking husbands. Although Cuban husbands appear to be rarely violent, the proportion of husbands that hit their wives more than triples when heavy drinking is taken into account.

2.10.4. Alcohol as a Temporal Antecedent of Wife Assault. Unlike most of the research discussed thus far, we also examined the extent to which intoxication was a component of the aggressive episode against a wife. Figure 3 shows the proportion of family members who report actual drinking or intoxication of self or partner at the time of a spousal assault. The findings are generally consistent with the relationships shown in the previous figures; that is, the likelihood of intoxication or drinking by one or both partners at the time of a wife assault is greatest among mainland Puerto Rican family members. This was the case in over half of the latter families where a wife assault had occurred. However, they also illustrate that drinking by wives contributes to alcohol-related assaults only in Puerto Rican and Anglo-American families. It should also be noted that the analyses presented in Fig. 3 were conducted only on families where wife assaults were reported. The small sample sizes, particularly for Puerto Rican and Cuban men, indicate that caution is needed in generalizing from these results. Nevertheless, with the exception of Cuban families (where both heavy drinking and violence are rare) and some variations in the role of drinking by wives, the results show similar patterns of alcohol-related marital assaults regardless of ethnicity.

2.10.5. Alcohol Cognitions. In additional analyses, the role of alcohol expectancies and norms legitimizing alcohol-related violence among Hispanic-American and Anglo-American men were explored. The findings showed that the main way in which Hispanic subgroups differed from Anglo subgroups is in the greater legitimation of alcohol-related behavior and in the acceptance of machismo drinking ("A real man can hold his liquor") by Hispanic Americans. Cubans differ significantly from all other groups with low expectancies about alcohol's ability to transform behavior. This is also consistent with Cuban's overall modest drinking habits. However, we concluded that the overall homogeneity of Hispanics, including Cubans, regarding acceptance of alcohol-related misbehavior is rather striking. We speculated that this may reflect a more forgiving and empathic standard among His-

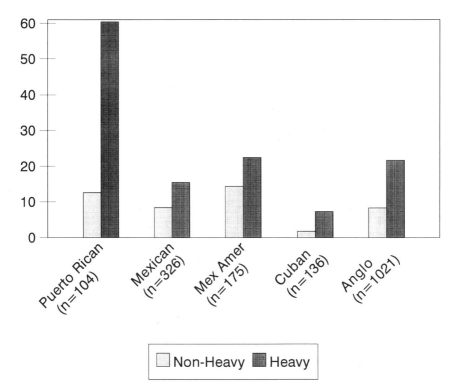

Figure 2. Percent husband-to-wife violence by ethnic group and husband's average drinking.

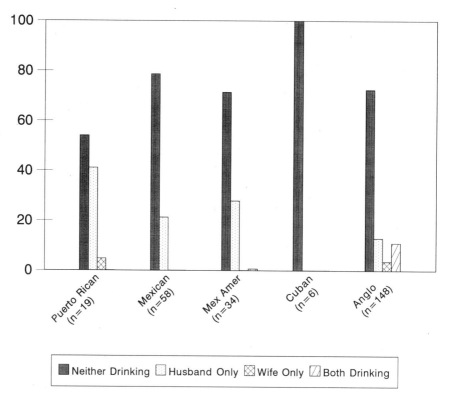

Figure 3. Drinking at the time of husband-to-wife violence by ethnic group.

panics compared with the sterner, more reproachful morality of Anglo-American men.

For Anglo-American men, further analyses using logistic regression indicated that aggressive expectancies in combination with youth significantly increased the likelihood of aggression toward wives, net of the effects of alcohol consumption patterns and socioeconomic factors. For Hispanic men, both disinhibition and aggressive expectancies affected the likelihood of wife assaults. Additionally, youth and unemployment added to the probability that Hispanic-American men would engage in assaults on wives. It should also be noted that both aggressive alcohol expectancies and unemployment each more than doubled the odds of wife assault among Hispanic-American husbands.

Anglo-American men in this study were considerably more economically advantaged than the Hispanic men and families studied. Yet their rate of high daily drinking was almost twice that of Cuban and less acculturated Mexican men. Despite the latter pattern for Anglo men, alcohol-related problems were less frequent. A significant linear association between alcohol consumption and husband-to-wife violence is evident only for Anglo husbands. The linearity of the alcohol–wife assault relationship for Anglos but not for Hispanics may be because binge-drinking patterns (at both lower- and higher-volume alcohol consumption) are more common to Hispanics, and the latter alcohol consumption pattern is linked to wife assaults among some Hispanic-American subgroups.

2.11. Evidence from Community and Clinical Samples of Multiethnic Groups

Unlike the analyses presented on data from the two national probability surveys, most research on alcohol and wife assaults in ethnic populations, albeit limited, has been conducted in particular geographical areas or among clinical samples of battered women. A recent study by Neff, Holamon, and Schluter[83] investigated wife assaults among Anglos, African Americans, and Mexican Americans residing in San Antonio, Texas. The study respondents differed from the currently partnered sample described in the 1992 national study in that respondents included previously partnered individuals. The study by Neff and associates also used a more limited measure of violence (one item) in contrast to the multiple-item measure used in the national surveys. This study considered the moderating effects of financial stress rather than acculturation or specific socioeconomic indicators such as unemployment. Additionally, the moderating effects of sex roles, partner drinking, and social desirability effects were taken into account by Neff and associates.

Neff and associates[83] concluded that females, the formerly married, and African-American females were most likely to report being beaten by and beating a partner. High rates of partner assaults persisted among married African-American females, even after taking into account the potential moderating variables discussed above and the drinking quantity of the partner. In fact, even while violence rates were highest among African Americans, drinking was least important.

No significant differences in violence were found in comparisons of Mexican-American and Anglo-American respondents. Sex role traditionalism, the principal sociocultural indicator, did not emerge as a significant predictor of spousal assaults. However, the authors note the limitation of the absence of data on the partner's sex role orientation. The authors also suggest that a curvilinear relationship exists between alcohol and violence such that the highest-quantity drinkers are less violent than lighter drinkers. Furthermore, among Mexican-American females, quantity of alcohol consumption by the wife or husband was not directly related to spousal assaults. The authors find little support for minority stress explanations of wife assault. They conclude that future research must pay more attention to relationship dynamics as a means of explaining alcohol-related wife assaults in differing ethnic groups.

A second study examining cultural explanations of wife assault among abused Latinas also considered the contributions of alcohol and sex role orientation, along with acculturation and family communication patterns. Perilla, Bakeman, and Norris[84] interviewed a sample of 60 women in a Southeastern city, including 30 battered women seeking help for abuse and 30 other women who sought other services from a Catholic hospital. Multivariate analyses found no significant effects of acculturation or sex role orientation. The authors did find that frequent drunkenness of the partner was associated with higher levels of abuse. However, they also concluded that the relationship was largely mediated by their measure of mutuality (items measuring "empathy, engagement, authenticity, empowerment, zest, and diversity"). Indirect evidence for the importance of culture related to male machismo was inferred by the finding that women's contributions to family income were positively associated with abuse. The authors argue that this is due to the husband's perceived loss of competency as a provider.

3. Summary and Conclusions

3.1. Examining the Theoretical Framework

The evidence examined in this chapter provided some support for utilizing an integrated theoretical framework, including individual, structural, and cultural constructs, in examining alcohol-related wife assaults. In particular, structural factors emerged as dominant in their influence on wife assaults. However, support for all of the constructs identified here cannot be unqualified because the available empirical evidence on ethnic differences in alcohol-related consequences largely omits personality correlates and family history factors. The only intraindividual characteristic examined in the studies reviewed here was the husband's alcohol use. Although alcohol use is central to our thesis of wife assaults because of its psychopharmacological effects and individual expectancies about the effects of alcohol, other factors such as aggressive personality style,[85] communication patterns, or family history of violence[86] may influence the likelihood that any one individual will engage in wife beating. Additionally, it is important to emphasize the need for caution in drawing firm conclusions about all of the questions considered here. This is necessary because research regarding the structural–cultural patterning of alcohol-related wife assaults in different ethnic groups is in its infancy.

3.2. Does Alcohol Influence Wife Beating Equivalently across Ethnic Groups?

The empirical evidence shows that the linkages between drinking and wife beating are not just a problem of poor, ethnic minorities. Research based on two large national probability samples of American families with Hispanic oversamples support the contention that heavy drinking per se is associated similarly in Hispanic-American and Anglo-American families. However, we also identified differences among Hispanic subgroups. Additionally, the study by Perilla and associates[84] found that husbands' frequent drunkenness increases assaults against Latina wives. Evidence from the two national studies also demonstrates that cultural variations in drinking patterns differentially affect wife assaults. For example, among Anglo men, alcohol-related problems were less frequent, but such problems were linearly and significantly associated with husband-to-wife violence. The linearity of the alcohol–wife assault relationships for Anglos and not Hispanics may occur because binge-drinking patterns (at both lower- and higher-volume alcohol consumption) are more common to Hispanics, and the latter alcohol consumption pattern is linked to wife assaults among some Hispanic-American subgroups. This phenomenon may be a function of where drinking takes place. That is, if men drink away from home, this may in turn create conflict between spouses that is fueled by the husband's intoxication and then escalates into violence. There also may be physiological differences in tolerance or metabolism between high daily drinkers and episodic drinkers that increase the likelihood of aggressive responding under the influence. Although Neff and associates[83] failed to find significant effects of alcohol quantity on wife assaults in Mexican-American families, this may be related to their use of alcohol quantity per se rather than volume-variability-based patterns such as binge drinking.

Experimental studies[87] do find greater negativity of alcoholic couples (more disagreements by wives) on "drink night" compared with normal couples. But there may also be differences in communication patterns depending on the drinking pattern of the husband. When binge and steady drinkers were compared, binge drinkers were found to have more negative communications when drinking, while steady drinkers had more positive communications when drinking during the experimental manipulation. Such effects may occur because partners can better cope with the predictability of steady-drinking behaviors, or possibly because binge drinkers may themselves have other characteristics such as greater aggressiveness that are confounded with drinking.

3.3. The Importance of Race and Social Structure

We found very limited empirical data on the relationship between alcohol and wife assaults in African-American families. However, the two studies that examined this relationship[67,83] found little or no net effect of drinking by African-American men after taking other variables into account. Rather, the effects of race dominated those of other variables examined. We believe that the effects of race represent variables unmeasured by these studies such as marginalization and the sequelae of years of segregation and discrimination. Additionally, studies demonstrating significant alcohol effects also show that these effects are moderated by relationship, structural, and cultural factors.

Structural factors were strongly predictive of wife assaults in minority and Anglo families, net of drinking. The greater importance of structural factors among minority families occurs because unemployment and poverty are disproportionately experienced by minority individuals. Additionally, minority individuals often reside in urban communities characterized by high rates of drug dependence, poverty, and substandard housing and plagued by high levels of predatory and violent crimes. The social pathology of such environments and the inequalities relative to the dominant culture can influence stress and, subsequently, assaultiveness in families. However, to a large extent many of these indicators of urban poverty went unmeasured in the studies examined. Although we have focused on net effects of structural variables in the models examined, variables do not exist in isolation in reality, and empirically the additive effects of alcohol, unemployment, and poverty sum up to greatly increased risks of wife assaults.

3.4. The Importance of Gender Roles

None of the studies examining gender role effects found significant associations with wife assaults. This may reflect the inability to measure central aspects of gender role conflicts between spouses or male dominance, or it may be that shifting gender roles with women's necessary entry into the work force may render many gender-role measures irrelevant in today's society. However, loss of the male provider role, traditionally defined as central to concepts of masculinity, does appear to affect the likelihood of wife abuse. Some argue that this is due to the husband's perceived loss of competency as a provider or loss of self-esteem when the wife must become the primary breadwinner. Additionally, some assert that violence by African-American men against women may occur because some aspect of the woman's behavior threatens his masculinity.[87]

3.5. The Importance of Culture and Acculturation

There was little evidence supporting a relationship between acculturation and wife assaults when linguistic measures of acculturation were used. On the other hand, acculturation as measured by country of birth did show a positive and significant association with wife assaults, such that being US (mainland) born increased the risk of wife assault in Puerto Rican- and Mexican-American families. The reasons for the latter effects are unclear. However, we[68] have previously hypothesized several explanations, such as abandonment of cultural norms of familialism and religiosity, or greater candor about disclosing violent behavior, or even the adoption of violent norms from exposure to the cultural or structural patterns of the United States.

There was no evidence that the saliency of particular cultural beliefs favoring violence toward women was intrinsic to any one ethnic group. Additionally, aggressive expectancies about alcohol characterized both violent Anglo and Hispanic men, suggesting a similar cultural framework for violence against women across ethnic groups. The major evidence for cultural differences was in the greater legitimation of alcohol-related behavior and in the acceptance of machismo drinking ("A real man can hold his liquor") and alcohol-related misbehavior by Hispanic Americans.

3.6. Implications

Our review suggests that more empirical testing is needed to assess the possibilities of cultural patterning and the dynamics of alcohol-related violence among different social groups. Longitudinal examination of the processes and empirical data based on both partners in an intimate relationship would improve our understanding of causal relationships.

Minority women do experience a disproportionate and unacceptable level of violence at the hands of their partners. However, they may be less willing to use formal social services and have fewer resources to escape from abusive situations. Similarly, minority men may be uncomfortable seeking help from formal treatment programs or may find treatment providers hostile or insensitive to their needs.[88] Prevention efforts and improved outreach to heavier-drinking subgroups are needed to counter normative beliefs about alcohol. Additional outreach and greater resources should be made available to women and families at risk. Additionally, both alcohol treatment and batterer treatment programs need to develop sensitivity and expertise in working with minority clients in order to improve treatment outcomes.

ACKNOWLEDGMENTS. Our research reported here was supported by Research Grant No. RO1AA09070 from the National Institute on Alcohol Abuse and Alcoholism. We are grateful to Mary Austin, Kelly Foster, and Jana Jasinski for their assistance in manuscript preparation.

References

1. Hampton RL: Family violence and homicide in the black community: Are they linked? in Hampton RL (ed): *Violence in the Black Family: Correlates and Consequences.* Lexington, MA, Lexington Books, 1987, pp 135 –156.
2. Straus MA, Gelles RJ, Steinmetz SK: *Behind Closed Doors: Violence in the American Family.* Newbury Park CA, Sage, 1980.
3. Straus MA, Smith C: Violence in Hispanic families in the United States: Incidence rates and structural interpretations, in Straus MA, Gelles RJ (eds): *Physical Violence in American Families: Risk Factors and Adaptations to Violence in 8,145 Families.* New Brunswick, NJ, Transaction Publishers, 1980, pp 341–367.
4. Cahalan D: *Problem Drinkers.* San Francisco, CA, Jossey-Bass, 1970.
5. Collins JJ: Drinking and violence: An individual offender focus, in: *Alcohol and Interpersonal Violence: Fostering Multidisciplinary Perspectives,* NIH Publication No. 93-3496. Rockville MD, 1993, pp 221–235.
6. Kaufman Kantor G, Straus MA: The "drunken bum" theory of wife beating. *Social Problems* 34(3):213–230, 1987.
7. Smith C: Status discrepancies and husband-to-wife violence. Paper presented at the Annual Meetings of the Eastern Sociological Society, 1988.

8. US Bureau of the Census, Current Population Reports: *Hispanic Americans Today*. (P23-183) Washington, DC, US Government Printing Office, 1993.
9. Levinson D: Family violence in cross-cultural perspective, in Van Hasselt VB, Morrison RL, Bellack AS, Hersen M (eds): *Handbook of Family Violence*. New York, Plenum Press, 1988, pp 435–455.
10. Gottheil E, Druley KA, Skoloda TE, Waxman HM: Aggression and addiction: Summary and overview, in Gottheil E, Druley KA, Skoloda TE, Waxman HM (eds): *Alcohol, Drug Abuse and Aggression*. Springfield, IL, Charles C. Thomas, 1983, pp 333–356.
11. Bennett LA, Ames GM (eds): *The American Experience with Alcohol: Contrasting Cultural Perspectives*. New York, Plenum Press, 1985.
12. Block CR: Lethal violence in the Chicago Latino community, 1965 to 1981. Paper presented at Research Conference on Violence and Homicide in Hispanic Communities, Los Angeles, CA, 1987.
13. Caetano R: *Drinking Patterns and Alcohol Problems in a National Sample of US Hispanics*. Prepared for presentation at the National Institute on Alcohol Abuse and Alcoholism conference on Epidemiology of Alcohol Use and Abuse among US Minorities, Bethesda MD, 1985.
14. Cahalan D, Cisin IH, Crossley HM: *American Drinking Practices: A National Study of Drinking Behavior and Attitudes*. New Brunswick, NJ, Rutgers Center for Alcohol Studies, 1969.
15. Cahalan D, Room R: *Problem Drinking among American Men*. New Brunswick, NJ, Rutgers Center for Alcohol Studies, 1974.
16. Clark W, Midanik L: Alcohol use and alcohol problems among US adults: Results of a 1979 national survey, in: *Alcohol and Health Monographs No. 1: Alcohol Consumption and Related Problems*, DHHS Publication No. ADM 82-1190. Washington, DC, US Department of Health and Human Services, 1982.
17. Herd D: Ambiguity in black drinking norms: An ethnohistorical interpretation, in Bennett LA, Ames GM (eds): *The American Experience with Alcohol: Contrasting Cultural Perspectives*. New York, Plenum Press, 1985, pp. 149–169.
18. Greeley AM, McCready WC, Theisen G: *Ethnic Drinking Subcultures*. New York, JF Bergin Publishers, 1980.
19. MacAndrew C, Edgerton RB: *Drunken Comportment: A Sociological Explanation*. Chicago, Aldin, 1969.
20. Levinson D: Alcohol use and aggression in American subcultures, in Room R, Collins G (eds): *ADAMHA 1981 Alcohol and Disinhibition: Nature and Meaning of the Link*, Monograph-12, DHHS Publication No. (ADM) 83-1246. Washington, DC, DHHS, 1981, pp 306–322.
21. Roizen J: Alcohol and criminal behavior among blacks: The case for research on special populations, in Collins JJ Jr. (ed): *Drinking and Crime: Perspectives on the Relationships between Alcohol Consumption and Criminal Behavior*. New York, Guilford Press, 1981, pp 207–251.
22. Barr KM, Farrell MP, Barnes GM, Welte JW: Race, class, and gender differences in substance abuse: Evidence of middle-class/underclass polarization among black males. *Social Problems* 40(3):314–327, 1993.
23. Stern MW: Drinking patterns and alcoholism among American Negroes, in Pittman DJ (ed): *Alcoholism*. New York, Harper & Row, 1967.
24. Harper FD (ed): *Alcohol Abuse and Black America*. Alexandria, VA, Douglass Publishers, 1976.
25. Bourne P: Alcoholism in the urban black population, in Harper FD (ed): *Alcohol Abuse and Black America*. Alexandria, VA, Douglass Publishers, 1976.
26. Fagan JA, Stewart DK, Hansen KV: Violent men or violent husbands? Background factors and situational correlates, in Finkelhor D, Gelles RJ, Hotaling GT, Straus MA (eds): *The Dark Side of Families*. Beverly Hills, CA, Sage Publications, 1983, pp 49–68.
27. Lewis BY: Psychosocial factors related to wife abuse. *J Fam Viol* 2(1):1–10, 1987.
28. Lockhart LL: A reexamination of the effects of race and social class on the incidence of violence: A search for reliable differences. *J Marriage Fam* 49:603–610, 1987.
29. Lockhart L, White B: Understanding marital violence in the black community. *J Interp Viol* 4(4):421–436, 1989.

30. Lockhart L: Spousal violence: A cross-racial perspective, in Hampton RL (ed): *Black Family Violence: Current Research and Theory.* Lexington, MA, Lexington Books, 1991, pp 85–102.
31. Hampton RL, Gelles RJ, Harrop JW: Is violence in black families increasing? A comparison of 1975 and 1985 national survey rates. *J Marriage Fam* 51:969–980, 1989.
32. Cazenave NA, Straus MA: Race, class, network embeddedness and family violence: A search for potent support systems. *J Comp Fam Stud* 10:280–299, 1979.
33. Hampton RL, Gelles RJ: Violence toward black women in a nationally representative sample of black families. *J Comp Fam Stud* 25:105–120, 1994.
34. Asbury J: African-American women in violent relationships: An exploration of cultural differences, in RL Hampton (ed): *Violence in the Black Family: Correlates and Consequences.* Lexington, MA, Lexington Books, 1987, pp 89–105.
35. Roy M (ed): *The Abusive Partner.* New York, Van Nostrand Reinhold, 1982.
36. Merton RK: *Social Theory and Social Structure.* New York, Free Press, 1968.
37. Johnson LV, LeMatre M: Anomie and alcohol use: Drinking patterns in Mexican American and Anglo neighborhoods. *J Stud Alcohol* 39(5):894–902, 1978.
38. Gray-Little B: Marital quality and power processes among black couples. *J Marriage Fam* 44(3):633–646, 1982.
39. Caetano R: Self-reported intoxication among Hispanics in northern California. *J Stud Alcohol* 45(4):349–354, 1985b.
40. Gilbert MJ: Mexican-Americans in California: Intracultural variation in attitudes and behavior related to alcohol, in Bennett LA, Ames GM (eds): *The American Experience with Alcohol: Contrasting Cultural Perspectives.* New York, Plenum Press, 1985, pp 255–277.
41. Paine HJ: Attitudes and patterns of alcohol use among Mexican Americans. *J Stud Alcohol* 38(3):544–553, 1977.
42. Trotter RT: Mexican-American experience with alcohol: South Texas examples, in Bennett LA, Ames GM (eds): *The American Experience with Alcohol: Contrasting Cultural Perspectives.* New York, Plenum Press, 1986, pp 279–296.
43. Mirande A: The Chicano family: A reanalysis of conflicting views. *J Marriage Fam* 44:851–873, 1977.
44. Anderson RM, Giachello AL, Aday L: Access of Hispanics to health care and cuts in services: A state-of-the-art overview. *Publ Health Rep* 101(3):238–265, 1986.
45. Linsky AS, Straus MA, Colby JJ Jr. Stressful events, stressful conditions and alcohol problems in the United States: A partial test of Bales' theory of alcoholism. *J Stud Alcohol* 46:72–80, 1985.
46. Abad V, Suarez J: *Machismo Alcoholism: Cross-Cultural Aspects of Alcoholism among Puerto Ricans.* Proceedings of the Fourth Annual Alcoholism Conference, NIAAA, 1975.
47. Caetano R: Alcohol use among Hispanic groups in the United States. *Am J Drug Alcohol Abuse* 14(3):293–308, 1988.
48. Trevino ME: *Machismo Alcoholism: Mexican-American machismo drinking.* Proceedings of the Fourth Annual Alcoholism Conference NIAAA, 1975.
49. Kaufman Kantor G, Aldarondo E, Jasinski JL: Incidence of Hispanic drinking and intrafamily violence. Paper presented at the Annual Meetings of the Research Society on Alcoholism, San Antonio, TX, 1993.
50. Levinson D: Social setting, cultural factors, and alcohol-related aggression, in Gottheil E, Druley KA, Skoloda TE, Waxman HM (eds): *Alcohol, Drug Abuse and Aggression.* Springfield, IL, Charles C. Thomas, 1983, pp 41–58.
51. Aviles-Roig CA: Aspectos Socioculturales del Problema de Alcoholismo en Puerto Rico, in Tongue E, Lambo RT, Blair B (eds): *Report of the Proceedings of the International Conference on Alcoholism and Drug Abuse.* Puerto Rico, 1977, pp 78–85.
52. Jacob T, Leonard KE: Alcoholic–spouse interaction as a function of alcoholism subtype and alcohol consumption interaction. *J Abnormal Psychol* 97(2):231–237, 1988.
53. Alcocer AM: Alcohol use and abuse among the Hispanic American population, in: *Alcohol and Health Monograph No. 4: Special Population Issues.* (ADM) 82-1193, Rockville, MD, US Department of Health and Human Services, 1982, pp 361–382.

54. Caetano R: Ethnicity and drinking in northern California: A comparison among whites, blacks, and Hispanics. *Alcohol Alcoholism* 19(1):31–44, 1984.
55. Gordon AJ: Hispanic drinking after migration: The case of Dominicans. *Med Anthropol* 2(4):61–84, 1978.
56. Gondolf EW, Fisher E, McFerron JR: Racial differences among shelter residents: A comparison of Anglo, black, and Hispanic battered women. *J Fam Violence* 3(1):39–51, 1988.
57. Mirande A, Perez P: *Ethnic and Cultural Differences in Domestic Violence: A Test of Conflicting Models of the Chicano Family.* Proceedings of the Research Conference on Violence and Homicide in Hispanic Communities California, UCLA Publications Services, 1988.
58. Torres S: Hispanic American battered women: Why consider cultural differences? *Response* 10(3):20–21, 1987.
59. Carroll JC: A cultural consistency theory of family violence in Mexican-American and Jewish-ethnic groups, in Hotaling GT, Straus MA (eds): *The Social Causes of Husband–Wife Violence.* Minneapolis, University of Minnesota Press, 1980, chapter 5.
60. Eberstein I, Frisbie WM: Differences in marital instability among Mexican Americans, blacks, and Anglos: 1960 and 1970. *Social Problems* 23(5):609–621, 1976.
61. Panitz DR, McConchie RD, Suaber SR, Fonseca JA: The role of machismo and the Hispanic family in the etiology and treatment of alcoholism in Hispanic American men. *J Family Ther* 11:31–44, 1983.
62. Becerra R: The Mexican American family, in Mindel CH, Habenstein RW, Wright Jr R (eds): *Ethnic Families in America: Patterns and Variations.* New York, Elsevier, Co., 1988, pp. 141–159.
63. Fernandez-Mariña R, Maldonado-Sierra ED, Trent RD: Three basic themes in Mexican and Puerto Rican family values. *J Social Psychol* 48:167–181, 1958.
64. Peñalosa F: Mexican family roles. *J Marriage Fam* 30(4):680–689, 1968.
65. Szapocznik J, Hernandez R: The Cuban American family, in Mindel CH, Habenstein RW, Wright R Jr. (eds): *Ethnic Families in America: Patterns and Variations.* New York, Elsevier, 1988, pp. 160–172.
66. Loya R, Mercy JA, *et al: The Epidemiology of Homicide in the City of Los Angeles, 1970–79.* University of California at Los Angeles and Centers for Disease Control, Department of Health and Human Services, Public Health Service, Centers for Disease Control, 1985.
67. Kaufman Kantor G: Ethnicity, drinking and wife abuse: A structural and cultural interpretation. Paper presented at the 42nd Annual Meeting of the American Society of Criminology, Baltimore, MD, 1990.
68. Kaufman Kantor G, Jasinski JL, Aldarondo E: Socioeconomic status and incidence of marital violence in Hispanic families. *Violence Victims* 9(3):207–222, 1994.
69. Gordon M: *Assimilation in American life: The Role of Race, Religion and National Origins.* New York, Oxford University Press, 1964.
70. Szapocznik J, Scopetta MA, Kurtines W, Aranalde M: Theory and measurement of acculturation. *Interam J Psychol* 12:113–130, 1978.
71. Burnam AM, Hough RL, Karno M, *et al:* Acculturation and lifetime prevalence of psychiatric disorders among Mexican Americans in Los Angeles, *J Health Soc Behav* 28:89–102, 1987.
72. Holck SE, Warren CW, Smith JC, Rochat RW: Alcohol consumption among Mexican American and Anglo women: Results of a survey along the US–Mexico border *J Stud Alcohol* 45(2):149–154, 1984.
73. Vega W, Warheit G, Buhi-Auth J, Meinhardt K: The prevalence of depressive symptoms among Mexican Americans and Anglos. *Am J Epidemiol* 120:592–607, 1984.
74. Griffith J, Villavicencio S: Relationships among acculturation, sociodemographic characteristics and social supports in Mexican American adults. *Hispanic J Behav Sci* 7(1):75–92, 1985.
75. Caetano R, Medina Mora ME: Acculturation and drinking among people of Mexican descent in Mexico and the United States. *J Stud Alcohol* 49(5):462–471, 1988.
76. Galan RJ: *Alcohol Use among Chicanos and Anglos: A Cross-Cultural Study.* Unpublished doctoral dissertation, Waltham, MA, Brandeis University, 1978.
77. Neff JA, Hoppe SK, Perea P: Acculturation and alcohol use: Drinking patterns and problems among Anglo and Mexican American male drinkers. *Hispanic J Behav Sci* 9:151–181, 1987.

78. Gordon AJ: The cultural context of drinking and indigenous therapy for alcohol problems in three migrant Hispanic cultures, in Gottheil E, Druley KA, Skoloda TE, Waxman HM (eds): *Alcohol, Drug Abuse and Aggression*. Springfield, IL, Charles C. Thomas, 1983, pp 41–58.

79. Torres S: *A Comparative Analysis of Wife Abuse among Anglo-American and Mexican-American Battered Women: Attitudes, Nature, Severity, Frequency, and Response to the Abuse*. Unpublished doctoral dissertation, Austin, University of Texas, 1986.

80. Sorenson SB, Telles CA: Self-reports of spousal violence in a Mexican-American and non-Hispanic white population. *Violence Victims* 6(1):3–15, 1991.

81. Portes A: The rise of ethnicity: Determinants of ethnic perceptions among Cuban exiles in Miami. *Am Soc Rev* 49:383–397, 1984.

82. Kaufman Kantor G, Straus MA: Substance abuse as a precipitant of wife abuse victimizations. *Am J Drug Alcohol Abuse* 15(2):173–189, 1989.

83. Neff JA, Holamon B, Schluter TD: Spousal violence among Anglos, blacks, Mexican Americans: The role of demographic variables, psychosocial predictors, and alcohol consumption. *J Fam Violence* 10(1):1–21, 1995.

84. Perilla JL, Bakeman R, Norris FH: Culture and domestic violence: The ecology of abused Latinas. *Violence Victims* 9(4):325–339, 1994.

85. O'Leary KD: Physical aggression between spouses: A social learning perspective, in Van Hasselt VB, Morrison RL, Bellack AS, Hersen M (eds): *The Handbook of Family Violence*. New York, Plenum Press, 1988, pp 31–56.

86. Kaufman Kantor G, Asdigian N: Socialization to alcohol-related family violence: Disentangling the effects of family history on current violence. Paper presented at the Annual Meetings of the American Society of Criminology, Phoenix, AZ, 1993.

87. Campbell DW, Campbell J, King C, *et al*: The reliability and factor structure of the index of spouse abuse with African-American women. *Violence Victims* 9(3):259–274, 1994.

88. Williams OJ, Becker RL: Domestic partner abuse treatment programs and cultural competence: The results of a national survey. *Violence Victims* 9(3):287–296, 1994.

4

Longitudinal Perspective on Alcohol Use and Aggression during Adolescence

Helene Raskin White

Abstract. While there is general agreement that alcohol use and aggression are related, few studies have examined this relationship among youth. This chapter reviews the literature on rates of alcohol use, aggression, and alcohol-related aggression among adolescents, as well as the cross-sectional and longitudinal associations among these behaviors. In general, the literature does not provide strong support for a unique association between alcohol use and aggressive behavior during adolescence. The observed relationship between alcohol use and aggression appears to be spurious because both behaviors are predicted by a similar set of individual, family, and environmental factors. Prevention programs that reduce these common risk factors should decrease both behaviors. Interventions with aggressive individuals, especially aggressive individuals who drink heavily, may be most indicated.

1. Introduction

The association between alcohol use and aggression is well documented.[1] Numerous correlational and laboratory studies support the notion that individuals are more aggressive while under the influence of alcohol.[1,2] Statistics indicate that alcoholics are overrepresented among persons convicted of violent crimes, and in clinical and nonclinical populations alcohol consumption is often reported immediately prior to violent offenses.[3,4] There is a paucity of similar statistics on adolescent samples, especially noninstitutionalized samples. The purpose of this chapter is to examine the relationship between

Helene Raskin White • Center for Alcohol Studies, Rutgers University, Piscataway, New Jersey 08855-0969.

Recent Developments in Alcoholism, Volume 13: Alcoholism and Violence, edited by Marc Galanter. Plenum Press, New York, 1997.

alcohol use and aggression among adolescents. First, I briefly discuss models advanced for explaining the nature and direction of the relationship. Then, I examine the prevalence of alcohol use, aggression, and alcohol-related aggression in community and institutionalized samples. Next, I present a broad overview on the degree of association and developmental trends in the relationship between alcohol use and aggression. I go on to discuss the spurious nature of the relationships among problem behaviors in adolescence. Finally, I describe prevention approaches that address alcohol use and aggression in youth.

Before I begin, let me clarify the scope of the chapter. This review is limited to research on adolescents. Adolescence, for the purposes of this review, encompasses approximately the ages of 12 to 18 years, unless otherwise noted. Aggression is defined as the "intent to harm or create a noxious condition for the target" (ref. 5, p. 313), whereas violence is defined as "behaviors by individuals that intentionally threaten, attempt or inflict physical harm on others" (ref. 6, p. 2.). Violent behaviors are considered a subset of aggressive behaviors; the use or threat of *physical* harm is a necessary ingredient in the definition of violence, but not necessary for aggression. In this chapter, I focus on the more general category of aggressive behavior and do not include acts directed at oneself (i.e., suicide). (I also do not discuss laboratory studies because they do not include adolescents as subjects. Interested readers are referred to refs. 2,7 for reviews.) I try to limit this review to alcohol use. However, much of the research on adolescents focuses on drug use including alcohol and usually excludes separate analysis on alcohol use alone. Therefore, I will also discuss other psychoactive drugs when appropriate. There are several methodological problems and issues that affect the interpretation of the empirical studies on alcohol and aggression. These issues relate to definition, operationalization, and measurement of variables, analysis strategies, sample selection, and experimental design characteristics. Due to space limitations these issues are not discussed here; the interested reader is referred to refs. 1,4,8.

2. Explanatory Models

While it is agreed that aggressive behavior and alcohol use are related, the extent of a direct causal relationship remains in question. Three primary theoretical frameworks have been advanced to account for the nature and direction of the relationship. The first model postulates that alcohol use causes aggressive behavior due primarily to the psychopharmacological effects of the drug. This psychopharmacological model proposes that the effects of intoxication (including disinhibition, cognitive–perceptual distortions, attention deficits, bad judgment, neurochemical changes, etc.) cause aggressive behavior.[5,9,10] It also assumes that situational factors accompanying occasions of intoxication, such as interpersonal interactions in certain bars, may contribute to aggression.[11] In addition, chronic intoxication may contribute to subsequent aggression due to factors such as withdrawal, sleep deprivation, nutritional deficits, impairment of neuropsychological functioning, or enhancement of psychopathological personality disorders.[12] (For greater detail on the psychopharmacological model, see refs. 1,5,10.)

A second model postulates that aggressive behavior leads to heavy alcohol use. This model is based on the assumption that aggressive individuals are more likely than nonaggressive individuals to select (or be pushed into) social situations and subcultures in which heavy drinking is condoned or encouraged. For example, several aspects of the professional crime lifestyle are conducive to heavy drinking, such as working periodically, partying between jobs, being unmarried, and being geographically mobile.[13] Aggression can also lead to heavy drinking because aggressive individuals may drink heavily in order to self-medicate.[14] Alternatively, aggressive individuals may drink to give themselves an excuse to act aggressively. That is, individuals hold expectations that alcohol use causes aggression,[15] and that if they act aggressively when they are drunk, they will be held less accountable for their behavior (deviance disavowal) and sanctions will be more lenient.[3,11]

It is also possible that both of the above models are correct so that the relationship between alcohol use and aggression is reciprocal. Drinking problems may lead to more aggression and aggressive behavior may lead to more drinking.[5]

The third model is the spurious model, which postulates that alcohol use and aggression are related either coincidentally or because they share common risk factors rather than a direct causal link.[16] For example, young males account for a disproportionate share of violent incidents and are also the heaviest drinkers. Also, common causes (such as genetic or temperamental traits, antisocial personality disorder, parental modeling of heavy drinking and aggression, and poor relations with parents) have been shown to predict both aggression and heavy drinking.[17] In addition, subcultural norms may reinforce both aggression and substance use. Certain subcultures may promote both aggression and heavy drinking as proof of masculinity, which would spuriously inflate the relationship.[5] Thus, a spurious model argues that alcohol and aggression are related because similar factors promote both behaviors. (This model is discussed in greater detail below.)

A routine activities perspective can also explain the spuriousness of the relationship between alcohol use and aggression. Aggressive behavior occurs most often when and where people are drinking, such as at bars and sports stadiums, at night, and on weekends.[11] Proponents of this perspective argue that bars are "ideal" places for violent crime because customers carry cash and are often too intoxicated to defend themselves, there are weakened social controls, and the bar atmosphere intensifies competition. Thus, situational factors also contribute to a spurious relationship between alcohol use and aggression.[11,18]

Clearly, no one model can account for all individuals or all types of aggression. Each of these models may be applicable to different subgroups of the population or to different incidents of alcohol-related aggression. Other more complicated models such as interactive, conditional, and conjunctive models have been described by Pernanen.[19] These models suggest that alcohol will cause aggression only for certain individuals and only under some conditions and situations. (For greater detail on these models, see refs. 1,5,19.) Before examining the empirical studies of youth that shed light on these models, I first examine the prevalence of alcohol use and aggression in adolescence.

3. The Extent of Alcohol Use and Aggression in Adolescence

In this section, I present data on the prevalence of alcohol use and aggression from early adolescence into young adulthood. The data that are presented in Fig. 1 come from the Rutgers Health and Human Development Project (HHDP), a prospective longitudinal study of adolescent development. A community sample of New Jersey adolescents was tested initially between 1979 and 1981 (time 1, T1) at the ages of 12, 15, and 18 ($N = 1380$). These subjects returned 3 years later in 1982–1984 (time 2, T2), again in 1985–1987 (time 3, T3), and finally in 1992–1994 (time 4, T4). Over 90% of the original sample returned at T4 ($N = 1257$). The data presented here are based on subjects who were tested at all four points in time ($N = 1201$). The sample of participants is most representative of white, working- and middle-class adolescents living in a metropolitan environment. Results of analyses on validity and reliability of the data indicate that the sample has a satisfactory degree of representativeness and that empirical findings have an acceptable degree of generalizability. (For more extensive details on the methodology of this study as well as sample recruitment and description, see ref. 20.)

Figure 1a presents the last-year prevalence rates for alcohol use by age and sex. There is a marked increase in alcohol use from age 12 to age 18 and then rates remain fairly steady from age 18 to age 31. Prevalence rates for males and females are remarkably similar, which is consistent with other research on young populations.[21]

Figures 1b and 1c depict age and sex differences in typical quantity (10-point scale from none to more than two six-packs of beer, a gallon of wine, or a fifth of hard liquor) and last-year frequency (10-point scale from never to daily) of drinking, respectively. Frequency increases throughout adolescence, then peaks in the mid-20s (at a mean of once a week for males and two to three times a month for females), and declines slightly thereafter (to a mean of two to three times a month for men and once a month for women). Quantity appears to peak somewhat earlier (at approximately five drinks per sitting for males and three drinks for females between ages 18 and 21) and declines in the late 20s (to an average of three to four drinks for men and two to three for women. (For greater detail on prevalence of drinking and heavy drinking over time and sociodemographic differences in a nationally representative sample, see ref. 22.)

Age and sex differences in rates of (any) aggressive behavior (including assault, vandalism, using a weapon in a fight, hitting parents, and robbery at T1–T3 and assault, vandalism, attacking someone, gang fighting, and robbery at T4) are shown in Fig. 1d. Males are more aggressive than females; at all age levels, male 3-year prevalence rates are at least two to three times greater than female rates. Aggressive behavior appears to peak at age 15 for females and ages 15 or 18 for males and then there is a large drop after age 18. These findings are consistent with other studies.[23] Yet our data indicate a slight increase in aggressive behavior in adulthood, which is inconsistent with most self-report studies.[24] This slight increase probably reflects the difference in the way the assault question was phrased at T1–T3 (hurt someone badly) as compared to T4 (hit or threatened to hit someone).

As stated above, the HHDP sample is primarily a white, middle- and working-class sample. While rates of alcohol use are comparable to those found in national studies (e.g., ref. 22), rates of aggressive behavior are fairly low and composed of primarily nonserious offenses. Data from the National Youth Survey (NYS)[25] indicate that self-reported rates of serious violent offending (i.e., robbery, rape, and atrocious assault) peak at age 17 at which time 36% of the African-American and 25% of the white males report one or more offense. Peaks for females occur between ages 15 and 16, with approximately 20% of the African-American and 10% of the white females reporting at least one offense. Not only do females peak earlier, but their decline is much steeper and the gender differential becomes greater over time. Interestingly, arrest data indicate a later peak than self-report data, and gender and ethnic differentials are substantially higher in official record studies.[25]

The NYS data indicate that after age 17 rates of serious violent offending drop dramatically, and approximately 80% of those who were violent during adolescence terminate by age 21.[24] Nearly twice as many African Americans as compared to whites continue their offending after age 21. In general, if a person has not initiated violence by age 20, it is unlikely that she or he will ever become a serious violent offender (ref. 24, pp. 1–2).

Arrest data indicate that about 6% of juvenile arrests are for violent crimes.[26] Between 1988 and 1992, the number of violent crime index arrests for juveniles increased by 47%, more than twice the increase for individuals age 18 and older. In this same time span, juvenile arrests for murder increased by 51% as compared to 9% for adults (ref. 26, p. 1). (For greater detail on the increases in juvenile violent crime by crime type, see ref. 27.) It should be noted that juvenile rates for violent offenses are still much lower than adult rates, so even a large percentage increase does not necessarily translate to a large contribution to the overall rate of violence.[27] Data from the National Crime Victimization Survey indicate that in 1991, 19% of all violent crimes were committed by juveniles.[27] Nine out of 10 of these crimes were committed by males.

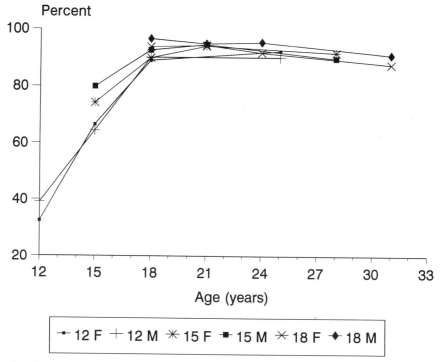

1a: Last year prevalence of alcohol use

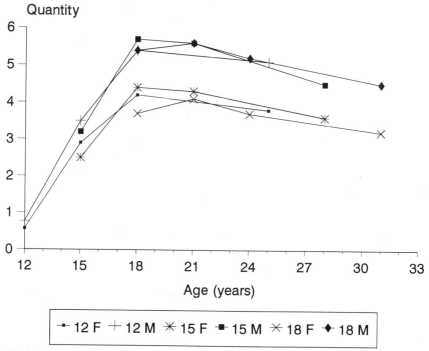

1b: Typical quantity of alcohol use

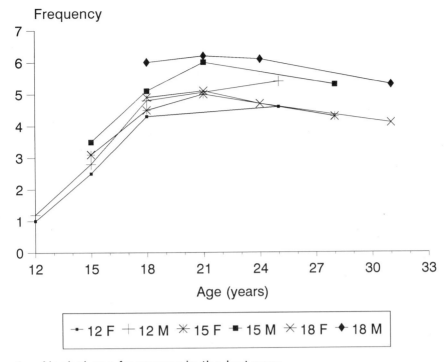

1c: Alcohol use frequency in the last year

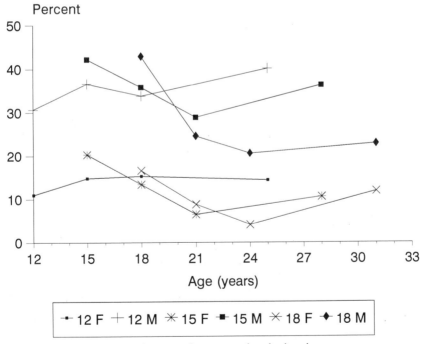

1d: Three-year prevalence of aggressive behavior

Figure 1. Longitudinal patterns in alcohol use and aggression by age and sex. (a) Last year prevalence of alcohol use. (b) Typical quantity of alcohol use. (c) Alcohol use frequency in the last year. (d) Three-year prevalence of aggressive behavior.

While this chapter focuses on involvement in aggressive behavior rather than on victimization, it should be noted that teenagers and young adults have the highest rates of victimization for crimes of violence.[26,28] Half of all rape victims are females under age 18, and homicides of teenagers have doubled from 1984 to 1991, with rates especially high for African-American males. Persons most likely to be victimized by juveniles are also juveniles.[27]

When one examines demographic variable differences in the patterns of aggression and alcohol use, several discrepancies emerge. First, alcohol use tends to peak later than violence and declines more steadily. Second, there are large gender differences in violence but not in the use of alcohol. In addition, African Americans as compared to whites have higher rates of violence yet lower rates of alcohol use. Thus, to some extent, these differences in trends argue against a direct causal relationship between alcohol use and violence.[29] Data that specifically address the relationship between alcohol use and aggression are discussed below.

4. The Association between Alcohol Use and Aggression in Adolescence

4.1. Acute Incidents of Alcohol-Related Aggression

The HHDP study is one of the few that directly assesses acute incidents of alcohol-related aggression. Subjects were asked to indicate the number of times they engaged in aggressive behaviors (including fighting or acting mean, vandalism, fire setting, forcing sex, and hurting someone badly) while they were drinking or because of their drinking. Except for fighting (around one fourth of females users), very few females have engaged in any type of alcohol-related aggression (1 to 2% of the users for most categories). Rates for fighting while intoxicated are very high for males and appear to increase with age from about 30% of the 15-year-old users, to about one third to one half of the 21-year-old users, and then drop off slightly at age 24 and continue to drop off into the 30s (to about one fifth of the users). Rates for alcohol-related vandalism among males are relatively high in late adolescence and early adulthood (around 20% of the users) and then drop off considerably. Forced sex (around 3% of the users or less), fire setting (2% or less), and hurting someone badly (7% or less) while drinking are relatively rare (see ref. 20).

Mitic[30] found that approximately 6% of junior high and 15% of high school students reported engaging in vandalism or violence toward others while drinking. Elliott and colleagues[23] examined self-reported alcohol use immediately prior to committing an offense. When subjects were 11–17 years old, 23% of the aggravated assaults (including gang fights) and 10% of the robberies were committed under the influence of alcohol only. In comparison, 20% of the motor vehicle thefts were also committed under the influence of alcohol. As these subjects entered young adulthood, however, alcohol use was more likely to precede an offense characterized by physical violence than one characterized by a profit motive. The NYS data suggest that the nature of the relationship between alcohol use and violent offenses may change over the life course. Taken together, the above studies do not suggest that rates of alcohol-related aggressive behaviors (except perhaps fighting) are especially high during adolescence.

Similarly, research on adolescent offenders indicates relatively low rates of alcohol use at the time of violent offenses.[3] Only 8% of all youth in custody in state institutions reported that they were under the influence of only alcohol when they committed a violent offense.[31] On the other hand, 24% committed violent offenses while under the influence of both alcohol and other drugs. Yet this percentage is the same as that for property crimes committed under the influence of alcohol and drugs (23%). Thus, it appears that some youth are committing crimes while under the influence of alcohol (just as they are engaging in all sorts of other activities while intoxicated); however, a unique effect of alcohol on violent crime is not borne out by these statistics. In fact, studies of youth gangs suggest that alcohol plays a role in facilitating intragroup cohesion as well as intergroup conflict (for greater detail on alcohol use among gang members, see ref. 11).

When adolescents are questioned about the contribution of alcohol intoxication to their aggression, mixed findings emerge. In a community interview study, most adolescents held expectancies that alcohol/drug use causes crime (due to disinhibition, economics, etc.) and attributed other people's crime to their drug use.[32] These same adolescents did not attribute their own crime to their drug use. The subjects said that they kept their drug use under control and it did not interfere with or cause their participation in delinquency. The researchers concluded that alcohol and drug use was incidental to and not a contributing factor for crime. Although they found that heavy drug users were most involved in violence, most of the violent incidents occurred while subjects were not using alcohol or drugs. A recent study of inner-city adolescents[33] supports these findings. Very few adolescents admitted that they used drugs while committing offenses or that they committed an offense in order to obtain drugs or money for drugs. Unfortunately, alcohol use was not included as a measure in this study.

In contrast, in a study of adolescents who were adjudicated for a violent crime, over half of the youths said that taking alcohol (29%) or drugs (33%) contributed to their acting violently, and almost half had used either alcohol (17%) or drugs (34%) immediately prior to their adjudicated violent offense.[34] Note, however, that the rates were higher for other drugs than for alcohol. In a study of incarcerated adolescents, it was found that over two thirds of the incidents of physically assaultive crime involved acute drug intoxication.[35] Almost all of the cases of acute intoxication involved alcohol either alone or in combination with another drug. Similarly, a large majority of the drug-related sexually assaultive crimes involved alcohol use. On the other hand, marijuana use was underreported in offenses against persons. Secobarbital (a sedative drug) was selected over alcohol as the drug most likely to lead to a fight, while marijuana was selected as the drug most likely to decrease assaultiveness. It is possible in both these studies that arrested juveniles overreported alcohol or drug use prior to their offense in order to justify their behavior.[3]

The above studies on degree of association looked at acute incidents of alcohol-related aggression. Many other studies have examined the associations between patterns of alcohol and aggression either through correlations or typologies, and some of these will be reviewed below.

4.2. Associations between Patterns of Alcohol Use and Aggression

Using the HHDP data, we examined the correlations between alcohol use (typical quantity times frequency) and aggression (sum of the five behaviors included in the prevalence analysis above). The cross-sectional correlations at each test occasion indicated that the two behaviors were significantly related with an average correlation (r) of .23. These correlations were higher for males (mean $r = .22$) than females (mean $r = .13$) and also higher for quantity (mean $r = .22$) than frequency (mean $r = .15$). Finally, it should be noted that the correlations between alcohol use and property crime (mean $r = .30$) were higher than those for alcohol use and aggression. Thus, these data do not support a unique relationship between alcohol as opposed to other drugs and aggression.

Several other studies have looked at the correlations between alcohol use and aggression. Most of these studies have been cross-sectional, although a few have been longitudinal. Cohen et al.[7] conducted a meta-analysis of the cross-sectional studies. In these analyses they did not separate studies of adolescents from studies of adults. They found that the average correlation for criminal (as compared to domestic) violence and alcohol use at the time of the offense was .12, while that for criminal violence and general pattern of alcohol use (not necessarily at the time of the offense) was .16. In practical terms, a mean correlation of .12 is equivalent to a contrast between a low-alcohol-use group that is 10% violent and a high-use group that is 15% violent (ref. 7, p. 27). While this difference may appear substantial, correlations of less than .2 are relatively weak and indicate that about three fourths of the variation in each behavior is not accounted for by the other. Cohen and colleagues concluded that greater alcohol use is associated with higher levels of violent behavior. They were careful to note that this association in no way supports a causal connection between alcohol use and violence and may be due to confounding factors. Further, while the correlations between criminal violence and drug use patterns were lower than the alcohol–violence correlations for most drugs, the correlation was higher for multiple drug use. Of greater interest is that the mean correlation for alcohol–nonviolent crime was higher than the mean alcohol–violence correlation, and this finding was obtained across studies of primarily adolescent samples. All of the studies reviewed identified control variables that accounted for a significant portion of the variance in violence independent of the effect of alcohol. In fact, in about half of the studies, once these other factors were statistically controlled, the relationship between alcohol use and criminal violence was no longer significant. In examining differences in samples, Cohen *et al.* found that the criminal violence–alcohol correlation was higher in adolescent (under age 21) than in adult samples.

Similarly, Osgood[29] examined correlations between self-reported substance use and various types of delinquency from the Monitoring the Future Study. He found that the correlations between violence and other drugs were generally the same as between violence and alcohol use (all coefficients around .2), but were lower than for alcohol/other drugs and theft. In an inner-city sample, Fagan and his colleagues[36] reported higher correlations between alcohol use and the incidence of violent crime than those reported above (coefficients around .3). However they also found that the correlations between alcohol and violent offenses were generally lower than those between alcohol and property crime.

In sum, the correlational studies reviewed above indicate that the association between alcohol use and aggression is similar to or weaker than the association between alcohol use and other forms of delinquency. Thus, both correlation studies, as well as self-reports of attribution, do not provide strong support for a unique association between alcohol use and aggression in community samples. In fact, after a review of the literature on alcohol, drugs, and violence among youth, Osgood[29] (p. 33) concluded that there is little evidence that substance use makes an independent contribution to adolescent violence.

While research on adolescents does not provide strong support for a direct relationship between alcohol and aggression, the data suggest that alcohol and drug users as opposed to nonusers are more likely to be delinquent and more likely to be involved in aggression.[29] Carpenter and colleagues[32] found that those youth involved in violence were also more involved in delinquency and alcohol/drug use than their peers. Not only were those heavily involved individuals more often perpetrators, but also they were more often victims of violence. Major assaults were committed by the heaviest drug users, while alcohol-only users had few felony violence offenses. Those subjects most involved in gang fights were also the heaviest drug users.

In studies of inner-city students, Fagan and his colleagues[36,37] found that substance use was prevalent regardless of level of delinquency. They found that prevalence of alcohol use did not vary across delinquency types, although frequency did. On the other hand, prevalence of marijuana and other illicit drugs increased from nondelinquents to multiple-index offenders. In the NYS data, Elliott *et al.*[23] found that level of violence increased across groups from nonusers to alcohol users to marijuana users to polydrug users. Thus, there were greater levels of violence among polydrug users and marijuana users (who also used alcohol) than among those who only used alcohol.

Similarly, the level of alcohol use increased from nondelinquents to exploratory delinquents to nonserious delinquents to serious delinquents.

A US national study found that drug (including alcohol) users were more likely than nonusers to fight, to take risks that predisposed them to assault, and to be victimized both in school and outside school supervision.[38] A study of high school juniors and seniors found that binge drinking was a strong predictor of fighting and that alcohol use was a strong predictor of carrying a weapon.[28] The authors noted that both behaviors may have been caused by a common factor.

Watts and Wright[39] studied white, African-American, and Hispanic adjudicated delinquents and high school students. They found that, across ethnic groups, the best predictor of violent delinquency was use of illegal drugs. In the multivariate analyses including all drug types, alcohol use was not a significant predictor of violent delinquency for any of the three ethnic groups, and, in fact, the beta weight was negative.

After reviewing the literature on the relationship between alcohol use and crime during adolescence, Collins[40] concluded that alcohol use by itself is not important to the occurrence of serious criminal involvement. Although those who drink and drink heavily are more likely to be involved in other forms of deviance, the association is probably spurious due to common etiologies. The spurious model is discussed in greater detail below. First, however, I review findings on the longitudinal associations between alcohol use and aggression.

4.3. Developmental Trends

Research suggests that involvement in delinquency occurs prior to or simultaneous with the first drink.[23,25] Elliott and colleagues[23] found that minor delinquency almost always came first in the sequence of delinquency and drug use, and, in fact, no one initiated marijuana or polydrug use before minor delinquency. Alcohol use came second; however, a substantial percentage of subjects initiated index offenses prior to alcohol use. In general, however, after alcohol use came marijuana use, then index offending, and finally polydrug use. Among subjects who initiated both marijuana use and index offending, index offending was more likely to precede marijuana use than vice versa. The researchers concluded that the onset of minor delinquency leads to the onset of drug use and not vice versa. Further, they stressed that while this sequence represents the dominant pattern, many adolescents do not adhere to it. More recent analyses of these data[25] indicate that for a substantial majority of adolescents, minor delinquency and alcohol use occurred simultaneously. In general, marijuana use followed next, and most adolescents who engaged in both index offending and multiple drug use engaged in index offending first. In terms of serious violent offending, the typical sequence was first aggravated assault, then robbery, and then rape.[25]

Although research indicates that conduct disorders and delinquency precede the initiation into drug and usually alcohol use, studies also show that increases in property crime and acquisitive violence occur subsequent to regular use of hard drugs among adolescents.[41] Elliott and colleagues[23] found that while delinquency is more likely to influence the onset of alcohol/drug use than the reverse, serious drug use (repeated polydrug use) is more likely to influence the maintenance of serious delinquency than the reverse. This result suggests the possibility that if alcohol/drug use does influence delinquency, it may be by reducing the probability of terminating rather than by increasing the probability of initiating delinquent behavior. Collins[40] also stated that while problem drinking may not be important for the onset of a criminal career, problem drinking may intensify or prolong serious involvement in criminal behavior in young adulthood. In sum, the longitudinal research indicates that initiation into aggressive behavior generally precedes alcohol/drug use; however, changes in drug and maybe alcohol use affect changes in aggression (see also ref. 42).

Longitudinal research has demonstrated that childhood antisocial behavior (usually defined as conduct disorders, delinquency, or aggressive behavior) is consistently related to the later development of alcohol problems in adolescence and adulthood.[43,44] However, Loeber's[41] review of the literature on antisocial behavior indicated that nonaggressive rather than aggressive antisocial behaviors are predictive of later substance use or abuse, while aggression is more strongly predictive of other forms of delinquency such as theft, burglary, and fraud. Similarly, White[45] found that alcohol and drug problems in late adolescence were predicted by nonaggressive delinquent behavior but not by aggressive behavior in early adolescence.

McCord[46] followed a cohort of 390 males over four decades and divided the sample into four groups based on aggression in childhood (high or low) and alcoholism at follow-up (present or absent). She found that both early aggressiveness and later alcoholism contribute to the probability of later antisocial behavior, but she was not able to ascertain the relationship between early alcohol use and aggressive behavior.

Using the HHDP data, White and colleagues[17,47] examined the longitudinal associations among alcohol use, aggression, and incidents of acute alcohol-related aggression from early adolescence into adulthood. They found that aggressive behavior was very stable for males from age 12 to age 24, while alcohol use was not very stable from age 12 to age 15 but became highly stable from age 15 on. Other longitudinal studies also attest to the stability of aggressive behavior over the life course (e.g., refs. 48,49). Farrington[50] found that boys who were aggressive in childhood or adolescence tended to be more violent in adulthood and to engage more often in violent and nonviolent offenses. In addition, as adults these boys were more likely to be heavier drinkers and smokers, drunk drivers, and drug takers. Farrington suggested that this continuity is probably not specific to aggression, but rather part of a general continuity in antisocial behavior from childhood to adulthood. On the other hand, several longitudinal studies in the alcohol field have shown that alcohol involvement or alcohol problems remain steady for some individuals, whereas they are constantly shifting or changing for others (e.g., refs. 44,51).

White and colleagues[17,47] found that early aggressive behavior predicted later alcohol use, but alcohol use was not related to subsequent increases in aggressive behavior. The findings also indicated that prior alcohol use was a better predictor of alcohol-related aggression for females, while prior aggression was a better predictor for males.

Cohen and colleagues[7] conducted a meta-analysis of the relationship between alcohol use and criminal violence over time from the few longitudinal studies that met their criteria. The meta-analysis indicated fairly weak associations across time. The average correlation between time 1 alcohol use and time 2 violence was .01 and between time 1 violence and time 2 alcohol use was .09. The fact that the latter was stronger than the former is consistent with the data presented above from the HHDP. Given the small number of studies, the researchers were unable to draw any conclusions about temporal sequencing. Overall, the results of the meta-analysis suggested that the evidence was insufficient to establish a causal relationship between alcohol use and violence.[7]

The studies reviewed above suggest that, in general, aggression occurs prior to alcohol use in the life course, and aggression is a better predictor of alcohol use than alcohol use is of aggression. In contrast, a study of juvenile offenders in Finland found that those juveniles who had arrests for drunkenness were more likely to have arrests for both violent and property crimes 5 to 10 years later.[52] Also, Dembo and colleagues[53] found that early alcohol use was an important predictor of later violent behavior among juvenile detainees.

While victimization is not the focus of this chapter, from a developmental perspective research on the consequences of childhood exposure to violence provides some interesting results. For example, studies indicate that alcoholic females have significantly higher rates of childhood sexual and physical abuse than nonalcoholic females.[54] (For greater detail on victimization and alcohol use, see refs. 54,55). It has also been demonstrated that exposure to violence in the family in childhood leads to greater participation in violence in adolescence. In one study, both maltreatment in childhood (i.e., physical abuse, sexual abuse, or neglect), as well as growing up in a home with violence (e.g., spouse abuse, family hostility, maltreatment of siblings), significantly increased the chances of an individual engaging in violent behavior in adolescence.[56] In addition, children who grew up in families with multiple forms of violence had twice the risk of engaging in violence in adolescence as compared to children who grew up in nonviolent families (for a review, see ref. 57). Similarly, studies have found that children who grew up in alcoholic homes were at a greater risk for exhibiting aggressive behavior in adolescence.[58]

The above studies suggest that parental violence and alcoholism can increase the risk for later violence and alcoholism. Therefore, a negative family background is indicated as one common cause of both aggression and heavy drinking. Other common causes are discussed in the next section.

5. A Common-Cause Model

The general consensus is that the relationship between alcohol use and aggression in adolescence is spurious.[16] As discussed above, developmentally, aggressive behavior generally precedes alcohol use initiation and early aggressive behavior predicts later alcohol use, but in most studies early alcohol use does not predict later aggression. Further, most acts of aggression by adolescents occur in the absence of alcohol use. Thus, alcohol use does not appear to cause aggressive behavior, but rather both are probably caused by a similar set of factors.

Evidence supporting a common-cause model has been derived from adolescent samples where relatively nonserious forms of substance use appeared to occur simultaneously with relatively minor and infrequent forms of delinquent behavior. This association led Jessor and Jessor[59] to identify a problem behavior syndrome in which cigarette use, precocious sexual behavior, problem drinking, use of marijuana and other drugs, stealing, and aggression clustered together. This cluster of behaviors was explained by the same set of environmental and personality variables and was negatively related to conventional behavior.

It appears, therefore, that alcohol use and aggressive behavior are related to each other during adolescence because of a tendency for adolescents, who share a similar set of risk factors, to experiment with a wide range of deviant behaviors. Nevertheless, not all adolescents who engage in one behavior engage in the others. Further, the risk factors may not have equal effects on each behavior. Hence, the generality versus specificity of deviance has been debated throughout the literature (e.g., refs. 45,60). According to one position, alcohol use and aggression serve similar functions and are, therefore, conceptualized as constituent behaviors of a more general problem behavior syndrome[59] or a general criminal propensity.[61] The alternative position views alcohol use and aggression as different and relatively independent manifestations of deviance.[36] Although the notion of common causes and common functions may apply to some individuals and help to account for the observed relationships among deviant behaviors, specific forms of deviance are equally likely to be shaped by causes and functions that are specific to each of the various problem behaviors. In other words, it may be reasonable to assume that the concept of a problem behavior syndrome applies only to a minority of adolescents. Some adolescents may be undifferentiated "generalists," others more differentiated "specialists" in deviance. That is, some adolescents may engage in a wide variety of deviant behavior including alcohol use and aggression (see ref. 61). At the same time, other groups of adolescents may drink heavily without engaging in aggressive behavior and vice versa (see refs. 36,62,63). In discussing this debate, Osgood[64] noted that a single set of explanatory factors might account for a large portion of the variance in each of a strongly related subset of problem behaviors. However, there are also important unique features of each behavior that require separate explanations.

White and Labouvie's[60] findings support the notion that the expression of deviance is not necessarily undifferentiated. Instead, their results indicated that a considerable number of individuals seem to specialize in particular problem behaviors. As compared to a group of generalists, both delinquent specialists and drug use specialists displayed a more differentiated pattern of coping reactions and all three groups differed in terms of psychological problems and personality traits. Subjects who were high in both drug use and delinquency (i.e., generalists) had significantly higher levels of mental health problems than all other subjects.

Most studies of young violent offenders indicate that they are generalists and only a small proportion of their annual offenses are violent offenses (e.g., refs. 25,33,34). In the NYS data, serious violent offenders constituted less than 5% of the entire sample, and yet they accounted for 83% of all the reported index offenses and more than 50% of all offenses.[25] In another analysis of these data, it was found that less than 5% of all youth reported serious crimes and used hard drugs. This small group accounted for approximately 40% of all delinquencies, 60% of all index offenses, over 50% of all felony assaults, over 60% of all felony thefts, 75% of all robberies, over 80% of all drug sales, 30% of all marijuana use occasions, and 60% of all other drug use occasions.[65]

The relationship between alcohol use and aggression in adolescence, which we have seen is relatively weak, is best explained by a common-cause model. Nevertheless, we cannot assume that both behaviors are caused by the exact same set of predictors, or that individuals who have certain risk factors will necessarily engage in both behaviors. In fact, having any specific risk factor or set of factors is not a guarantee that an individual will engage in either behavior. Rather, there are life experiences and opportunities as well as protective factors that can mediate the relationship between risk factors and problem outcomes (see ref. 66).

With these caveats in mind, an examination of the most often-cited predictors of violence and alcohol use reveals considerable overlap. For example, the National Research Council Report[6] identified numerous risk factors for violence, including hyperactivity, impulsivity, attention deficit disorder, restlessness, lack of concentration, risk taking, inability to delay gratification, low empathy and low IQ, abnormal frequency of viewing television violence, bullying in early years, harsh and erratic discipline, abuse or rejection in family, lack of parental nurturance, low income, large family, familial criminal behavior, early school failure, peer rejection, poor housing, and growing up in a high-crime neighborhood. Interestingly, almost every one of these risk factors (except, perhaps, violence on television, low income, low IQ, and poor housing) have also been identified in the literature as risk factors for teenage alcohol/drug use or for adult alcohol and drug problems.[66,67] (For other reviews of risk factors, see refs. 68–71.)

In addition to common risk factors, the same theories have been applied successfully to explain delinquency/violence and alcohol/drug use. The most often-tested theories are control theory,[72] differential association theory,[73] and integrations of the two (e.g., ref. 74). However, a social learning model that takes into account both person and environmental factors may provide the most comprehensive explanation for the specific relationship between alcohol use and aggression. Such a model has been applied to each behavior separately.[48,75–77] According to Bandura's[78] social learning model, human behavior is explained in terms of a continuous reciprocal interaction between the person, the environment, and behavior. The person brings to the environment a unique endowment (including genetic makeup, temperament, personality, expectancies) that imposes certain limits on what and how things are learned and influences the person's selection of various environments. Observational learning (i.e., modeling) and reinforcement (i.e., reward and punishment) are the two primary social learning processes by which influences from the environment are transmitted. Individuals in the proximal (e.g., family and peers) and distal (e.g., social milieu, media) environments model and reinforce behavior either directly or vicariously, and thus teach individuals the appropriate manner in which to behave.[76] Based on a social learning model, one would hypothesize that alcohol use and aggression will be related in certain individuals who have expectancies that alcohol use causes aggression, have genetic or temperamental traits that foster aggressive behavior (e.g., impulsivity, hyperactivity, etc.), and have been exposed to significant others who separately or simultaneously model and reinforce aggressive behavior and heavy drinking.[17] Thus, research on risk factors will need to address the interactions among individual and environmental variables.

In sum, this review of the literature suggests that the relationship between alcohol use and aggression among youth is spurious, and both aggressive behavior and heavy drinking may be caused by a third factor or set of factors. Individual, family, peer, and environmental factors account for a clustering of risk factors for both behaviors. This common-cause model has certain implications for prevention strategies, and in the following section these strategies are discussed.

6. Preventing Alcohol Abuse and Aggression

Because the risk factors for violence overlap with those for substance abuse, several of the prevention programs in each area have similar goals and approaches. Youth prevention programs for both alcohol abuse (for reviews, see refs. 79–81) and violence (for reviews, see refs. 6,68,70,71) target the individual, the family, peers, and/or the community. Hawkins and colleagues[71] have argued that efforts to prevent violence and substance abuse should be combined because of the overlap of risk factors.

The general consensus is that prevention approaches need to be developmental because risk factors differ over the life course.[69] For example, in the infant and preschool period, programs appear most effective that address parenting skills and needs, as well as healthy physical and cognitive development of the child.[71] As children become school-age, in addition to parent programs, selected school programs have also had positive results (e.g., reducing kindergarten and first-grade class sizes, improving instructional strategies, and monitoring behavior) (for a complete list, see ref. 70). Overall, most of the reviews agree that early prevention is needed, that working with parents or soon-to-be parents is advantageous, that programs should be aimed at multiple risk factors, and that continuity of programs from birth into adolescence is important.[69-71] Although less evaluated, some societal-level approaches seem worthwhile, including reducing exposure to violence in the media, reducing access to lethal firearms, and changing norms regarding alcohol use.[68,79] On the other hand, reviews consistently have found that most peer programs (e.g., resistance skills, peer mediation, guided group interaction, recruiting out of gangs) are ineffective for both violence[68,70] and substance abuse.[80]

The current trend in prevention is toward encouraging community-wide approaches,[71] although evaluations of community interventions for alcohol abuse have not demonstrated positive results.[81] Several prevention specialists stress the need to increase protective factors (e.g., resilience and a positive social orientation, social bonding to prosocial individuals and institutions, and healthy beliefs and standards for behavior) in addition to decreasing risk factors.[70,71]

Many of the current prevention programs have not been properly evaluated, and when they have been, data have been weak.[68] Thus, more sophisticated evaluation designs need to be implemented (see ref. 68 for suggestions). However, the existing data from well-evaluated programs show that some of these programs can be effective. That is, early childhood prevention has had a positive impact on reducing the risk factors for later violence and substance abuse.[69]

7. Conclusions

The empirical evidence suggests that aggressive behavior is highly stable during adolescence[17,47] and into adulthood[48,49] and that many adult violent offenders were aggressive as youth.[24] Thus, an aggressive behavior pattern is formed at an early age and sets the stage for later violence as well as later alcohol use and alcohol-related aggression.[17] Further, it has been demonstrated that intoxication facilitates aggression most in those individuals already inclined to aggression.[1] Thus, early intervention with aggressive children (especially males) would help prevent later violence as well as later alcohol problems and alcohol-related aggression.

It should be kept in mind, however, that many adolescents mature out of aggressive behavior and heavy drinking as they reach young adulthood. Therefore, efforts should be made to identify those individuals who will persist in deviant behaviors. Research identifying these individuals is currently underway and suggests that persistence may be related to early onset as well as cognitive dysfunctions, impulsivity, and undercontrol.[82]

Obviously, the group of adolescents high in both alcohol use and aggressive behavior clearly stands out as in need of attention. White and Labouvie[60] found that cumulative involvement in a range of problem behaviors during adolescence was coupled with the highest levels of distress and negative affect as well as the highest levels of impulsivity, undercontrol, and emotional instability. Thus, it is reasonable to expect that generalists (i.e., those adolescents who engage in a wide range of problem behaviors) will be least likely to make successful transitions into adulthood and most likely to develop full-blown substance abuse and/or psychopathology in adulthood. For these reasons, adolescent generalists in deviance would seem to constitute an important target for intervention programs. Such programs would require strategies that address a multitude of problem behaviors and a multitude of underlying psychological problems as well as other risk factors. At the same time, heavy drinkers or aggressive behavior specialists may benefit more from specific interventions designed to address their individual problems.

ACKNOWLEDGMENTS. Preparation of this chapter was supported, in part, by grants from the National Institute on Drug Abuse (#DA/AA-03395) and the Alcoholic Beverage Medical Research Foundation. The author thanks Patricio Calderon for his assistance with preparation of the manuscript and Drs. Carl Danziger and Allan Horwitz for their comments on an earlier draft of this manuscript.

References

1. White HR: Alcohol, illicit drugs, and violence, in Stoff D, Brieling J, Maser JD (eds): *Handbook of Antisocial Behavior*. New York, John Wiley & Sons, in press.
2. Bushman BJ, Cooper HM: Effects of alcohol on human aggression: An integrative research review. *Psychol Bull* 107:341–354, 1990.
3. Collins JJ: Drinking and violence: An individual offender focus, in Martin SE (ed): *Alcohol and Interpersonal Violence: Fostering Multidisciplinary Perspectives*. Rockville, MD, National Institute of Health, NIAAA Research Monograph No. 24, 1993, pp 221–235.
4. Roizen J: Issues in the epidemiology of alcohol and violence, in Martin SE (ed): *Alcohol and Interpersonal Violence: Fostering Multidisciplinary Perspectives*. Rockville, MD, National Institute of Health, NIAAA Research Monograph No. 24, 1993, pp 3–36.
5. Fagan J: Intoxication and aggression, in Tonry M, Wilson JQ (eds): *Drugs and Crime*. Chicago, University of Chicago Press, 1990, vol 13, pp 241–320.
6. Reiss AJ, Roth JA (eds): *Understanding and Preventing Violence*. Washington DC, National Academy Press, 1993.

7. Cohen MA, Lipsey MW, Wilson DB, *et al:* The role of alcohol consumption in violent behavior: Preliminary findings. Nashville, TN, Vanderbilt University, 1994.

8. Fagan J: Interactions among drugs, alcohol, and violence. *Health Affairs* 12:65–79, 1993.

9. Collins JJ (ed): *Drinking and Crime.* New York, Guilford, 1981.

10. Pihl R, Peterson J: Alcohol and aggression: Three potential mechanisms of the drug effect, in Martin SE (ed): *Alcohol and Interpersonal Violence: Fostering Multidisciplinary Perspectives.* Rockville, MD, National Institute of Health, NIAAA Research Monograph No. 24, 1993, pp 149–159.

11. Fagan J: Set and setting revisited: Influences of alcohol and illicit drugs on the social context of violent events, in Martin SE (ed): *Alcohol and Interpersonal Violence: Fostering Multidisciplinary Perspectives.* Rockville, MD, National Institute of Health, NIAAA Research Monograph No. 24, 1993, pp 161–191.

12. Virkkunen M, Linnoila M: Brain serotonin, type II alcoholism and impulsive violence. *J Stud Alcohol* (Suppl 11): 163–169, 1993.

13. Collins JJ, Messerschmidt PM: Epidemiology of alcohol-related violence. *Alcohol Health Res World* 17:93–100, 1993.

14. Khantzian EJ: The self-medication hypothesis of addictive disorders: Focus on heroin and cocaine dependence. *Am J Psychiatry* 142:1259–1264, 1985.

15. Lindman RE, Lang AR: The alcohol–aggression stereotype: A cross-cultural comparison of beliefs. *Int J Addict* 29:1–13, 1994.

16. White HR: The drug use-delinquency connection in adolescence, in Weisheit R (ed): *Drugs, Crime and the Criminal Justice System.* Cincinnati, OH, Anderson Publishing, 1990, pp 215–256.

17. White HR, Brick J, Hansell S: A longitudinal investigation of alcohol use and aggression in adolescence. *J Stud Alcohol* (Suppl 11): 62–77, 1993.

18. Roncek DW, Maier PA: Bars, blocks and crimes revisited: Linking the theory of routine activities to the empiricism of "hot spots." *Criminology* 29:725–753, 1989.

19. Pernanen K: Theoretical aspects of the relationship between alcohol use and crime, in Collins JJ (ed): *Drinking and Crime.* New York, Guilford Press, 1981, pp 1–69.

20. White HR, Hansell S, Brick J: Alcohol use and aggression among youth. *Alcohol Health Res World* 17:144–150, 1993.

21. White HR, Huselid RF: Gender differences in alcohol use during adolescence, in Wilsnack R, Wilsnack S (eds): *Gender and Alcohol.* New Brunswick, NJ, Rutgers Centers of Alcohol Studies, 1977, 176–198.

22. Johnston LD, O'Malley PM, Bachman JG: *National Survey Results on Drug Use from the Monitoring the Future Study, 1975–1993.* Rockville, MD, National Institute on Drug Abuse, 1994.

23. Elliott DS, Huizinga D, Menard S: *Multiple Problem Youth: Delinquency Substance Use and Mental Health Problems.* New York, Springer-Verlag, 1989.

24. Elliott DS: *Youth Violence: An Overview.* Boulder, CO, The Center for the Study and Prevention of Violence, 1994.

25. Elliott DS: Serious violent offenders: Onset, developmental course, and termination—the American Society of Criminology 1993 Presidential Address. *Criminology* 32:1–21, 1994.

26. Allen-Hagen B, Sickmund M, Snyder HN: *Juveniles and Violence: Juvenile Offending and Victimization.* Washington, DC, Office of Juvenile Justice and Delinquency Prevention, US Department of Justice, 1994.

27. Snyder HN, Sickmund M: *Juvenile Offenders and Victims: A Focus on Violence* (Statistics summary). Washington, DC, Office of Juvenile Justice and Delinquency Prevention, US Department of Justice, 1995.

28. Valois RF, Vincent ML, McKeown RE, *et al:* Adolescent risk behaviors and the potential for violence: A look at what's coming to campus. *J Am College Health* 41:141–147, 1993.

29. Osgood DW: Drugs, alcohol, and adolescent violence. Presented at the American Society of Criminology annual meeting, Miami, FL, 1994.

30. Mitic WR: Adolescent drinking problems: Urban vs. rural differences in Nova Scotia. *Cand J Commun Mental Health* 8:5–14, 1989.

31. Bureau of Justice Statistics: *Fact Sheet: Drug-Related Crime.* Washington DC, US Department of Justice, 1994.
32. Carpenter C, Glassner B, Johnson BD, *et al: Kids, Drugs, and Crime.* Lexington, MA, Lexington Books, 1988.
33. Altschuler DM, Brounstein PJ: Pattern of drug use, drug trafficking, and other delinquency among inner-city adolescent males in Washington, DC. *Criminology* 29:589–622, 1991.
34. Hartstone E, Hansen KV: The violent juvenile offender: An empirical portrait, in Mathias RA, DeMuro P, Allison RS (eds): *Violent Juvenile Offenders: An Anthology.* San Francisco, CA, National Council on Crime and Delinquency, 1984, pp 83–112.
35. Tinklenberg JR, Murphy P, Murphy PL, *et al:* Drugs and criminal assaults by adolescents: A replication study. *J Psychoactive Drugs* 13:277–287, 1981.
36. Fagan J, Weis J, Cheng YT, *et al:* Drug and alcohol use, violent delinquency, and social bonding: Implications for theory and intervention. Washington, DC, National Institute of Justice Drug and Crime Research Program, 1987.
37. Fagan J, Weis JG, Cheng Y-T: Delinquency and substance use among inner city students. New York, New York City Criminal Justice Agency, 1988.
38. Kingery PM, Pruitt BE, Hurley RS: Violence and illegal drug use among adolescents: Evidence from the US National Adolescent Student Health Survey. *Int J Addict* 27:1445–1464, 1992.
39. Watts WD, Wright LS: The relationship of alcohol, tobacco, marijuana, and other illegal drug use to delinquency among Mexican-American, black, and white adolescent males. *Adolescence* 25:171–181, 1990.
40. Collins JJ: The relationship of problem drinking to individual offending sequences, in Blumstein A, Cohen J, Roth J, *et al* (eds): *Criminal Careers and "Career Criminals."* Washington DC, National Academic Press, 1986, vol 2, pp 89–120.
41. Loeber R: Natural histories of conduct problems, delinquency, and associated substance use, in Lahey BB, Kazdin AE (eds): *Advances in Clinical Child Psychology,* New York, Plenum, 1988, vol 11, pp 73–124.
42. Chaiken J, Chaiken M: Drugs and predatory crime, in Tonry M, Wilson JQ (eds): *Drugs and Crime.* Chicago, The University of Chicago Press, 1990, vol 13, pp 203–239.
43. Robins LN: The adult development of the antisocial child. *Semin Psychiatry* 2:420–434, 1970.
44. Zucker RA: The concept of risk and the etiology of alcoholism: A probablistic–developmental perspective, in Pittman DJ, White HR (eds): *Society, Culture and Drinking Patterns Reexamined.* New Brunswick, NJ, Rutgers Center of Alcohol Studies, 1991, pp 513–532.
45. White HR: Early problem behavior and later drug problems. *J Res Crime Delinq* 29:412–429, 1992.
46. McCord JF: Alcohol in the service of aggression, in Gottheil E, Druley KA, Skoloda TE, *et al* (eds): *Alcohol, Drug Abuse and Aggression.* Springfield, IL, Charles C. Thomas, 1983, pp 270–279.
47. White HR, Hansell S: The moderating effects of gender and hostility on the alcohol-aggression relationship. *J Res Crime Delinq* 33:451–472, 1996.
48. Huesmann LR, Eron LD, Lefkowitz MM, *et al:* Stability of aggression over time and generations. *Dev Psychol* 20:1120–1134, 1984.
49. Olweus D: The stability of aggressive reaction patterns in human males: A review. *Psychol Bull* 85:852–875, 1979.
50. Farrington DP: The development of offending and antisocial behavior from childhood: Key findings from the Cambridge study in delinquent development. *J Child Psychol Psychiatry* 36:1–36, 1995.
51. Fillmore KM: Drinking and problem drinking in early adulthood and middle age: An exploratory 20-year follow-up study. *Q J Stud Alcohol* 35:819–840, 1974.
52. Virkkunen M: Arrests for drunkenness and recidivism in juvenile delinquents. *Br J Addict* 72:201–204, 1977.
53. Dembo R, Williams L, Getreu A, *et al:* A longitudinal study of the relationships among

marijuana/hashish use, cocaine use, and delinquency in a cohort of high risk youths. *J Drug Issues* 21:271–312, 1991.

54. Miller BA: Investigating links between childhood victimization and alcohol problems, in Martin SE (ed): *Alcohol and Interpersonal Violence: Fostering Multidisciplinary Perspectives*. Rockville, MD, National Institute of Health, 1993, NIAAA Research Monograph No. 24, pp 3–36.

55. Widom CS: Child abuse and alcohol use and abuse, in Martin SE (ed): *Alcohol and Interpersonal Violence: Fostering Multidisciplinary Perspectives*. Rockville, MD, National Institute of Health, 1993, NIAAA Research Monograph No. 24, pp 291–314.

56. Thornberry TP: Violent families and youth violence. Office of Juvenile Justice and Delinquency Prevention, US Department of Justice, December, 1994.

57. Widom CS: The cycle of violence. *Science* 244:160–166, 1989.

58. Johnson JL, Perez-Bouchard L, Rebeta JL: Parental reports of behavior problems and stress in sons of alcoholics. *Alcohol Clin Exp Res* 18:472, 1994.

59. Jessor R, Jessor S: *Problem Behavior and Psychosocial Development—A Longitudinal Study of Youth*. New York, Academic Press, 1977.

60. White HR, Labouvie EW: Generality versus specificity of problem behavior: Psychological and functional differences. *J Drug Issues* 24:55–74, 1994.

61. Gottfredson MR, Hirschi T: *A General Theory of Crime*. Standford, CA Standford University Press, 1990.

62. White HR, Pandina RJ, LaGrange RL: Longitudinal predictors of serious substance use and delinquency. *Criminology* 25:715–740, 1987.

63. White HR: Marijuana use and delinquency: A test of the "independent cause" hypothesis. *J Drug Issues* 21:231–256, 1991.

64. Osgood DW: Covariation among adolescent problem behaviors. Presented at American Society of Criminology annual meeting, Baltimore, MD, 1990.

65. Johnson BD, Wish E, Schmeidler J, et al: The concentration of delinquent offending; Serious drug involvement and high delinquency rates, in Johnson BD, Wish E (eds): *Crime Rates among Drug Abusing Offenders*. New York, Interdisciplinary Research Center, Narcotic and Drug Research, 1986, pp 106–143.

66. Hawkins JD, Catalano RF, Miller JY: Risk and protective factors for alcohol and other drug problems in adolescence and early adulthood: Implications for substance abuse prevention. *Psychol Bull* 112:64–105, 1992.

67. Kandel D: Drug and drinking behavior among youth, in Inkeles A, Smelser NJ, Turner RH (eds): *Annual Review of Sociology*. Palo Alto, CA, Annual Reviews, 1980, vol 6, pp 235–285.

68. Tolan P, Guerra N: *What Works in Reducing Adolescent Violence: An Empirical Review of the Field*. Boulder, CO, Center for the Study and Prevention of Violence, 1994.

69. Tremblay RE, Craig WM: Developmental crime prevention, in Tonry M, Farrington DP (eds): *Building a Safer Society: Strategic Approaches to Crime Prevention*. Chicago, The University of Chicago Press, 1995, vol 19, pp 151–236.

70. Brewer DD, Hawkins JD, Catalano RF, et al: Preventing serious, violent and chronic juvenile offending: A review of evaluations of selected strategies in childhood, adolescence and the community, in Howell JC, Krisberg B, Hawkins JD, et al (eds): *Sourcebook on Serious, Violent, and Chronic Juvenile Offenders*. Thousand Oaks, CA, Sage, in press, 1995, pp 61–141.

71. Hawkins JD, Catalano RF, Brewer DD: Preventing serious, violent and chronic delinquency and crime: Effective strategies from conception to age six, in Howell JC, Krisberg B, Hawkins JD, et al (eds): *Sourcebook on Serious, Violent, and Chronic Juvenile Offenders*. Thousand Oaks, CA, Sage, 1995, pp 47–60.

72. Hirschi T: *Causes of Delinquency*. Berkeley, University of California Press, 1969.

73. Sutherland EH, Cressey DR: *Criminology*. Philadelphia, Lippincott, 1978.

74. Elliott DS, Huizinga DH, Ageton SS: *Explaining Delinquency and Drug Use*. Beverly Hills, CA, Sage, 1985.

75. Bandura A: *Aggression: A Social Learning Analysis*. Englewood Cliffs, NJ, Prentice-Hall, 1973.

76. White HR, Bates ME, Johnson V: Social reinforcement and alcohol consumption, in Cox WM

(ed): *Why People Drink: Parameters of Alcohol as a Reinforcer*. New York, Gardner Press, 1990, pp 233–261.

77. Abrams DB, Niaura RS: Social learning theory, in Blane HT, Leonard KE (eds): *Psychological Theories of Drinking and Alcoholism*. New York, Guilford Press, 1987, pp 131–178.
78. Bandura A: *Social Learning Theory*. Englewood Cliffs, NJ, Prentice-Hall, 1977.
79. Hawkins JD, Arthur MW, Catalano RF: preventing substance abuse, in Tonry M, Farrington DP (eds): *Building a Safer Society: Strategic Approaches to Crime Prevention*. Chicago, The University of Chicago Press, 1995, vol 19, pp 343–427.
80. Gorman DM: Do school-based social skills training programs prevent alcohol use among young people? *Addict Res*, 4:191–210, 1996.
81. Gorman DM, Speer PW: Preventing alcohol abuse and alcohol-related problems through community interventions: A review of evaluation studies. *Psychol Health* 11:95–131, 1995.
82. Moffitt TE: Adolescence-limited and life-course-persistent antisocial behavior: A developmental taxonomy. *Psychol Rev* 100:674–701, 1993.

Alcohol and Violence-Related Injuries in the Emergency Room

Cheryl J. Cherpitel

Abstract. This chapter reviews data on estimated blood alcohol concentration (BAC), self-reported consumption, and drinking patterns and problems from emergency room (ER) studies of alcohol and violence-related injury. These studies used probability samples of all injured patients that were representative of the population served by the ER where the data were collected. Those with violence-related injuries were more likely to be admitted to the ER with a positive BAC, to report drinking prior to the event, and to report more frequent heavy drinking and alcohol-related problems than those admitted to the same ER during the same time period with injuries from other causes. Limitations to these ER studies, including representativeness of samples, alcohol's presence and role in violence perpetration compared to violence victimization, the presence of other psychoactive substances, and the actual risk at which alcohol places the individual for injuries resulting from violence are discussed.

1. Introduction

Alcohol consumption has been found to be associated with both fatal and nonfatal injuries resulting from violence.[1–3] Data documenting alcohol's presence in nonfatal injuries have come primarily from studies of patients admitted to hospital emergency rooms (ERs) for treatment. Emergency rooms are the primary source of treatment for all types of injuries including those related to violence. Injuries resulting from violence that are serious enough to require emergency room treatment are thought to account for over 20 times as many cases as violence-related (nonsuicide) fatal injuries.[4] While studies in ERs provide more information on victims of violence than on perpetrators

Cheryl J. Cherpitel • Alcohol Research Group, Western Consortium for Public Health, Berkeley, California 94709

Recent Developments in Alcoholism, Volume 13: Alcoholism and Violence, edited by Marc Galanter. Plenum Press, New York, 1997

(unless the perpetrator also sustains injuries requiring treatment), these studies can provide data on the estimated prevalence of alcohol's presence in events involving violence, drinking characteristics of those involved, and other information on alcohol's role in such events. This chapter will review findings from ER studies of violence-related injuries in relation to prevalence estimates of alcohol's involvement in such injuries, as well as alcohol's role in the event and drinking patterns and problems of those with injuries resulting from violence. The present work updates and expands upon an earlier review article on the same topic.[5]

Alcohol is thought to be positively associated with severity of injury, including injuries resulting from violence,[6] although findings have been found to vary considerably across studies. One study found 29% of those with severe injuries related to violence reported drinking more than 10 drinks in the 12 hr prior to the event, compared to 18% of those with minor injuries.[7] Additionally, 30% of those with multiple injuries reported drinking at this level compared to 19% of those with single injuries. These authors suggest that loss of judgment induced by alcohol may prolong the violent event or the victim may be less able to avoid the encounter, both of which would result in more serious injury. To further explore alcohol's association with severity of violence-related injury, data will be compared on alcohol's presence from representative samples of fatal and nonfatal injuries resulting from violence, both occurring in the same county during the same time from two regions of the United States where per capita consumption of alcohol differ greatly—the South and the West. These data will provide information on alcohol's involvement in violence-related events resulting in injury in relation to severity of injury and typical drinking patterns that may influence the occurrence of such events.

2. Prevalence Estimates of Blood Alcohol Concentration

Emergency room studies that are the most informative regarding alcohol's presence in violence-related injuries are those which have obtained a measure of estimated blood alcohol level (BAC) from blood, breath, saliva, or urine soon after arrival in the ER. A number of these studies have included representative samples of patients both with and without injuries related to violence admitted to the ER during the same period of time (see Table I).

Among those studies in Table I that meet these criteria, the proportion of patients with violence-related injuries who had positive BACs ranged from 17% (in a health maintenance organization) to 70% (in a rural district general hospital in Scotland). While a large amount of variation exists, both in the prevalence of positive BACs and in the proportion of those legally intoxicated (BACs of 0.08 or higher), across all of these studies, those with violence-related injuries were from two to five times more likely to be positive for alcohol (and to be intoxicated) at the time of the ER visit than those with other injuries. This also has been found to be true when age and gender are con-

Table I. ER Studies Measuring BAC[a] Among Probability Samples of Patients

Study (year, location)	Age	Alcohol measure	Violent injuries: % pos BAC (N)	Nonviolent injuries: % pos BAC (N)
1. Wechsler et al (1967)[8] (US—MA)	≥16	Breath	56 (188) 39 ≥ .05	22[f] (2701) 11[f] ≥ .05
2. Peppiatt et al. (1976/77)[9] (UK)	≥15	Blood	45 (29)	10[f] (671)
3. Walsh & Macleod (1980)[10] (Scotland)	≥15	Breath	70 (56) 50 ≥ .08	14[f] (698) 8[f] ≥ .08
4. Papoz et al (1982/83)[11] (France)	≥15	Blood within 6 hr	64 (544) 50 ≥ .08	32[f] (4245) 18[f]
5. Yates et al [12] (UK)	≥16	Blood or breath	60 (59) 9 ≥ .08	14[f] (946) 3
6. Cherpitel (1984/85)[13] (US—CA)	≥18	Breath within 6 hr	44 (57) 30 ≥ .10	16[f] (148) 11[f] ≥ .10
7. Cherpitel (1985)[b] (US—CA)	≥18	Breath within 6 hr	26 (102) 12 ≥ .10	9[f] (764) 3 ≥ .10
8. Cherpitel (1986)[c] (Mexico)	≥18	Breath within 6 hr	38 (438) 21 ≥ .10	15[f] (1113) 8[f] ≥ .10
9. Cherpitel (1986/87)[16] (US—CA)	≥18	Breath within 6 hr	25 (142) 14 ≥ .10	14[f] (591) 6[f]
10. Cherpitel (1987/88)[d] (Spain)	≥18	Breath within 6 hr	25 (81) 16 ≥ .10	10[f] (1520) 4[f] ≥ .10
11. Cherpitel (1989)[e] (US—CA)	≥18	Breath within 6 hr	17 (12) 0 ≥ .10	7 (355) 2 ≥ .10
12. Cherpitel (1992)[19] (US—MS)	≥18	Breath within 6 hr	35 (54) 11 ≥ .10	7[f] (210) 5

[a]BAC is recorded as mg %: Positive is ≥0.01 (10 mg. of alcohol per 100 ml of blood). .05, .08, .10 are BACs as indicated.
[b]Reanalysis of data from ref. 14.
[c]Reanalysis of data from ref. 15.
[d]Reanalysis of data from ref. 17.
[e]Reanalysis of data from ref. 18.
[f]$P < 0.05$ Comparison of positive breathalyzer readings between injured and noninjured in the same sample using tests of significant difference between proportions.

trolled. One study that compared violence-related injuries with all other injuries, separately for males and females under 30 and those 30 and older, found those with injuries resulting from violence were significantly more likely to be heavy problem drinkers than those with other injuries in each of the gender–age groups.[20] A study of representative samples of ER patients in Acapulco, Mexico found those with positive breathalyzer readings less than 0.10 were almost 13 times more likely than those with negative readings to have injuries related to violence as opposed to injuries resulting from animal bites or workplace or recreational accidents, when age, gender, other demographic characteristics, and time of occurrence (weekday vs. weekend) were controlled.[21] Surprisingly, those with breathalyzer readings over 0.10, however, were no more likely to have sustained injuries resulting from violence.

Other ER studies of nonrepresentative samples of patients among whom one might expect a larger proportion to be alcohol positive, e.g., those admitted to the ER on weekend evenings[22] or those so seriously injured as to require blood typing,[23] have generally found higher rates of alcohol's presence among both those with and without violence-related injuries (86 vs. 46% and 71 vs. 33%, respectively) than studies of representative samples of patients.

These data suggest that while a substantial association appears to exist between alcohol consumption and violence-related injuries treated in the ER, the estimated prevalence of positive BACs at the time of arrival in the ER varies considerably, even among representative samples of patients. Measures of both blood and breath were used to obtain BAC estimates; however, this would not be expected to affect prevalence rates reported, since breath analysis for alcohol has been found to be highly correlated with chemical analysis of blood among cooperative patients ($r = .96$).[24] As seen in Table I, however, the age criteria for inclusion in samples of patients varied across studies, from 15 and older to 18 and older, which may have influenced reported prevalence estimates. The length of data collection in each site, which varied from 1 week in each of eight ERs in Mexico City (Study 8)[25] to 1 year in one ER in California (Study 9),[16] may also have influenced prevalence rates, since a shorter length of data collection would have a higher probability of being less representative of all patients attending the ER than a longer period of data collection. The degree of ascertainment for obtaining BAC estimates may also affect prevalence rates, particularly if patient refusal or severity of injury are related to drinking in the event (for both those with violence-related injuries and those with other injuries). While data were not available on injury severity in these studies, completion rates for obtaining an estimated BAC ranged from 99% (Study 3)[10] to 72% (Study 9)[16] (no ascertainment rate was reported for Study 4). One ER study found that among those injured who were not interviewed because of refusal, severity of injury, or for other reasons, but on whom a BAC estimate was obtained, a larger proportion tested positive than those who did participate in the study.[26]

Another factor that could influence the proportion of positive BACs found is the time that elapsed between the injury and admission to the ER, as well as the time that elapsed between admission to the ER and when the BAC estimate was obtained. Although a BAC estimate was obtained within 6 hr of ER admission for many of the studies listed in Table I, the length of time between the event that resulted in injury and arrival in the ER is not known. Blood alcohol concentration has been found to be negatively correlated with the length of time between injury and arrival in the ER among all of those seeking treatment for injuries, with those arriving at the ER within 3 hr of injury over twice as likely to be alcohol positive as those arriving more than 6 hr after the event, when drinking after the event was controlled.[8] Another study, however, found no association between the likelihood of being alcohol positive and the time elapsed between injury and arrival in the ER when drinking after the event was controlled.[13]

The prevalence of alcohol-positive cases in an ER (across all types of injury) has also been found to vary by the type of ER facility and the associated sociodemographic characteristics of the clientele served by the facility.[27] For example, in Table I, the US studies in which the largest proportion of alcohol-positive violence-related injuries was found were those carried out in large urban level 1 trauma centers, where considerable proportions of those attending the ER were indigent and heavier drinkers (Studies 1, 2, and 6). On the other hand, the smallest proportion of alcohol-positive violence-related injuries was found among those attending suburban county and community hospital ERs (Studies 7 and 9) and a health maintenance organization (HMO) emergency room (Study 11).

3. Self-Reports of Alcohol Consumption Prior to Injury

The last seven studies in Table I also obtained data on self-reported drinking within 6 hr prior to the injury event (see Table II). In each of the studies in Table II except one, the proportion of those with violence-related injuries was significantly more likely to report drinking prior to the event than those with other injuries. In the one study that did not find a significant difference (perhaps due to the small number of patients with violence-related injuries) those with injuries resulting from violence were still three to four times more likely to report drinking prior to the event than those with other injuries. Additional analyses of data from a combined California sample of patients from Studies 2 and 4 in Table II found that among those with violence-related injuries who reported drinking within the 6 hr prior to injury, 35% reported consuming more than six drinks during this time (compared to 23% of those with other injuries), and well over half (67%) reported less than an hour

Table II. Self-Reported Consumption Prior to Injury

Year of study	Violent injuries: % positive BAC (N)	Nonviolent injuries: % positive BAC (N)
1. 1984/85[13]	55 (158)	27[e] (397)
2. 1985[a]	52 (116)	14[e] (826)
3. 1986[b]	52 (448)	18[e] (1136)
4. 1986/87[16]	49 (160)	22[e] (622)
5. 1987/88[c]	36 (87)	0[e] (1327)
6. 1989[d]	27 (15)	8 (361)
7. 1992[19]	56 (57)	14[e] (214)

[a]Reanalysis of data from ref. 14.
[b]Reanalysis of data from ref. 15.
[c]Reanalysis of data from ref. 17.
[d]Reanalysis of data from ref. 18.
[e]$P < 0.05$ Comparison of positive breathalyzer readings between injured and non-injured in the same sample using tests of significant difference between proportions.

Table III. Drinking Patterns and Problems among Drinkers (in percent)

	San Francisco, CA[a]		Contra Costa County, CA[19]		Jackson, MS[19]	
	Violence (141)	No violence (337)	Violence (84)	No violence (1007)	Violence 48)	No violence (139)
Heavy drinkers	41	25[b]	22	15	17	12
Drunk > 1 time per month	37	24[b]	20	13	27	9[b]
2 or more consequences	34	18[b]	11	7	8	3
3 or more dependence experiences	35	21[b]	13	6	17	9

[a]Reanalysis of data from ref. 14.
[b]$P < 0.05$ Comparison of positive breathalyzer readings between injured and noninjured in the same sample using tests of significant difference between proportions.

lapsed between their last drink and the event.[20] Of those who reported drinking, 45% reported feeling drunk at the time of injury, and almost half of these (46%) believed the event would not have happened if they had not been drinking. Similar analyses of data from Mississippi (Table I, Study 12) found 32% of those with violence-related injuries who reported drinking during the 6 hr prior to the event consumed more than six drinks during this time (compared to 11% of those with other injuries), and three fourths reported less than an hour between the last drink and the event.[19] A third of those with violence-related injuries who had been drinking reported feeling drunk, and of these, 60% believed the event would not have happened had they not been drinking.

    Also of interest in Table II is the fact that a larger proportion of both those with and those without violence-related injuries reported drinking within 6 hr prior to the event than were positive for estimated blood alcohol at the time of ER arrival (see Table I). Several of these same studies have compared the concordance of positive estimates for blood alcohol and self-reported consumption prior to the event for those who arrived at the ER within 6 hr of injury. While relatively small proportions of those who deny drinking prior to injury register positive for estimated blood alcohol, ranging from 0.5%[28] to 3.6%[13] in US studies across all causes of injury, substantial proportions of those who report drinking prior to the event have been found to register negative for estimated blood alcohol. A comparison of violence-related injuries among those from whom a BAC estimate was obtained within 6 hr of injury and who reported no drinking following the event in comparable studies carried out in United States, Mexico, and Spain found that while no patients who denied drinking were positive for estimated BAC in the US sample, 4% in Mexico and 12% in Spain denied drinking while registering positive.[28] However, 42% of those in the United States, 13% in Mexico, and 27% in Spain reported drinking prior to the event involving violence while registering negative for estimated BAC. The validity of self-reports has been found to be high even when BAC estimates have been obtained after self-reported consumption was obtained.[29] While self-reports of alcohol use have generally been found to be reasonably valid when compared to objective measures, some variation in accuracy has been found, leading to both under-reporting and overreporting.[30–32] The social desirability of responses has been found to affect validity of self-report drinking[33]; thus, differences in self-reported consumption between those with and those without injuries resulting from violence may be conservative. Interestingly, in the Spain sample (mentioned above), those with violence-related injuries were more likely than those with injuries from falls or vehicular or other accidents to deny drinking while having a positive BAC, while in the Mexico and US samples, those with violence-related injuries were no more likely to deny drinking than those with injuries from other causes.

4. Drinking Patterns and Alcohol-Related Problems

Findings from ER studies have also suggested that those with injuries related to violence are more likely to be frequent heavy drinkers with more alcohol-related problems compared to those with other injuries as well as to those in the general population from which these patients come.[12,20,34,35] One study that compared representative samples of patients seen in the same emergency rooms during the same period of time found those with violence-related injuries twice as likely (30 vs. 15%) to report frequent heavy drinking (drinking at least once a week and reporting five or more drinks at a sitting at least weekly).[20] These patients were also found to report more frequent drunkenness, social consequences of drinking, alcohol-dependence experi-

Table IV. BAC[a] in Fatal Compared to Nonfatal
Violence-Related Injuries

| BAC | Contra Costa County | | Hinds County | |
	ER (47)	Coroner (38)	ER (46)	Coroner (37)
Positive	19	47[b]	37	54
≥.10	15	34[b]	11	27

[a]BAC is recorded as mg %: Positive is ≥0.01 (10 mg of alcohol per 100 ml of blood).
[b]$P < 0.05$ Comparison of proportions between those breathalyzed with 6 hr of ER admission and reported no drinking after the event and blood toxicology screen for those whose blood was drawn or who died within 6 hr of injury, using tests of significant difference between proportions.

ences, and treatment for alcohol problems than those with injuries not resulting from violence, and these differences were found within gender-by-age (less than 30 and 30 and older) categories.

Table III shows the proportion who report heavy drinking, at least monthly drunkenness, two or more social consequences of drinking, and three or more dependence experiences among drinkers with and without violence-related injuries from three ER studies, which, using similar methods, obtained representative samples of all patients admitted to the ER. In this table, heavy drinking is defined as reporting drinking at least three times per week with 12 or more drinks on at least one occasion during the last year. Social consequences included reporting any of the following problems related to drinking during the last year: problems with personal relationships, work, police or other authorities, physical health, psychological health or mental well-being. Experiences related to alcohol dependence included blackouts, relief drinking, hands shaking alot the morning after drinking, binge drinking, and feeling that one should cut down on his or her drinking or quit altogether.

As seen in Table III, those with violence-related injuries were more likely to report heavy drinking, more frequent drunkenness, social consequences of drinking, and alcohol-dependence experiences than those with other injuries within the same ER sample, although the proportion of those reporting heavy and problem drinking varies considerably across the three studies. While differences between those with and without injuries resulting from violence were statistically significant only for the San Francisco sample, differences were substantial in the other two samples, although not significant, possibly due to the relatively small numbers of those with violence-related injuries in these two samples. A comparison of those in the Contra Costa sample (which is a merged sample of the county hospital, three of the six community hospitals, and the three HMO ER, all of which were weighted to be representative of those admitted to the ER in the entire county) to a general population sample of the same county found both those with and without injuries resulting from violence significantly more likely to report heavy and problem drinking.[36]

Because high rates of frequent heavy drinking and alcohol-related problems have been found among those with violence-related injuries in ER studies, it has been suggested that presenting to the ER with injuries resulting from violence may be a sign of excessive alcohol consumption, particularly among males over 25.[35]

Although, as a group, those with violence-related injuries in the ER have high rates of heavy and problem drinking, estimated BAC at the time of ER admission often fails to identify most problem drinkers across all injury causes, ranging from 16[37] to 31%.[12] One study found that while two thirds of injured patients who were BAC positive met criteria for alcohol dependence, almost half of those who were BAC negative also met criteria for alcohol dependence.[38]

5. Regional Comparisons of ER and Coroner Data

While alcohol is thought to be positively associated with severity of injury, including those resulting from violence,[7] few data are available that have compared representative samples of both fatal and nonfatal injuries resulting from violence occurring in the same geographic locality during the same period of time. Additionally, alcohol's association with both fatal and nonfatal injury may be expected to vary from one region of the country to another as regional drinking patterns vary.[39] Table IV shows the proportion of those with nonfatal (ER sample) and fatal (coroner sample) injuries who were alcohol positive and intoxicated for two diverse regions of the United States: Contra Costa County, California[16] and Hinds County, Mississippi.[40] Emergency room and coroner data in each region included representative samples and covered the same geographic area during the same period of time.

Similar data on fatal and nonfatal injuries from two geographically diverse regions of the United States are of interest because national alcohol surveys consistently have found distinct regional differences in drinking patterns and associated problems. The "dryer" regions of the United States (those which have traditionally supported a strong pro-temperance sentiment), particularly the South, have been found to report higher rates of abstention but also higher rates of frequent heavy drinking among those who do drink and more problems related to drinking (e.g., alcohol-related aggression) at a given level of consumption compared to the "wetter" regions of the country.[39,41] Mississippi has had the strongest pro-temperance sentiment of any of the Southern states, as evidenced by their being the last state to repeal prohibition (in 1966) and allow for local county option for selling alcoholic beverages. Presently, 44% of Mississippi's counties are dry (representing a 25% increase since 1988) compared to an average of 15% for the four surrounding states.[42] Mississippi reports a lower per capita consumption, based on gallons of absolute alcohol per person aged 14 years and older (2.09) than the Southern region as a whole (2.28), which is lower than the United States (2.28) and California (2.55).[43]

As seen in Table IV, those with violence-related fatalities were more likely to be alcohol positive and to be legally intoxicated than those with nonfatal injuries in both samples; however, differences were statistically significant only in the Contra Costa County sample. Both those with fatal and nonfatal injuries were more likely to be alcohol positive, but less likely to be intoxicated in the Mississippi sample compared to the California sample. These data suggest that, while alcohol may have a greater association with violence-related fatal than nonfatal injuries, the difference may be less pronounced in dryer regions of the country. The data also suggest that alcohol may have a greater association with both fatal and nonfatal violence-related injuries in dryer areas than in wetter areas, but not at high levels of consumption. While various explanations have been offered for the reasons for regional differences in drinking patterns and problems in the United States,[44,45] the possibility that areas of the United States that have relatively low rates of per capita consumption have higher rates of alcohol-related injuries resulting from violence than areas with greater per capita consumption presents an interesting paradox in relation to prevention of alcohol-related violent injuries. This is in contrast to the positive temporal association that has been found between per capita consumption and aggregate-level violence in a number of Scandinavian countries.[46] It is important to note, however, that the counties compared here are not necessarily representative of the larger geographic area from which they come. As seen in Table I, a great deal of variation exists in the proportion of ER patients who are BAC positive, even in adjacent geographic areas (e.g., Studies 7 and 11), and this may also be true of coroner cases from adjacent counties.

6. Limitations to ER Studies

While this review of alcohol and violence-related injuries in the ER strongly supports the supposition that alcohol is related to such injuries treated in the ER, there are several limitations to ER studies that affect their usefulness for understanding alcohol's presence and role in injuries resulting from violence. Even given representative samples of patients treated in the ER, many victims of violence may obtain treatment from other sources or may not have injuries severe enough to require any treatment. Comparisons of ER data with data from the general population from which these patients come, however, have shown that, while injured ER patients are more likely to be frequent heavy and problem drinkers as compared to the general population as a whole, they are similar in demographic and drinking characteristics to those in the general population who have used the ER for treatment for an injury during the last year.[20,36] The greatest difference between the two groups is the frequency of ER use, as might be expected, since those sampled in an ER would tend to be more frequent users of the ER than those sampled elsewhere. While factors associated with frequency of ER use may differ between these two groups, comparative findings between ER samples and the general population are reassuring in relation to the representativeness of ER samples to their counterparts in the general population. Another potential bias in ER data is that of misclassification, in which an unknown proportion of those with injuries related to violence may go unrecognized or be deliberately misclassified by either the patient or ER staff because of the stigma that may be associated with such injuries.

As mentioned earlier, ER studies, by their nature, are limited to victims of violence, and little may be learned from these studies about the perpetrator of the violent event unless the perpetrator is also injured and obtains ER treatment. A review of both ER patients as well as those known to the criminal justice system in Great Britain found a substantial association of alcohol with both violence perpetration and violence victimization, with both increasing as alcohol consumption increased.[3] Additionally, alcohol's involvement may vary by the nature of the event, e.g., whether family members or nonfamily members are involved. One study of perpetration of violence-related events during the preceding 3 months among patients admitted to a psychiatric ER found those who reported such events were over twice as likely to report alcohol abuse when the event involved nonfamily members as when the event involved family members (45 vs. 22%).[47]

While estimated BAC at the time of admission to the ER provides quantitative data on alcohol consumption prior to the ER visit, this may actually have little to do with alcohol consumption prior to or at the time of the violence-related injury event, depending on the length of time between the event and arrival at the ER, as well as drinking after the injury event. One study found that only 56% of injury patients reported to the ER within 6 hr of the event.[26] Therefore, a positive BAC at the time of ER admission is not necessarily an indication that a patient had been drinking prior to the violent event, and conversely a negative BAC at the time of the ER visit does not mean the patient had not been drinking. Although ER studies that obtain an estimate of BAC may document the presence of alcohol at the time of the event, the actual role that alcohol may have played in the event is not known, i.e., whether alcohol was related to or caused the event, or whether alcohol use was just coincidental to the event. While alcohol is thought to act as a social disinhibitor[48] leading to aggressive behavior in certain individuals,[39] and alcohol is also known to affect motor coordination and reaction time and to alter judgment—all of which could result in injury—the actual causative mechanism for the association of alcohol and violence-related injury is not known. Further, alcohol's role in perpetrating a violence-related event may be different than alcohol's role in becoming the victim of such an event. Additionally, many individuals who drink also use psychoactive drugs, which makes determining the independent role of alcohol in the event more difficult. In the Contra Costa County study in Table IV, of those in the ER sample who were positive for alcohol, 31% were also positive for drugs, while 39% of those in the coroner sample who were alcohol positive were also drug positive. It is also possible that associations of alcohol consumption and violence may be the result of their co-occurrence in relation to time of day and day of week. Drinking patterns have been found to vary in the United States, with higher rates of heavier drinking occurring during weekend evening hours.[49,50] If violent-related events are also more likely to occur during weekend evenings than at other times, the association of alcohol consumption and violence may be the result of a temporal association rather than a causal association. One ER study found, however, that regardless of the time of admission to the ER, those with violence-related injuries were more likely to be positive for estimated BAC and to report drinking prior to the event than those with other injuries.[20]

While this review of ER studies suggests that alcohol may be a major risk factor for injuries resulting from violence, the actual risk at which various levels of drinking, or any drinking, places the individual for violence-related injuries cannot be determine from these studies. One study of alcohol and injury in the general population suggests that an individual's risk for injury may increase at relatively low levels of drinking.[51] Emergency room studies that have found those with violence-related injuries more likely to be frequent, heavy, and problem drinkers compared with those with other injuries may actually underestimate alcohol's involvement in violence, since those injured from other causes have also been found to report higher rates of heavy and problem drinking than the noninjured as well as those in the general population. We are also not able to determine the proportion of violence resulting in injury that can be attributed to alcohol consumption, since we do not know whether the perpetrator of the event had also been drinking at the time. Only studies of alcohol and injury in representative samples from the general population can begin to provide data to address these concerns. Nevertheless, ER studies do provide a useful window for observing alcohol's association with injuries that are treated in this setting, and they also provide an important arena for the identification of those with alcohol-related problems who could benefit from an intervention or referral for problem drinking.

ACKNOWLEDGMENTS. This work was supported by the US National Institute of Alcohol Abuse and Alcoholism Alcohol Research Center Grant (AA 05595).

References

1. Roizen J: Estimating alcohol involvement in serious events, in: *Alcohol Consumption and Related Problems*. Washington, DC, US National Institute on Alcohol Abuse and Alcoholism, 1982, pp 179–219.
2. Roizen J: Alcohol and trauma, in Giesbrecht N, Gonzales R, Grant M, *et al* (eds): *Drinking and Casualties: Accidents, Poisonings and Violence in an International Perspective*. London, Tavistock/Helm, 1989, vol 1, pp 21–66.
3. Norton RN, Morgan MY: The role of alcohol in mortality and morbidity from interpersonal violence. *Alcohol Alcoholism* 24:565–576, 1989.
4. Barancik J, Chatterjee B, Greene YC, *et al*: Northeastern Ohio Trauma Study: 1. Magnitude of the problem. *Am J Public Health* 73:746–751, 1983.
5. Cherpitel CJ: Alcohol and injuries resulting from violence: A review of emergency room studies. *Addiction* 89:157–165, 1994.
6. Honkanen R, Smith GS: Impact of acute alcohol intoxication on the severity of injury: A cause-specific analysis of non-fatal trauma. *Injury* 21:353–357, 1990.
7. Shepherd J, Irish M, Scully C, Leslie I: Alcohol intoxication and severity of injury in victims of assault. *Br Med J* 296:1299, 1988.
8. Wechsler H, Kasey E, Thum D, Demone H: Alcohol level and home accidents. *Public Health Rep* 84:1043–1050, 1969.
9. Peppiatt R, Evans R, Jordan P: Blood alcohol concentrations of patients attending an accident and emergency department. *Resuscitation* 6:37–43, 1978.
10. Walsh ME, Macleod D: Breath alcohol analysis in the accident and emergency department. *Injury* 15:62–66, 1983.
11. Papoz L, Weill J, Gate C, *et al*: Biological markers of alcohol intake among 4,796 subjects injured in accidents. *Br Med J* 292:1234–1237, 1986.

12. Yates D, Hadfield J, Peters K: The detection of problem drinkers in the accident and emergency departments. *Br J Addict* 82:163–167, 1987.

13. Cherpitel CJ: Breathalyzer and self-reports as measures of alcohol-related emergency room admission. *J Stud Alcohol* 50:155–161, 1989.

14. Cherpitel CJ: Alcohol consumption and casualties: A comparison of two emergency room populations. *Br J Addict* 83:1299–1307, 1988.

15. Cherpitel CJ, Rosovsky H: Alcohol consumption and casualties: A comparison of emergency room populations in the United States and Mexico. *J Stud Alcohol* 51:319–326, 1990.

16. Cherpitel CJ: Alcohol and casualties: A comparison of emergency room and coroner data. *Alcohol Alcoholism* 29:211–218, 1994.

17. Cherpitel CJ, Parés A, Rodés J: Drinking patterns and problems: A comparison of emergency room populations in the United States and Spain. *Drug Alcohol Depend* 29:5–15, 1991.

18. Cherpitel CJ: Alcohol consumption among emergency room patients: Comparison of county/community hospitals and an HMO. *J Stud Alcohol* 54:432–440, 1993.

19. Cherpitel CJ: *Alcohol and Injuries Resulting from Violence: A Comparison of Emergency Room Samples from Two Regions of the US. J Addict Dis,* in press.

20. Cherpitel CJ: Alcohol and violence-related injuries: An emergency room study. *Addiction* 88:79–88, 1993.

21. Borges G, Garcia G, Gill A, Vandale S: Casualties in Acapulco: Results of a study of alcohol use and emergency room care. *Drug Alcohol Depend* 36:1–7, 1994.

22. Holt S, Stuart I, Dixon J, et al: Alcohol and the emergency service patient. *Br Med J* 281:638–640, 1980.

23. Honkanen R, Visuri T: Blood alcohol levels in a series of injured patients with special reference to accident and type of injury. *Ann Chir Gynaecol* 65:287–294, 1976.

24. Gibb K, Yee A, Johnson C, et al: Accuracy and usefulness of a breath alcohol analyzer. *Ann Emerg Med* 13:516–520, 1984.

25. Rosovsky H, Lopez J, Narvaez A: Trauma and acute medical problems in emergency rooms: Two dimensions of alcohol involvement? The International Workshop on Alcohol and the Emergency Room, Trieste, Italy, 1990, October 15–17.

26. Cherpitel CJ: A study of alcohol use and injuries among emergency room patients, in Giesbrecht N, Gonzales R, Grant M, et al (eds): *Drinking and Casualties: Accidents, Poisonings and Violence in an International Perspective.* London: New York, Tavistock/Routledge, 1989, pp 288–299.

27. Cherpitel CJ: Alcohol and injuries: A review of international emergency room studies. *Addiction* 88:923–937, 1993.

28. Cherpitel CJ, Parés A, Rodés J, Rosovsky H: Validity of self-reported alcohol consumption in the emergency room: Data from the U.S., Mexico and Spain. *J Stud Alcohol* 53:203–207, 1992.

29. Cherpitel CJ: Timing of the breath analyzer: Does it make a difference? *J Stud Alcohol* 54:517–519, 1993.

30. Midanik LT: Validity of self-reported alcohol use: A literature review and assessment. *Br J Addict* 83:1019–1029, 1988.

31. Midanik LT: Perspectives on the validity of self reported alcohol use. *Br J Addict* 84:1419–1424, 1989.

32. Babor TF, Stephens RS, Marlatt GA: Verbal report methods in clinical research on alcoholism: Response bias and its minimization. *J Stud Alcohol* 48:410–424, 1987.

33. Embree BG, Whitehead PC: Validity and reliability of self-reported drinking behavior: Dealing with the problem of response bias. *J Stud Alcohol* 54:334–344, 1993.

34. Cherpitel CJ: Drinking patterns and problems associated with injury status in emergency room admissions. *Alcoholism Clin Exp Res* 12:105–110, 1988.

35. Shepherd J, Irish M, Scully C, Leslie I: Alcohol consumption among victims of violence and among comparable UK populations. *Br J Addic* 84:1045–1051, 1989.

36. Cherpitel CJ: Alcohol and casualties: Comparison of county-wide emergency room data with the county general population. *Addiction* 90:343–350, 1995.

37. Redmond AD, Richards S, Plumhett PK: The significance of random breath alcohol sampling in the accident and emergency department. *Alcohol Alcoholism* 22:341–343, 1987.
38. Soderstrom CA, Dischinger PC, Smith GS, *et al:* Psychoactive substance dependence among trauma center patients. *JAMA* 267:2756–2759, 1992.
39. Hilton ME: Regional diversity in United States drinking practices. *Br J Addic* 83:519–532, 1988.
40. Cherpitel CJ: Alcohol in fatal and non-fatal injuries: A comparison of coroner and emergency room data from the same county. *Alcoholism Clin Exp Res* 20:338–342, 1996.
41. Midanik LT, Clark WB: The demographic distribution of US drinking patterns in 1990: Descriptions and trends from 1984. *Am J Public Health* 84:1218–1222, 1994.
42. Holder H, Cherpitel C: The end of US prohibition: A case study of Mississippi. *Contemp Drug Problems*, 23:301–330, 1996.
43. Williams GD, Clem DA, Dufour MC: *Apparent per Capita Consumption: National, State and Regional Trends: 1977–1992.* Rockville, MD, National Institute on Alcohol Abuse and Alcoholism, Alcohol Epidemiologic Data System, 1994.
44. Room R: Normative perspectives on alcohol use and problems. *J Drug Issues* 5:358–368, 1975.
45. Room R: Ambivalence as a sociological explanation: The case of cultural explanations of alcohol problems. *Am Sociol Rev* 41:1047–1065, 1976.
46. Lenke L: Alcohol and crimes of violence: A causal analysis. *Contemp Drug Problems* 11:355–365, 1982.
47. Gondolf EW: Characteristics of perpetrators of family and nonfamily assaults. *Hosp Community Psychiatry* 41:191–193, 1990.
48. Room R, Collins G (eds): *Alcohol and disinhibition: Nature and meaning of the link,* NIAAA Research Monograph No. 12, Publication No. (ADM) 83-1246. Washington D.C.: Government Printing Office, 1983.
49. Arfken CL: Temporal pattern of alcohol consumption in the United States. *Alcoholism Clin Exp Res* 12:137–142, 1988.
50. Cherpitel CJ, Flaminio D, Poldrugo F: Alcohol and casualties in the emergency room: A US–Italy comparison of weekdays and weekend evenings. *Addic Res* 1:223–238, 1993.
51. Cherpitel CJ, Tam TW, Midanik LT, *et al:* Alcohol and non-fatal injury in the US general population: A risk function analysis. *Accident Anal Prevent* 27:651–661, 1995.

II

Neurobiology

Richard A. Deitrich, Section Editor

Overview

Richard A. Deitrich

All of us have seen the "mean drunk" in which the entire personality of the individual seems to change under the influence of alcohol. It is frightening to realize that such an easily acquired substance can rip the veneer from an individual's behavior to expose the violent base underneath.

This section covers some of the basic data obtained from studies of animals regarding the relationship between ethanol and aggression. Chapter 6, by Yudko et al., outlines the preclinical research on alcohol and aggression. They point out how difficult such research can be and they establish the link between the influence of ethanol on animal and human aggressive behavior.

Chapter 7, an excellent chapter by Miczek et al., reviews some of the same material and then concentrates on the relationship between $GABA_A$–benzodiazepine receptor complex and aggression. A recurring theme in these chapters is the individual variability and the need to recognize this in animal experimentation. The specter that the genetic makeup of an individual may alter their aggressive tendencies either in the drug-free condition or under the influence of alcohol or other drugs is raised by these findings. This is a controversial subject; however, the recent identification of a gene that influences risk-taking behavior in humans is a good example of how such studies can be carried out.[1,2,3]

Chapter 8, by Virkkunen and Linnoila, details the evidence that there is a relationship between early-onset alcoholism, violent behavior, and serotonin mechanisms in the brain.

Finally, moving from rodent studies to higher animal models, Higley and Linnoila outline in Chapter 9 the development of a nonhuman primate model

Richard A. Deitrich • Department of Pharmacology, Alcohol Research Center, University of Colorado Health Sciences Center, Denver, Colorado 80262.

Recent Developments in Alcoholism, Volume 13: Alcoholism and Violence, edited by Marc Galanter. Plenum Press, New York, 1997

of excessive ethanol consumption that simulates many of the characteristics of alcoholism in humans.

Thus, these four chapters, while each reviews some of the ground to be found in others, provide a thorough review of the evidence that ethanol precipitates violent behavior in lower animals as well as in humans, and they begin to provide explanations at the biochemical and genetic level of how that may come about.

A major difference between human and animal ethanol-precipitated aggression may be that at high ethanol levels animals are less aggressive, perhaps because of the physical inability to attack others. However, with humans verbal abuse or use of a weapon is still possible, even at high ethanol levels.

The lack of tolerance development to ethanol in precipitating aggressive behavior may also be of importance here. It is critical to determine if this exists in humans as well as in laboratory animals.

The well-known tendency of males to be the aggressor and females to be the victim is covered in these chapters. The influence of testosterone or perhaps other steroids is important. However, the fact that victims, male or female, are also often intoxicated indicates that this may play a role in the ultimate outcome of an encounter with an intoxicated male.

References

1. Benjamin J, Li L, Patterson C, Greenberg, BD, Murphy DL, Hamer DH: Population and familial association between the D4 dopamine receptor gene and measures of Novelty Seeking. *Nat Genet* 12:81–84, 1996.
2. Cloninger CR, Adolfsson R, Svrakic NM: Mapping genes for human personality. *Nat Genet* 12:3–4, 1996.
3. Ebstein RP, Novick O, Umansky R, Priel B, Osher Y, Blaine D, Bennett ER, Nemanov L, Katz M, Belmaker RH: Dopamine D4 receptor (D4DR) exon III polymorphism associated with the human personality trait of Novelty Seeking. *Nat Genet* 12:78–80, 1996.

6

Emerging Themes in Preclinical Research on Alcohol and Aggression

Errol Yudko, D. Caroline Blanchard, J. Andy Henrie, and Robert J. Blanchard

Abstract. Animal research into the alcohol–aggression relationship is based on a need to understand this relationship in people, and its success depends on the degree to which animal models can provide appropriate parallels to relevant human phenomena. Comparisons of human and animal literature suggest that parallels may be found for the following: alcohol enhances aggression in some, but not all individuals; consumption increases the probability of victimization (being attacked by a conspecific); alcohol reduces anxiety, and socially stressed individuals show increased voluntary consumption; alcohol reduces avoidance of threatening situations or stimuli and may place individuals at greater risk of being attacked; both anxiety reduction and decreased avoidance of threat may increase the probability of involvement in violent situations. These findings suggest that a variety of mechanisms may be involved in alcohol enhancement of aggression.

Differences in effects of alcohol on human, as opposed to animal, aggression may reflect specific human capabilities. Although high doses of alcohol consistently reduce aggression in laboratory animals, this may reflect motoric and sedative effects that are not relevant for human behavior, in which verbal aggression and aggression involving the use of weapons make motor capability less important. Human voluntary alcohol consumption may also reflect response to stressors that also simultaneously promote aggression, a situation not paralleled by animal studies in which the drug is administered rather than voluntarily consumed. Nonetheless, obtained parallels suggest that animal experimentation using ecologically relevant situations can provide highly generalizable analyses of the alcohol–aggression relationship.

Errol Yudko • Department of Psychology, University of Hawaii at Manoa, Honolulu, Hawaii 96822.   **D. Caroline Blanchard** • Bekesy Laboratory of Neurobiology, Department of Anatomy and Reproductive Biology, University of Hawaii at Manoa, Honolulu, Hawaii 96822. **J. Andy Henrie** • Department of Chemistry, University of Hawaii at Manoa, Honolulu, Hawaii 96822.   **Robert J. Blanchard** • Department of Psychology, Bekesy Laboratory of Neurobiology, University of Hawaii at Manoa, Honolulu, Hawaii 96822.

Recent Developments in Alcoholism, Volume 13: Alcoholism and Violence, edited by Marc Galanter. Plenum Press, New York, 1997.

Animal research on alcohol and aggression reflects the need and desire to utilize a full spectrum of experimental methodologies in understanding the complex interrelationships of alcohol consumption, aggression, and violence in humans. These interrelationships have several different aspects, each of which may suggest specific phenomena that need to be modeled and in some cases have been modeled in animal research.

1. Alcohol Effects on Aggression and Violence

The existence of a strong positive correlational relationship between alcohol consumption, violence, and violent crime has been repeatedly demonstrated.[1–4] Moreover, this relationship also appears to be somewhat selective: alcohol is associated with violent crime at a significantly higher level than it is with nonviolent crime.[5] Miller and Potter-Efron[6] reported that alcohol is one of a small group of substances of abuse (others include PCP, amphetamines, and cocaine) that are regularly associated with aggressive patterns of behavior.

A number of recent studies also suggest that the involvement of alcohol in family violence may be particularly potent. O'Farrell and Choquette[7] reported that a sample of married alcoholic men had a five to six times greater prevalence of violent acts toward their wives than national norms. In a study of domestic homicide cases, 85% of the cases (70% of the suspects and 45% of the victims) had alcohol present,[8] while over 50% of maritally violent men self-reported that drinking accompanied their abusive events.[9] In comparisons of violent and nonviolent distressed families seeking counseling,[10] the maritally violent men consumed more alcohol than distressed but nonviolent men. Wesner et al.[11] found that alcohol played a role in 82% of male "explosive rage" episodes involving a spouse or girlfriend. In a study of violent lesbian relationships, 64% reported that alcohol or drugs were taken before or during incidents of battering, and the frequency of drinking significantly correlated with committing abusive acts.[12] Alcohol use is also a significant predictor of abuse toward children.[13]

One complicating factor in this relationship is that alcohol use is associated with victimization as well as with the commission of violent acts. The Slade et al.[8] report cited above notes that victims as well as perpetrators of domestic homicide are likely to have been drinking at the time. Both the incidence and severity of spousal violence is higher for women alcoholics,[14] even when other factors such as alcohol problems in the spouse, income, parental violence, and parental alcohol problems are controlled.[15] In a study of women jailed for killing their abusive husbands, daily alcohol use by the male victim was a particularly common finding.[16]

2. Effects of Aggression, Violence, and Other Stressors on Alcohol Use and Abuse

The alcohol–aggression relationship may also be bidirectional. A family history of violence[17] predicts alcohol abuse in individuals, and particularly the combination of alcohol problems and spouse abuse.[18] However, it seems likely that this effect is, at least in part, nonspecific, with a history of other types of severe stress such as childhood sexual exploitation[19] also leading to increased alcohol (and drug) abuse. Lindenberg et al.[20] reviewed nine relatively large-scale studies done between 1984 and 1991 on the relationship of the magnitude or intensity of social stress to one or more types of alcohol or drug use and abuse. Of these, six reported a positive relationship, two did not, and one reported mixed findings. In addition, analysis of studies failing to find a relationship between stress and substance use[21] suggests that factors such as the time span following stress, possible attrition from the sample of more affected individuals, and the use of a control group that had also been through stressful experiences may obscure this relationship. A number of recent studies have reported high rates of alcohol or drug use or abuse in subgroups that experience unusually high stress levels, such as firefighters,[22] homeless women,[23] and human immunodeficiency virus (HIV)-positive homosexual men.[24] It is notable that these groups are extremely divergent in characteristics (e.g., social and employment status) other than high stress levels, suggesting that stress is a major common factor in their alcohol or drug use.

In a recent longitudinal study that investigated the progressive use of alcohol in adolescents and their subsequent aggressive behaviors, White et al.[25] found that early aggressive behavior, as compared to alcohol use, is a better predictor of later alcohol use and alcohol-related aggression. The authors conclude from these data that "aggressive individuals become heavy drinkers because of subcultural norms, situational contexts, self-medication, or to give themselves an excuse to act aggressively" (p. 74). An additional view is also suggested. Both aggression and heavy alcohol consumption may be potentiated by a common factor such as stress. Thus, in addition to a possible general potentiation of both behaviors as a function of early or chronic stress, such a relationship could facilitate the expression of both behaviors simultaneously in response to acute stress. In a recent article,[26] the behavior patterns of 183 maritally violent men were compared to those of maritally nonviolent men. Maritally violent men consumed significantly more alcohol than did maritally nonviolent men. Moreover, the maritally violent men also reported that the major stressors in their lives were their wives and children. This is consonant with the interpretation that stress can elicit both alcohol consumption and violence, with these men both drinking in response to stress and simultaneously acting aggressively toward the perceived source of their stress.

These findings from research on humans, here only very briefly outlined, suggest several hypotheses in need of experimental attention. Over the past decade or so, quite a number of studies using laboratory animals have attempted to examine these suggested relationships.

3. Does Administration of Alcohol Increase Aggression in Animal Models?

In 1986, Berry and Smoothy[27] summarized the literature on alcohol effects on aggression in animal models, concluding, first, that the specific test situation used is a crucial factor in this relationship. Further, the potentiation of aggression by alcohol was seen almost exclusively at low-to-moderate doses, with higher doses attenuating this behavior. While some animals, notably fish, cats, and primates, did show this relationship, potentiation of aggression by alcohol was rare in rodents, although it did tend occur only at a low (0.3 g/kg) to moderate (1.0 g/kg) dose range such as is effective in other animals showing this relationship more strongly. Alcohol potentiation was more common in situations involving chronic rather than acute administration, and it appeared to reflect both individual subject variation and situational characteristics. Thus, in one study[28] isolate aggressive mice showed some enhancement of aggressive behavior at 0.3 g/kg alcohol and a decrease at 0.8 g/kg, while isolate timid/defensive mice showed an enhancement at 0.8 g/kg and sociable isolates showed no enhancement at any dose.

The individual difference variable in the alcohol–aggression relationship has received particular attention in recent work. One area of investigation relates to initial levels of attack. Blanchard et al.[29] reported that when rats were divided on the basis of pretest aggression screening with an intruder into their home cages into nonaggressive, moderately aggressive, and highly aggressive groups, only the moderately aggressive animals showed a potentiation of attack following alcohol (0.3 and 0.6 g/kg) administration.[29] Nonaggressive animals continued to fail to show attack, while the highly aggressive animals tended to show less aggression following alcohol administration.

This view that moderately but not highly aggressive rats show enhanced aggression in response to ethanol administration is consonant with findings in mice. When male mice were isolated (a treatment that increases aggression) for 10 days, ethanol (0.8 mg/kg) decreased their aggression, but in less aggressive 5-day isolates, the same dose of ethanol increased aggression.[30] When male mice of different weights—light, average, or heavy (heavy mice were significantly more aggressive than light mice but all were aggressive)— were paired with male mice of equivalent weight, no significant ethanol effect was evident.[31] However, the nonsignificant differences did tend in the predicted direction, with light animals showing a twofold increase in aggression at 0.8 mg/kg ethanol, while both average and heavy animals showed small nonsignificant decreases in aggression.

An additional and perhaps interacting individual difference factor is testosterone level. Miczek and his colleagues have reported a number of findings suggesting that testosterone levels may be important in the alcohol–aggression relationship, with higher testosterone levels tending to potentiate this relationship in male mice[32] and squirrel monkeys,[33] but not in females.[34] As aggression is an androgen-dependent behavior in male rodents,[35] testosterone deficiency may be an important factor in findings that alcohol does not increase aggression in nonaggressive rats.

A range of studies of the effects of situational and opponent-related factors in the alcohol–aggression relationship suggest that alcohol may enhance aggression because it reduces some type of inhibition on attack. Miczek and O'Donnell[36] reported that alcohol or chlordiazepoxide doses that failed to potentiate attack by Swiss-Webster mice on intruders in their home cages did so when tests were held in a neutral arena that tended to inhibit fighting relative to that of residents in their home cages. An additional type of inhibition may be involved in the sharply lower level of attack by males toward females in comparison to that seen to other males. In rat colonies acute alcohol administration produced a dramatic shift from male to female targets of attack during group formation (at 0.6 and 1.2 g/kg)[37] and increased attacks toward familiar (but not unfamiliar) females in an established group.[38] Inhibition based on size of opponent may also modulate the alcohol–aggression relationship. Alcohol potentiated attack by lactating females on small, but not large, male intruders into their nesting cages.[39] Since even the small intruders in this test were about the size of the females (and the large males about 50% heavier), this finding suggests that alcohol can reduce some degree of inhibition, but is less effective with extremely potent inhibitory factors. This is consonant with findings[40] that attack by male rats on a conspecific show a precipitous decline after cat exposure, and that alcohol doses in typical effective ranges (0.3–0.6), while tending to increase attack, fail to do so significantly.

4. Alcohol and the Recipient of Attack

As an increasing volume of human literature suggests, alcohol may influence aggression in part through its effect on the recipient of attack. Administration of alcohol to intruder mice and rats and to subordinate male squirrel monkeys increased attack seen toward these animals by resident or dominant male conspecifics.[41] This particular mechanism of potentiation of attack occurs at somewhat higher doses than does direct potentiation following administration of alcohol to the attacker. Most studies of alcohol–aggression relationships focus on attack by residents on intruders into their home cages or of dominant on subordinate animals, models that tend to produce offensive attack patterns. However, the recipient of attack by a conspecific typically responds with a pattern of defensive behavior that includes defensive or retaliatory attack components. The differentiation of offensive and defensive forms of attack is now relatively well accepted and it involves differences in virtually every component of these neurobehavioral systems. Offensive and defensive attack involve different antecedent conditions, behavior patterns, and specific targets for attack on the body of the opponent,[42] as well as, in many cases, differential response to drugs and other biological manipulations.[43,44] The question of the degree of fit between offensive (or defensive) attack and human aggression has never been satisfactorily resolved. Indeed, it has hardly been studied, and as yet there have not been any serious attempts to provide detailed descriptions of human aggression in terms that might be unequivocally related to either offensive or defensive attack modes. However, it has been suggested[45] that much of human aggression corresponds better to a defensive than to an offensive mode of attack. Certainly, given that fear tends to reduce offensive attack and promote defensive attack, it is to be expected that human aggression often contains at least some components of the latter.

The only direct test of the effect of alcohol on defensive attack measured a pattern of defensive threat vocalizations, jump-attacks, and bites to an approaching threat stimulus (the human experimenter) and to a terminally anesthetized conspecific.[44] These were potentiated by administration of moderate (0.6 g/kg) doses of alcohol. Peterson and Pohorecky[46] have reported that ethanol administration, while increasing the frequency and severity of biting attacks in a resident–intruder test, also shifts the distribution of wounds made by dosed residents on intruders from the normal upper-back target site for offensive attack (73% wounds for intruders bitten by vehicle control residents) to the lower back and ventrum (65% wounds made by ethanol-dosed residents). This finding suggests that alcohol may blur the distinction between offensive and defensive attack modes that is normally seen in an experienced resident male, perhaps by potentiating defensive attack patterns. Alternatively, since bites to the ventrum appear to be strongly inhibited in rats,[42] the finding of ventrum wounds may suggest again that alcohol acts to reduce a variety of inhibitions relevant to aggressive behavior.

5. Does Social Stress Enhance Voluntary Alcohol Consumption (VAC)?

The studies described above provide some indication that alcohol may promote aggression in laboratory rodents and other animals, either through direct effects on the attacker or, when administered to the target of an attack, by increasing conspecific attack on the dosed animal and through potentiation of defensive attack. However, consideration of the magnitude of the potentiation obtained in animal studies relative to the magnitude of the alcohol–aggression/violence conjunction outlined in the human literature suggests a considerable remaining discrepancy. Does this reflect a real limitation on the usefulness of animal studies to model alcohol effects on aggressive or violent behaviors, or does it indicate that the factors typically encountered in violent human situations have not yet been sufficiently analyzed and then duplicated in the animal work?

One aspect of the alcohol–aggression relationship that has as yet received relatively little attention in animal models concerns social stress. The human literature cited earlier strongly suggests that stress is a major risk factor for substance use and addiction (e.g., refs. 17–25). This possibility, difficult to test experimentally in people, may have extended implications for the observed effects of alcohol on aggression/violence in human populations.

The relationship between social stress and voluntary consumption of alcohol (and some other aggression-promoting substances) can be and has been examined in laboratory rats and mice. Social grouping reliably increases alcohol consumption in male rats,[47] and those males that show the greatest alcohol consumption are also characterized by withdrawal, inactivity, and lowered dominance.[48] A visible burrow system (VBS) providing tunnels and chambers to mimic the natural habitat of wild rats produces particularly high levels of fighting within rat groups, facilitating the development of a strong dominance hierarchy, and thus presumably stress, among males.[49] In rat groups housed in a VBS, subordinate males showed increased voluntary alcohol consumption (VAC).[50] When alcohol intake and defensive behaviors were measured prior to VBS grouping, subordinate but not dominant males showed an increase in VAC, indicating that the effect is not due to differential alcohol preference for animals that become subordinate in grouping situations.[51] This phenomenon is not restricted to rats. Hilakivi-Clark and Lister[31] have reported enhanced VAC in subordinate but not dominant mice.

Are these subordinate males truly stressed? While grouping per se is not likely to be a stressor in social animals such as rats, subordination reflects the results of fighting within groups, and the stress effects of VBS housing on subordinate males have been extensively documented. In the VBS, subordinates show greatly enhanced defensive behavior and reduced social, sexual, exploratory, and aggressive activity within the habitat.[52] They also suffer increased mortality,[53] a phenomenon that may be similar to the "social stress deaths" reported by Barnett[54,55] among wild rats introduced to an established colony. Early subordinate mortality increases with features that enhance group aggression levels such as the presence of females or the provision of a burrowing habitat.[53] Moreover, individual subordinate mortality appears to be related to the degree of stress experienced and expressed in individual behavior. In somewhat less stressful open-bin colonies in which subordinate mortality is spread out over the normal life span of rats, early-dying individuals can be predicted several hundred days in advance by a pattern of avoidance of the dominant male and reduced sexual behavior.[53] The period over which individual subordinate mortality could be predicted is so long (about one quarter of the life span of the rat) that it is highly unlikely that the animal died of any bodily disease or wound that was directly altering its behavior when the behavior change first appeared. Also, in behavioral tests of "emotionality" outside the colony, subordinates show changes that sometimes persist for weeks after the group is disbanded,[56] providing further confirmation of a severe behavioral stress response.

Subordinate males also show a number of physiological differences suggestive of stress, including adrenal and spleen enlargement and reductions in the weight of the thymus and testes.[57] Basal corticosterone (CORT) levels are increased and corticosterone-binding globulin (CBG) levels decreased, suggesting that free CORT levels may have been dramatically increased in these animals. Plasma testosterone levels are dramatically decreased and alterations of hypothalamic–pituitary–adrenal (HPA) axis functioning have been found in many subordinates.[57] A variety of brain system changes, including specific alterations of regional serotonin receptors,[58] mineralocorticoid and glucocorticoid receptors,[59] corticotropin-releasing hormone receptors,[60] and galanin levels[61] attest to widespread brain involvement in the chronic stress response of these animals.

6. Stress and Substance Abuse of Other Aggression-Impacting Substances

Alcohol is not the only substance for which stress facilitates self-administration. Stressful rearing conditions have been shown to increase cocaine[62] and amphetamine[63] self-administration in rats, and repeated tail pinch also enhanced vulnerability to self-administration of amphetamine. Offspring of mothers stressed by a heavy schedule of restraint during gestation days 14–21 also showed enhanced amphetamine self-administration,[64] suggesting that maternal hypersecretion of CORT may have lasting effects on the fetus. Consonant with this view, the restraint stress-based enhancement of locomotor response to amphetamine and morphine was not obtained in adrenalectomized animals with CORT implants.[65]

Rats vulnerable to amphetamine self-administration, either because of individual differences[66] or following prenatal stress,[64] also show enhanced locomotor response to amphetamine in a novel but not a familiar environment.[67] These animals have higher magnitude and longer-lasting stress-induced increases in nucleus accumbens concentrations of dopamine than do animals not showing the enhanced locomotory response to amphetamine.[68] The authors suggest that changes in these brain systems may constitute an important neurobiological substrate of the predisposition to acquire amphetamine self-administration as well as other addictive behaviors. Rats that developed self-administration also tended to be those that showed an enhanced locomotor response in a novel environment and acquired schedule-induced polydipsia. However, when tested for schedule-induced polydipsia first (an experience that is interpreted as having a coping function), the polydipsic rats subsequently failed to acquire self-administration and had a reduced locomotor response to novelty.[69] It is particularly notable that cocaine and amphetamine, like alcohol, are among the relatively few substances that do appear to be associated with aggression in people.[6] Again, however, individual difference factors are important, in addition to the effects of stressful experience. Taylor *et al.*[70] reported that rats that show a high plasma catecholamine response to stress show higher intake of a cocaine solution than do low catecholamine stress responders.

The specificity of this relationship is not yet clear. Pohorecky *et al.*[71] found that prenatal stress (gestational days 14–21) also increased sensitivity to caffeine on measures of corner activity and rearing. While some studies, notably those involving measures more clearly related to defensive attack,[72,73] have found that caffeine increases aggression, others typically involving offensive attack[74,75] have reported no effect.

7. The Relationship of Aggression to the Predisposition to VAC

Some of the human literature described above[26,76] suggests that aggressive individuals may be predisposed (in particular situations?) to both alcohol consumption and alcohol-related aggression. Laboratory animal research may again provide a parallel. Voluntary alcohol consumption measured prior to grouping in the VBS does not predict dominance–subordination status after grouping. However, a positive correlation between pregrouping biting of an intruder and postgrouping alcohol consumption for subordinates strongly suggests that it is the more aggressive males that are most stressed by the process of subordination. Notably, postgrouping VAC was not related to total attack times in pregrouping tests with the intruder, and additional analyses within this study strongly suggest that "aggressiveness" is better measured through terminal components of the attack process such as biting rather than overall attack times, which primarily measure lengthy but nondamage components such as the lateral attack or chasing.[51] In addition, behavioral analyses of those subordinate males (nonresponders) that show a particular change in HPA axis response, involving minimal or no CORT elevation to acute stress,[57] suggests that these are individuals that are both highly aggressive and highly defensive.[56] Rats bred to exhibit increased basal CORT[77] response and decreased CORT output in response to stress, a pattern similar to that of the nonresponder rats, spontaneously drink more ethanol than do control rats bred from the same line. These results suggest that VAC may be, at least in part, related to stress, and that in the VBS highly aggressive subordinates are particularly stressed animals.

A single study using mouse colonies has reported similar, although not identical, findings.[78] Subordinate male mice generally increased alcohol intake, and this was particularly marked in the most severely wounded subordinates, which showed an enhancement of the ratio of alcohol intake to total fluid intake compared to dominants and controls during a 2-week period following disbanding of the groups.[78] Overall correlations between pregrouping biting and postgrouping alcohol consumption for subordinates were not reported, and, as in the Blanchard *et al.*[51] study, total pregrouping attack times tended not to be reliably correlated to postgrouping VAC. However, the single reliable correlation (of 8 calculated) was in the opposite direction to what might be expected if total attack times and bites are valid measures of the same factor.

8. Is an Anxiolytic or Inhibition-Reducing Property of Alcohol an Important Component of the Relationship between Stress, Voluntary Alcohol Consumption, and Aggression?

The human literature suggests that stress increases voluntary alcohol consumption and the animal literature provides experimental confirmation of this. Alcohol also reduces the CORT response to a variety of stressors[79–81] and high-ethanol-consuming rats show greater preference for diazepam in comparison to rats with a lower preference for alcohol.[82] These findings suggest that anxiety reduction may be a mechanism in enhanced ethanol consumption.

Preclinical research provides strong support for the view that alcohol is an anxiolytic. In mice, alcohol produces an anxiolytic response in the black–white box[83] and in the elevated plus-maze.[84] Lister and Hilakivi[85] reported anxiolytic effects of alcohol in rats in both a hole-board test and in the elevated plus-maze. Alcohol withdrawal has anxiogenic effects that have been used to provide a model for analysis of anxiolytic drugs (e.g., File *et al.*[86]). In two defense test batteries measuring a range of natural defensive behaviors to potential predators and conspecifics, alcohol provided a profile of effects on proximate avoidance of potentially dangerous areas and risk assessment (investigation of possible danger) behaviors that was very similar to the profile obtained with diazepam. Alcohol also reduced the cat-induced inhibition of consummatory behavior.[40]

One aspect of these specific effects on defensive behaviors is particularly notable. The dose-dependent reduction in proximate avoidance by alcohol is so pronounced that alcohol-dosed rats may preferentially approach areas in which they have seen a highly dangerous stimulus (i.e., cat). The effect of this specific alteration of defensive behavior may be that alcohol produces an inclination to approach, rather than avoid, potentially dangerous situations, a factor that is likely to be involved in the findings of more conspecific attacks on alcohol-drugged animals,[41] as well as the enhanced levels of alcohol intake for victims of human violence.[6,8]

The previously described findings of an alcohol enhancement of the proportion of attacks by male rats toward females, and particularly toward familiar females, suggests a slightly different interpretation: that alcohol reduces a variety of inhibitions, some but possibly not all of which are associated with anxiety. Certainly the reduction in approach to a potentially dangerous stimulus can be viewed as reflecting inhibition, in this case an inhibition that responds to anxiolytic drugs.[87] Inhibition of attack on females has an obvious adaptive potential, but little is known of the mechanisms involved; and there is, in the absence of relevant data, no reason to assume that this is related to anxiety or indeed to other types of inhibition. Some commonality of neurobehavioral inhibitory systems is strongly suggested by the work of Bohus, Koolhaas, and their colleagues at Groningen, and some aspects of the biology of these systems are beginning to be described.[88–90] Nonetheless, an understanding of the relationships among different inhibitory systems and their response to alcohol is just beginning to develop.

9. Relationship of Preclinical Studies of Alcohol Effects to Human Alcohol–Aggression Phenomena

Briefly summarized, preclinical studies of alcohol and aggression, with consideration also of the potential interaction of these with stress and responses to stress suggest the following. Alcohol at low to moderate doses may potentiate both offensive and defensive attack. However, the former appears to be potentiated in only a subpopulation of animals. Moreover, alcohol strikingly reduces avoidance of potentially threatening or dangerous situations. These three findings suggest a particularly potent scenario for those situations in which both participants in a dyadic interaction have taken alcohol. If potentially hostile or aversive interactions arise, one or both participants fail to show a normal avoidance response but instead approach. The approach itself provides stimuli that may elicit either an offensive or a defensive attack, depending on the situation and other motivational/emotional factors of the individual responding. The attack by one participant then triggers a defensive (retaliatory) attack by the other, heightened by the effects of alcohol and triggering an escalating series of mutually aggressive acts.

There are differences, however, between the existing animal literature and human experience that may reduce or obscure the relevance of animal studies to an understanding of the effects on alcohol on human behavior. First, in the vast majority of animal studies when alcohol effects are to be evaluated, alcohol is administered to the animal, not taken voluntarily. If, as both animal and human literature suggest, aggressiveness and alcohol preference are positively correlated (under specific circumstances?), then the alcohol–aggression relationship may be more clearly seen when voluntary consumption is allowed.

An additional difference, of possibly immense importance, is that aggression or violence in humans reflects two factors that are not, and are not likely to be, of much significance in laboratory rodent studies. First, human aggressiveness is often, and quite reasonably, evaluated in terms of verbal rather than physical violence. Hostile, insulting, and denigrating speech is capable of doing lasting damage to relationships; to the mental well-being and development of children, in particular, who are exposed to it; and, it comprises an especially relevant stimulus for the elicitation of retaliatory hostility and sometimes physical violence from interacting individuals. Second, human aggression often involves weapon use. The reverse U-shaped dose–response relationship consistently obtained in those animal studies that do show an alcohol potentiation of aggression probably reflects both sedation and motor impairment at higher doses. Indeed, this effect may be involved in the finding that chronic rather than acute alcohol intake is more likely to produce enhanced aggression in animal studies,[27] if chronic administration reduces the motoric and sedative effects of a given dose of alcohol. Notoriously, the possession of a weapon can reduce or eliminate the effects of motor impairment and even sedation associated with high levels of alcohol intake, a common factor in human experience and one that is unlikely to be easily duplicated in laboratory animal studies.

Overall, however, the animal literature does hold the promise of providing relatively comprehensive models for experimental investigation of many aspects of the alcohol–aggression relationship. While relatively few, preclinical studies incorporating attention to mechanisms such as stress and inhibitory systems and their interactions with individual differences may provide a more detailed understanding of the bidirectional relationship between alcohol and aggression and may provide specific suggestions for improved control of some of the consequences of this relationship.

ACKNOWLEDGMENT. Support for this research was provided by a grant from the Howard Hughes Medical Institute through the Undergraduate Biological Sciences Education Program.

References

1. Shupe LM: Alcohol and crimes: A study of the urine alcohol concentration found in 882 persons arrested during or immediately after the commission of a felony. *J Criminal Law Criminol* 44:661–665, 1954.
2. Wolfgang ME, Strohm EB: The relationship between alcohol and criminal homicide. *Q J Stud Alcohol* 17:411–425, 1956.
3. Pernanen K: Alcohol and crimes of violence, in Kissin B, Begleiter H (eds.): *The Biology of Alcoholism: Social Aspects of Alcoholism.* New York, Plenum, 1976, pp 351–444.
4. Straus MA, Gelles RJ, Steinmetz SK: *Behind Closed Doors: Violence in the American Family.* New York, Anchor/Doubleday, 1980.
5. Murdoch C, Pihl RO, Ross D: Alcohol and crimes of violence: Present issues. *Int J Addict* 25:1065–1081, 1990.
6. Miller MM, Potter-Efron RT: Aggression and violence associated with substance abuse. *Chem Depend Treat* 3:1–36, 1989.
7. O'Farrell TJ, Choquette K: Marital violence in the year before and after spouse-involved alcoholism treatment. *Family Dynamics Addict Q* 1:32–40, 1991.
8. Slade M, Daniel LJ, Heisler CJ: Application of forensic toxicology to the problem of domestic violence. *J Forensic Sci* 36:708–713, 1991.
9. Fagan RW, Barnett OW, Patton JB: Reasons for alcohol use in maritally violent men. *Am J Drug Alcohol Abuse* 14:371–392, 1988.

10. Russell MN, Llpov E, Phillips N, White B: Psychological profiles of violent and nonviolent maritally distressed couples. *Psychotherapy* 26:81–87, 1989.
11. Wesner D, Patel C, Allen J: A study of explosive rage in male spouses counseled in an Appalachian mental health clinic. *J Counsel Dev* 70:235–241, 1991.
12. Schilit R, Lle G, Montagne M: Substance use as a correlate of violence in intimate lesbian relationships. *J Homosex* 19:51–65, 1990.
13. Suh EK, Abel EM: The impact of spousal violence on the children of the abused. *J Independ Social Work* 4:27–34, 1990.
14. Miller, BA: The interrelationships between alcohol and drugs and family violence. In: De La Rosa, M, Lambert, EY, and Gropper, BA (eds.), *Drugs and Violence: Causes, Correlates, and Consequences*. NIDA Research Monograph No. 103, DHHS Publication No. (ADM) 91–1721, Washington D.C.: Government Printing Office 1990, pp. 177–207.
15. Miller BA, Downs WR, Gondoli DM: Spousal violence among alcoholic women as compared to a random household sample of women. *J Stud Alcohol* 50:533–540, 1989.
16. Foster LA, Veale CM, Fogel CI: Factors present when battered women kill. Special issue: Family violence. *Issues Ment Health Nurs* 10:273–284, 1989.
17. Plutchik A, Plutchik R: Psychosocial correlates of alcoholism. *Integrative Psychiatry* 6:205–210, 1988.
18. Hastings Je, Hamberger LK: Personality characteristic of spouse abusers: A controlled comparison. *Violence Victims* 3:31–48, 1988.
19. Rew L: Long-term effects of childhood sexual exploitation. *Issues Ment. Health Nurs.* 10:229–244, 1989.
20. Lindenberg CS, Gendrop SC, Reiskin HK: Empirical evidence for the social stress model of substance abuse. *Res Nurs Health* 16:351–362, 1993.
21. Tennant C, Goulston K, Dent O: Clinical psychiatric illness in prisoners of war of the Japanese: Forty years after release. *Psychol Med* 16:833–839, 1986.
22. Boxer PA, Wild D: Psychological distress and alcohol use among fire fighters. *Scand J Work Environ Health* 19:121–125, 1993.
23. Smith EM, North CS, Spitznagel EL: Alcohol, drugs, and psychiatric comorbidity among homeless women: An epidemiologic study. *J Clin Psychiatry* 54:82–87, 1993.
24. Atkinson JH Jr, Grant I, Kennedy CJ, *et al:* Prevalence of psychiatric disorders among men infected with human immunodeficiency virus. A controlled study. *Arch Gen Psychiatry* 45:859–864, 1988.
25. White HR, Brick J, Hansell S: A longitudinal investigation of alcohol use and aggression in adolescence. *J Stud Alcohol* (Suppl 11):62–77, 1993.
26. Barnett OW, Fagan RW: Alcohol use in male spouse abusers and their female partners. *J Family Violence* 8:1–24, 1993.
27. Berry MS, Smoothy R: A critical evaluation of claimed relationships between alcohol intake and aggression in infrahuman animals, in Brain PF (ed): *Alcohol and Aggression*. London, Croom-Helm, 1986, pp 84–137.
28. Krsiak M, Elis J, Poschlova N, Masek K: Increased aggressiveness and lower brain serotonin levels in offspring of mice given alcohol during gestation. *J Stud Alcohol* 38:1696–1704, 1977.
29. Blanchard RJ, Hori K, Blanchard DC, Hall J: Ethanol effects on aggression of rats selected for different levels of aggressiveness. *Pharmacol Biochem Behav* 27:641–644, 1987.
30. Hilakivi LA, Lister RG: Effects of ethanol on the social behavior of group-housed and isolated mice. *Alcoholism Clin Exp Res* 13:622–625, 1989.
31. Hilakivi-Clarke LA, Lister RG: The role of body weight in resident–intruder aggression. *Aggressive Behav* 18:281–288, 1992.
32. DeBold JF, Miczek KA: Testosterone modulates the effects of ethanol on male mouse aggression. *Psychopharmacology* 86:286–290, 1985.
33. Winslow JT, Miczek KA: Naltrexone blocks amphetamine-induced hyperactivity, but not disruption of social and agonistic behavior in mice and squirrel monkeys. *Psychopharmacology* 96:493–499, 1988.

34. Lisciotto CA, Debold JF, Miczek KA: Sexual differentiation and the effects of alcohol on aggressive behavior in mice. *Pharmacol Biochem Behav* 35:357–362, 1990.

35. Matochik JA, Sipos ML, Nyby JG, Barfield RJ: Intracranial androgenic activation of male-typical behaviors in house mice: Motivation versus performance. *Behav Brain Res* 60:141–149, 1994.

36. Miczek KA, O'Donnell JM: Alcohol and chlordiazepoxide increase suppressed aggression in mice. *Psychopharmacology* 69:39–44, 1980.

37. Blanchard RJ, Hori K, Flannelly K, Blanchard DC: The effects of ethanol on the offense and defensive behaviors of male and female rats during group formation. *Pharmacol Biochem Behav* 26:61–64, 1987.

38. Blanchard RJ, Blanchard DC: The relationship between ethanol and aggression: Studies using ethological models, in Olivier B, Mos J, Brain PF (eds.): *Ethopharmacology of Agonistic Behavior in Animals and Humans.* Dordrecht/Boston/Lancaster, Martinus Nijhoff Publishers, 1987, pp 145–161.

39. Blanchard DC, Flannelly K, Hori K, *et al:* Ethanol effects on female aggression vary with opponent size and time within session. *Pharmacol Biochem Behav* 27:645–648, 1987.

40. Blanchard RJ, Blanchard DC, Flannelly KJ, Hori K: Ethanol effects on freezing and conspecific attack in rats previously exposed to a cat. *Behav Process* 16:193–201, 1988.

41. Miczek KA, Winslow JT, Debold JF: Heightened aggressive behavior by animals interacting with alcohol-treated conspecifics: Studies with mice, rats and squirrel monkeys. *Pharmacol Biochem Behav* 20:349–353, 1984.

42. Blanchard RJ, Blanchard DC: Aggressive behavior in the rat. *Behav Biol* 21:197–224, 1977.

43. Blanchard RJ, Kleinschmidt CK, Flannelly KJ, Blanchard DC: Fear and aggression in the rat. *Aggressive Behav* 10:309–315, 1984.

44. Blanchard R, Blanchard DC: Ethological models of fear and angry aggression. *Clin Neuropharmacol* 9(Suppl 4):383–385, 1986.

45. Albert DJ, Walsh ML, Jonik RH: Aggression in humans: What is its biological foundation? *Neurosci Biobehav Rev* 17:405–425, 1993.

46. Peterson JT, Pohorecky LA, Hamm MW: Neuroendocrine and beta-adrenoceptor response to chronic ethanol and aggression in rats. *Pharmacol Bichem Behav* 34:247–253, 1989.

47. Ellison G, Staugaitis S, Crane P: A silicone delivery system for producing binge and continuous ethanol intoxication in rats. *Pharmacol Biochem Behav* 14:207–211, 1981.

48. Ellison G, Levy A, Lorant N: Alcohol-preferring rats in colonies show withdrawal, inactivity, and lowered dominance. *Pharmacol Biochem Behav* 18(Suppl 1):565–570, 1983.

49. Blanchard RJ, Blanchard DC: Antipredator defensive behaviors in a visible burrow system. *J Comp Psychol* 103:70–82, 1989.

50. Blanchard RJ, Hori K, Tom P, Blanchard DC: Social structure and ethanol consumption in the laboratory rat. *Pharmacol Biochem Behav* 28:437–442, 1987.

51. Blanchard RB, Flores T, Magee L, *et al:* Pregrouping aggression and defense scores influences alcohol consumption for dominant and subordinate rats in the visible burrow systems. *Aggressive Behav* 18:459–467, 1992.

52. Blanchard DC, Sakai RR, McEwen B, *et al:* Subordination stress: Behavioral, brain, and neuroendocrine correlates. *Behav Brain Res* 58:113–121, 1993.

53. Blanchard RJ, Blanchard DC, Flannelly KJ: Social stress, mortality, and aggression in colonies and burrowing habitats. *Behav Process* 11:209–213, 1985.

54. Barnett SA: Physiological effects of "social stress" in wild rats. 1. The adrenal cortex. *J Psychosom Res* 3:1–11, 1958.

55. Barnett SA: Enigmatic death due to "social stress" a problem in the strategy of research. *Interdisciplinary Sci Rev* 13:40–51, 1988.

56. Yudko E, Bjorenson K, Blanchard RJ: Behavioral differences of dominant and subordinate rats in a visible burrow system. Abstracts of the Annual Meeting for the Society of Neuroscience 1993. (Abstract)

57. Blanchard DC, Spencer RL, Weiss SM, *et al:* Visible burrow system as a model of chronic

social stress: Behavioral and Neuroendocrine correlates. *Psychoneuroendocrinology* 20:117–134, 1995.

58. McKittrick CR, Blanchard DC, Blanchard RJ, *et al:* Serotonin receptor binding in a colony model of chronic social stress. *Biol Psychiatry* 37:383–393, 1995.

59. Chao HM, Blanchard DC, Blanchard RJ, *et al:* The effect of social stress on hippocampal gene expression. *Cell Mol Neurobiol* 4(6):543–560. 1993.

60. Albeck DS, McKittrick CR, Blanchard DC, *et al:* Chronic social stress inhibits corticotropin-releasing hormone mRNA in the paraventricular nucleus of a subpopulation of subordinates. Abstracts of the Society of Neuroscience 1994. (Abstract)

61. Holmes PV, Blanchard DC, Blanchard RJ, *et al:* Chronic social stress increases levels of preprogalanin mRNA in the rat locus coeruleus. *Pharmacol Biochem Behav* 50:655–660, 1995.

62. Schenk S, Hunt T, Klukowski G, Amit Z: Isolation housing decreases the effectiveness of morphine in the conditioned taste aversion paradigm. *Psychopharmacology* 92:48–51, 1987.

63. Maccari S, Piazza PV, Deminere JM, Lemaire V: Life events-induced decrease of corticosteroid type I receptors is associated with reduced corticosterone feedback and enhanced vulnerability to amphetamine self-administration. *Brain Res.* 574:7–12, 1991.

64. Deminiere JM, Piazza PV, Guegan G, Abrous N: Increased locomotor response to novelty and propensity to intravenous amphetamine self-administration in adult offspring of stressed mothers. *Brain Res* 586:135–139, 1992.

65. Deroche V, Piazza PV, Casolini P, Maccari S: Stress-induced sensitization to amphetamine and morphine psychomotor effects depend on stress-induced corticosterone secretion. *Brain Res* 598:343–348, 1992.

66. Deminiere JM, Piazza PV, le Moal M, Simon H: Experimental approach to individual vulnerability to psychostimulant addiction. *Neurosci Biobehav Rev* 13:141–147, 1989.

67. Piazza PV, Calza L, Giardino L, Amato G: Chronic thioridazine treatment differently affects DA receptors in striatum and in mesolimbo-cortical systems. *Pharmacol Biochem Behav* 35:937–942, 1990.

68. Rouge-Pont F, Piazza PV, Kharouby M, le Moal M: Higher and longer stress-induced increase in dopamine concentrations in the nucleus accumbens of animals predisposed to amphetamine self-administration: A microdialysis study. *Brain Res* 602:169–174, 1993.

69. Piazza PV, Mittleman G, Deminière JM, *et al:* Relationship between schedule-induced polydipsia and amphetamine intravenous self-administraiton. Individual differences and role of experience. *Behav Brain Res* 55:185–193, 1993.

70. Taylor J, Harris N, Vogel WH: Voluntary alcohol and cocain consumption in "low" and "high" stress plasma catecholamine responding rats. *Pharmacol Biochem Behav* 37:359–363, 1990.

71. Pohorecky LA, Roberts P, Cotler S, Carbone JJ: Alteration of the effects of caffeine by prenatal stress. *Pharmacol Biochem Behav* 33:55–62, 1989.

72. Eichelman B, Orenberg E, Hackley P, Barchas J: Methylxanthine-facilitated shock-induced aggression in the rat. *Psychopharmacology* 56:305–308, 1978.

73. Emley GS, Hutchinson RR: Unique influences of ten drugs upon post-shock biting attack and pre-shock manual responding. *Pharmacol Biochem Behav* 19:5–12, 1983.

74. Hansen S, Ferreira A: Food intake, aggression, and fear behavior in the mother rat: Control by neural systems concerned with milk ejection and maternal behavior. *Behav Neurosci* 100:64–70, 1986.

75. File SE, Guardiola Lemaitre BJ: I-Fenfluramine in tests of dominance and anxiety in the rat. *Neuropsychobiology* 20:205–211, 1988.

76. White HL, Ascher JA: Preclinical and early clinical studies with BW 1370U87, a reversible competitive MAO-A inhibitor. *Clin Neuropharmacol* 15(Suppl 1 Pt A):343A–344A, 1992.

77. Prasad C, Prasad A: A relationship between increased voluntary alcohol preference and basal hypercorticosteronemia associated with an attenuated rise in corticosterone output during stress. *Alcohol* 12:59–63, 1995.

78. Hilakivi Clarke LA, Lister RG: Social status and voluntary alcohol consumption in mice: Interaction with stress. *Psychopharmacology* 108:276–282, 1992.

79. Pohorecky LA, Rassi E, Weiss JM, Michalak M: Biochemical evidence for an interaction of ethanol and stress: Preliminary studies. *Alcoholism Clin Exp Res* 4:423–426, 1980.

80. Brick J, Horowitz GP: Alcohol and morphine induced hypothermia in mice selected for sensitivity in ethanol. *Pharmacol Biochem Behav* 16:473–479, 1982.

81. Thomas R, Beer R, Harris B, *et al:* GH responses to growth hormone releasing factor in depression. *J Affect Disord* 16:133–137, 1989.

82. Wolfgramme J, Heyne A: Social behavior, dominance, and social deprivation of rats determine drug choice. *Pharmacol Biochem Behav* 38:389–385, 1991.

83. Costall B, Kelly ME, Naylor RJ, Onaivi ES: Actions of buspirone in a putative model of anxiety in the mouse. *J Pharm Pharmacol* 40:494–500, 1988.

84. Melchior CL, Ritzmann RF: Dehydroepiandrosterone is an anxiolytic in mice on the plus maze. *Pharmacol Biochem Behav* 47:437–441, 1994.

85. Lister RG, Hilakivi LA: The effects of novelty, isolation, light and ethanol on the social behavior of mice. *Psychopharmacology* 96:181–187, 1988.

86. File SE, Zharkovsky A, Hitchcott PK: Effects of nitrendipine, chlordiazepoxide, flumazenil and baclofen on the increased anxiety resulting from alcohol withdrawal. *Prog Nuropsychopharmacol Biol Psychiatry* 16:87–93, 1992.

87. Blanchard DC, Veniegas R: Alcohol and anxiety: Effects on offensive and defensive aggression. *J Stud Aggression* (Supplement 11):9–19, 1993.

88. Roozendaal B, Wiersma A, Driscoll P, Koolhaas JM: Vasopressinergic modulation of stress responses in the central amygdala of the Roman high-avoidance and low-avoidance rat. *Brain Res* 596:35–40, 1992.

89. de Ruiter C, Cohon L: Persoonlijkheidskenmerken van patienten met agorafobie: een studie met het Comprehensive System voor de Rorschach. (Personality characteristics of patients with agoraphobia: A study with the comprehensive system for the Rorschach Test.) *Nederlands Tijdschrift voor de Psychologie en haar Grensgebieden* 48:35–42, 1993.

90. Compaan JC, Wozniak A, De Ruiter AJH, *et al:* Aromatase activity in the preoptic area differs between aggressive and nonaggressive male house mice. *Brain Res Bull* 35:1–7, 1994.

Alcohol, GABA$_A$–Benzodiazepine Receptor Complex, and Aggression

Klaus A. Miczek, Joseph F. DeBold, Annemoon M.M. van Erp, and Walter Tornatzky

Abstract. Neurobiological investigations have become productive since experimental protocols were developed that engender large increases in aggressive behavior after acute alcohol challenges in individual experimental animals. Recent developments extended the heightened aggressive behavior to rats that self-administered alcohol shortly before the social confrontation. Quantitative ethological analysis revealed that alcohol prolongs "bursts" of aggressive acts and displays and disrupts communication between the aggressive animal and the opponent who defends, submits, or flees. Pharmacological modulation of the GABA$_A$ receptor with benzodiazepine agonists and neuroactive steroids results in dose-dependent biphasic changes in aggressive behavior that mimic the dose–effect function of alcohol; benzodiazepines potentiate the aggression-heightening effects of alcohol as well as the behaviorally suppressive effects; and antagonists at benzodiazepine receptors prevented the aggression-heightening effects of alcohol. The maturational and experiential origins for potentially distinctive GABA$_A$ receptor characteristics in individuals who exhibit heightened aggressive behavior await identification.

1. Introduction

The dissection of the alcohol–aggression link remains a formidable challenge to the social and neurobiological scientific communities. How cultural and social conventions, sanctions, licensures, and expectations interact with an individual's drinking habits and social behavior and how the individual's physiological processes at the systems and cellular level are modified by alcohol's action on receptor molecules that are relevant to the drug's effect on

Klaus A. Miczek • Departments of Psychology, Psychiatry, and Pharmacology, Tufts University, Medford, Massachusetts 02155.   **Joseph F. DeBold, Annemoon M.M. van Erp, and Walter Tornatzky** • Department of Psychology, Tufts University, Medford, Massachusetts 02155.

Recent Developments in Alcoholism, Volume 13: Alcoholism and Violence, edited by Marc Galanter. Plenum Press, New York, 1997

aggressive behavior requires integration of information from anthropological, sociological, psychological, and neurobiological sources. An important characteristic of alcohol in a social context is the observation, portrayed artistically in Greek symposia, Renaissance bacchanales, party scenes by the Dutch masters of the Golden Age, or an intimate tete-à-tete by Picasso, that most alcohol drinking is associated with a convivial mood. Benchmark data on the amount and pattern of alcohol drinking on the one hand and the incidence of violent acts on the other are still lacking.[1] Conversely, the consistently high and persistent numbers of aggressive and violent acts that are associated with alcohol have been documented for decades in several communities throughout the world, as summarized in the first section of this volume.

The sheer magnitude of the public health problem of how alcohol is associated with aggressive and violent behavior is overwhelming, in most epidemiological analyses exceeding more than 50% of all incidences of these types of behavior.[2–4] From the perspective of violence research, it is most instructive that many different kinds of aggressive and violent behavior are linked to alcohol, ranging from murders, rapes, sexual violence, wife beatings, child abuse, incestuous offenses, and felonies. In human experimental research and in clinical studies, acute doses of alcohol have been shown to increase feelings of hostility and behavioral indices of competitive and retaliatory tendencies.[5–7] In recent reviews of the world literature on alcohol, drugs of abuse, aggression, and violence that also encompassed evidence from experimental laboratory research, alcohol was found to be "the drug that is most consistently and seriously linked to many types of aggressive and violent behavior" (ref. 4, p. 389).

In order to gain insight into the precise sequence of events at the behavioral, physiological, and neurobiological levels that characterize alcohol-heightened aggression, it is necessary to glean from epidemiological and criminal statistics whether or not the perpetrator or the victim of the violent and aggressive behavior was under the influence of alcohol. Detailed information is required to determine whether or not the alcohol-intoxicated individual provokes more aggressive behavior than a sober individual. And if so, how the alcohol intoxication contributes to the escalation of interactions that ultimately result in violent and aggressive acts. Epidemiological data rarely provide insight into these questions and they need to be complemented by information that stems from situations in which the details of alcohol and the social confrontation are specified.

Experimental research on alcohol and aggression has the advantages of being able to (1) specify the precise amount of alcohol that is in the individual who engages in aggressive behavior, as well as in the victim or target of aggressive behavior at the relevant times of the initiation, execution, and termination of the behavioral sequence; (2) delineate acute and chronic alcohol conditions; (3) disentangle the issue whether the perpetrator, victim, or both were under the influence of alcohol; and (4) analyze the proximal and triggering social events that are influenced by alcohol. Signals of provocation and appeasement characterize social confrontations in humans and other animal species.[8] In the escalation of social confrontations, alcohol appears to profoundly alter the communication of socially significant signals.[9] Detailed experimental analysis of the nature of the confrontation, the phases of escalation, and the sending and receiving of social signals reveals how alcohol modifies not only the sensations of sounds, smells, and movements, but distorts the communicative processes. For example, low alcohol doses, given orally to dominant squirrel monkeys confronting an opponent, increase aggressive vocalizations concurrently with the display of aggressive acts[10]; by contrast, the targets of these vocal and postural displays, when under the influence of increasing doses of alcohol, are more frequently attacked.[11] Rats that confront an aggressive resident typically emit certain types of ultrasonic vocalizations that reduce the probability of being attacked; when given increasing doses of alcohol, these vocalizations become less frequent, and it appears that this disruption of vocal signals may contribute to the higher frequency of being attacked (K.A. Miczek, unpublished observations).

A major challenge and dilemma for experimental research on alcohol and aggression continues to be the development and conduct of protocols that lead to increased aggression that is potentially injurious, harmful, and painful (e.g., ref. 12). Avoidance and reduction of pain, harm, and injury are the very principles that govern experimental research. How does one apply these principles to research protocols in which validity is achieved when the pharmacological manipulations and behavioral phenomena approximate the events that constitute the public health problem, namely alcohol-linked violence? At present, the most rational approach to this type of experimental research is to evaluate the significance of each protocol in terms of its neurobiological, pharmacological, and behavioral validity and to judge its relevance to the public health problem.

From an experimental viewpoint, one of the most perplexing facets of alcohol's impact on aggressive behavior is the enormous variability in outcome. Even under conditions that control for pharmacological, genetic, situational, behavioral, and social factors, across individuals alcohol may increase or decrease or leave aggressive behavior unaltered, and this individual variability extends from humans to other animal species. The study of individual alcohol effects on aggressive behavior represents a genuine experimental challenge necessitating experimental strategies that differ from the practice of randomly assigning individuals to a test sample and averaging the test results from all individuals in a sample. Such novel strategies have to capture relatively rare, episodic events in individuals.

2. Alcohol and Aggressive Behavior in Animals: Ethological Analysis

2.1. Individual Differences in Alcohol Effects on Aggressive Behavior

By now, it has become possible to identify major sources for apparently opposing conclusions that have been reached about alcohol and aggression in reviews of epidemiological, experimental human, and preclinical studies in various animal species. A decade ago, a survey of alcohol effects on animal aggression prompted the conclusion that alcohol is *not* a potent aggression-stimulating drug (e.g., ref. 13). Of course, this conclusion needs to be contrasted with the conclusion that alcohol does indeed cause aggression, based on a meta-analysis of human experimental studies[14] and on the overwhelming epidemiological findings (see Chapters 1 and 2, this volume). How can one explain these seemingly contradictory conclusions? It is difficult to accept the notion that animal studies on alcohol and aggression may not be informative on the human condition.

As in humans, alcohol affects aggressive behavior patterns in individual animals ranging in species from fish to nonhuman primates that differ from other individuals in terms of the direction and magnitude of effect. In addition to the critical alcohol parameters such as dose and time course, it has become apparent that environmental and behavioral determinants are of paramount significance in whether or not alcohol enhances aggressive behavior (e.g., refs. 3,4,15). When Siamese fighting fish or Cichlid fish confront a territorial intruder, when isolated male mice encounter another male mouse, when dogs or rats compete with a rival, when a resident rat opposes an intruder into the colony, when a dominant squirrel monkey or macaque threatens a rival, the administration of low acute doses of alcohol has been reported to *increase* these aggressive behaviors (e.g., refs. 16–30). These findings appear robust and impressive on account of their repeated demonstration in a wide range of animal species, yet only *suppressive* effects of alcohol on aggressive behavior were reported in several other studies with mice, rats, and monkeys (e.g., refs. 31–41). These contrasting effects appear particularly perplexing since the parameters of alcohol administration and the animal species are closely similar in reports of increased and decreased aggression. One source for these apparent inconsistencies derives from the practice of assigning subjects in experimental studies randomly to treatment groups and to schedule experimental treatments in a systematically varied sequence. In fact, most research samples of subjects contain individuals that show qualitatively opposite effects of alcohol on aggressive behavior, and pooling data from individuals with divergent effects prompts the conclusion that lower alcohol doses do not exert reliable effects on aggressive behavior.

During the past decade, studies with random-bred Swiss-Webster mice and hooded rats of the Long-Evans strain revealed that approximately 15–25% of the animals engage in significantly more aggressive behavior after being given low acute alcohol doses than they exhibit under drug-free conditions.[42,43] During the past two decades, appropriate laboratory procedures have been developed that engender a behavioral repertoire of agonistic behavior in rats and mice that represents all salient elements characteristic of the colonial cohesive social behavior in rats and dispersed territorial behavior of mice.[44,45] When given the opportunity to mark the boundaries of a specific locale and to establish residence, adult male mice and about two thirds of adult male rats of most common laboratory strains will investigate, pursue, threaten, and attack an adult intruder in a species-typical manner.[46–49] Intruder mice and rats may initially retaliate, then attempt to escape, and engage in defensive responses, and when escape is barred, mice will display a characteristic upright defeat posture or, alternatively, rats display a submissive supine posture.[50]

Quantitative ethological methods provide the means to adequately measure alcohol effects on the initiation, execution, and termination of aggressive interactions in terms of frequency, duration, and temporal and sequential pattern. These methods have supplanted the earlier used rating scales of "aggressiveness" or "aggressivity" and simple tallies of whether or not animals were fighting.[3] With the aid of microprocessor-based encoding programs, each behavioral element such as acts, postures, displays, and vocal signals during a confrontation between a resident and an intruder or between social rivals can be measured accurately and precisely in terms of initiation and termination (e.g., refs. 42,51).

Alcohol, when given in low acute doses, increased aggressive behavior by resident rats and mice confronting an intruding opponent. These aggression-heightening effects of alcohol were large and repeatable, but limited to a subgroup of individuals.[42,43] As illustrated in Fig. 1, the alcohol dose–effect curves for the entire population contained those for two subgroups that had qualitatively different types of alcohol effects on aggressive behavior both in rats and in mice. The highest proportion of mice and rats exhibiting heightened aggressive behavior was seen after administration of 1.0 g/kg ethanol, by mouth; typically this subgroup [alcohol-heightened aggression (AHA)] represents a quarter of animals in any given sample. Several behavioral elements of aggressive behavior, most prominently attack bites and sideways threats, are more frequent after alcohol administration, whereas in alcohol-suppressed animals (ASA) these behaviors are significantly decreased. When alcohol and water vehicle are administered over the course of alternating test days, the frequency of attack bites is significantly increased repeatedly in each individual mouse and rat of the AHA subgroups after the alcohol administration (Fig. 2). Whether the heightened aggression after alcohol is a phasic, spikelike phenomenon or a consistent characteristic for a specific individual has to await more detailed long-term analysis. Preliminary observations have not revealed any evidence for tolerance or sensitization to the aggression-heightening effects of alcohol.

Aggressive acts belong to those behavioral and biological functions that occur in an episodic fashion. In addition to seasonal peaks and troughs, a microanalysis of the temporal organization of aggressive behavior reveals bursts or epochs of rapidly succeeding aggressive acts that are separated by long gaps between bursts. Figure 3 depicts an event record of consecutive aggressive acts by a resident rat confronting an intruder and, in addition, summarizes more than 20,000 intervals between consecutive aggressive acts in a log-survivor plot. It is apparent that more than 85% of all aggressive acts are separated by very short intervals, i.e., they constitute aggressive bursts,

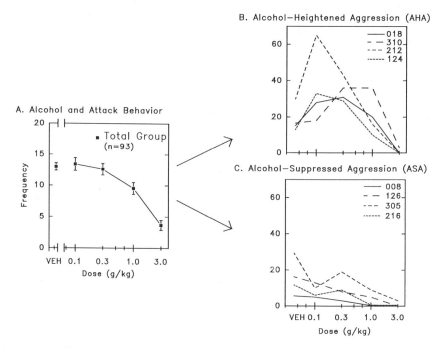

Figure 1. Effects of alcohol on frequency of attacks. (A) Alcohol dose–effect curve for the total population ($n = 93$). (B) Four selected individual alcohol dose–effect curves showing increases in attack frequency at several alcohol doses. (C) Four selected individual alcohol dose–effect curves showing suppression of attack behavior at all alcohol doses. (Data in part from Miczek et al.[42])

and the remaining intervals represent the gaps between aggressive bursts. In experimentally conducted resident–intruder confrontations, administration of alcohol to the resident aggressive animals lengthened the burst of aggressive behavior without affecting the latency to initiate nor the gaps between consecutive bursts (Fig. 4). At a behavioral level of analysis, prolonged aggressive bursts may be due to alcohol rendering the individual impaired in terminating highly energy-demanding exertions, diverting important energies from other behavioral demands, and unable to recognize signals of submission and appeasement.

By contrast to the effects on the burstlike characteristics of aggressive behavior, administration of alcohol did not modulate the intricate sequential organization of aggressive behavior in resident–intruder confrontations. As depicted in Fig. 5, a lag sequential analysis of the salient elements of aggressive behavior by resident rats reveals a sequence of the elements "pursuit" → "sideways threat" → "attack bite" → "aggressive posture" that is two to four times more probable than chance. Neither low, activating doses of ethanol nor higher sedating doses altered this high-probability sequence of behavioral

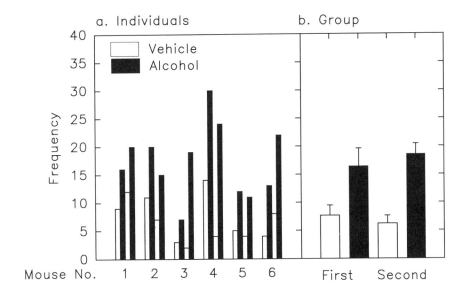

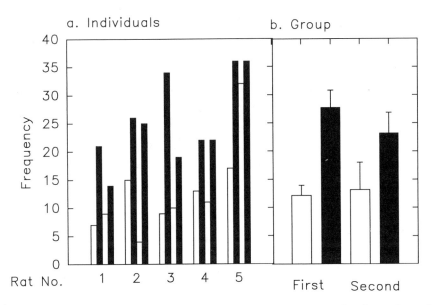

Figure 2. A subgroup of rats ($n = 5$) and mice ($n = 6$) that showed enhanced attack bites upon repeated administration of alcohol. (Top) All mice received 1.0 g/kg alcohol in both tests. (Bottom) Rats no. 1, 2, and 4 showed peak effects at 0.1 g/kg alcohol, and rats no. 3 and 5 showed peak effects at 0.3 g/kg alcohol. (a) Individual alcohol and vehicle tests. (b) Group means for first and second administration of peak aggression-heightening dose of alcohol. (Data in part from Miczek *et al.*[42])

A. Time Line

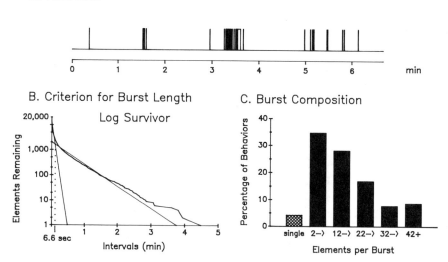

B. Criterion for Burst Length   C. Burst Composition

Figure 3. Temporal analysis of aggressive behavior. (A) The start and end times of all elements of aggressive behavior (pursuit, sideways threat, attack bite, aggressive posture) by a resident rat directed toward an intruder in real time during a selected confrontation. Each behavioral event is depicted as an upward deflection from the time line. (B) Burst criterion. Log survivor plot of all intervals between consecutive occurrences of aggressive behavior as a function of interval size. Note the logarithmic scale on the y-axis. Regression lines are fitted against the steep and flat portions of the data curve. The intersection of the two regression lines defines the maximal interval size that is considered to be part of a "burst." The burst criterion in the present studies was 6.6 seconds. (C) Definition of "burster." The ratio between behavioral elements within an aggressive bursts (i.e., within 6.6 seconds or less since a previous aggressive element) to those elements outside of the burst criterion. Ratios that are smaller than 10 identify 77 out of 389 5-min confrontations with the least clear burst characteristics. (Miczek *et al.*[42])

elements in a burst. It is most remarkable that individuals who fight at a rate more than twice than normal or who are barely capable of fighting emit aggressive behavior in a sequentially organized fashion.

In primates, individual differences in the effects of alcohol on aggression have become apparent in studies with multigenerational groups of squirrel monkeys (Fig. 6). Acute alcohol doses increase a dominant monkey's aggressive behavior toward rivals within the social group as well as from unfamiliar groups; however, this effect is not seen in lower-ranking group members.[10,29,30,52,53] The aggression-heightening effects extend behaviorally from dominance displays such as bipedal stances and shaking of branches to threats in the form of chin thrusts and genital displays as well as aggressive vocalizations.[9,10] Increases in aggressive behavior after alcohol did not de-

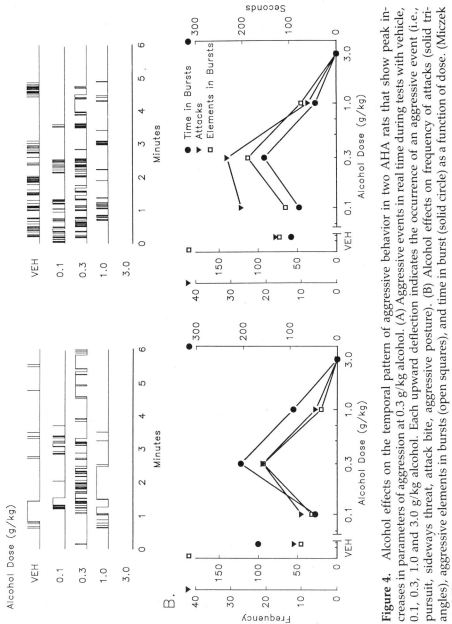

Figure 4. Alcohol effects on the temporal pattern of aggressive behavior in two AHA rats that show peak increases in parameters of aggression at 0.3 g/kg alcohol. (A) Aggressive events in real time during tests with vehicle, 0.1, 0.3, 1.0 and 3.0 g/kg alcohol. Each upward deflection indicates the occurrence of an aggressive event (i.e., pursuit, sideways threat, attack bite, aggressive posture). (B) Alcohol effects on frequency of attacks (solid triangles), aggressive elements in bursts (open squares), and time in burst (solid circle) as a function of dose. (Miczek et al.[42])

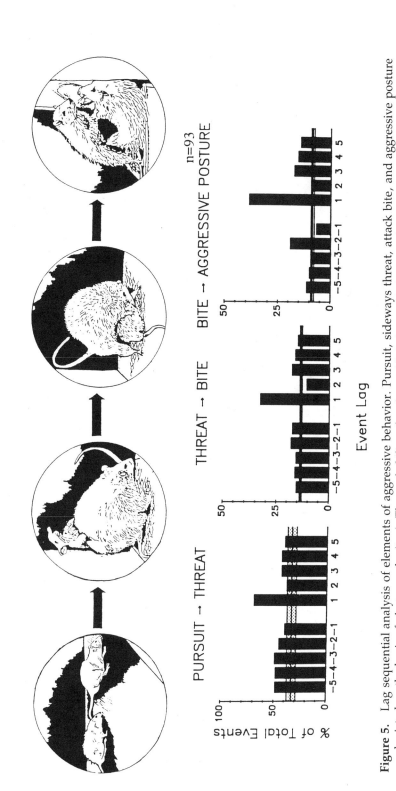

Figure 5. Lag sequential analysis of elements of aggressive behavior. Pursuit, sideways threat, attack bite, and aggressive posture are depicted on the basis of photographs (top). The probability of each specific behavioral element following (lag +1, +2 . . . +n) and preceding (lag −1, −2 . . . −n) as the first, second, third, fourth, and fifth next behavioral element is shown with the expected level of random sequence (stipled horizontal lines). Each probability is determined according to the rate of its occurrence. Specifically, the expected mean of the transition from pursuit to threat is 33.0 + 4.4% (mean + 95% confidence levels), while the actual occurrence of this transition at lag 1 is 68.8%; the expected mean of the transition from pursuit to threat at lag 1 is 13.3 + 0.6%, while the actual occurrence at lag 1 is 32.6%; the expected mean of the transition from threat to attack bites is 13.3 + 0.6%, while the actual occurrence at lag 1 is 32.6%; the expected mean of the transition from threat to attack bites to aggressive posture is 8.4 + 0.8%, while the actual occurrence at lag 1 is 38.5%. (Miczek et al.[42])

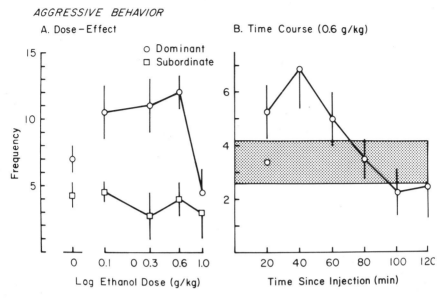

Figure 6.   (A) The frequency of aggressive behavior (grasps, display, displacements) during the 40-min period starting 5 min after alcohol administration to dominant ($n =$ 5) and subordinate ($n = 6$) members of groups of captive, free-ranging squirrel monkeys. Vertical lines in each data point indicate ±SEM. (B) The frequency of aggressive behaviors measured in consecutive 20-min segments of a 2-hr observation. The data represent the effects of 0.6 g/kg alcohol on the aggressive behavior of dominant male squirrel monkeys ($n = 5$). The shaded area represents the mean ± 1 SEM of five water vehicle control tests for each of the five dominant monkeys. (Reprinted from Winslow and Miczek[30])

pend on the baseline rate of this behavior in a particular individual monkey; as a matter of fact, the very low level of aggressive displays in subordinate monkeys failed to be "disinhibited" by alcohol, whereas the markedly higher rates of dominant monkeys were even further increased by alcohol. Pharmacologically, the aggression-heightening effects are seen at low acute ethanol doses (0.3, 0.5, 0.6 g/kg, by mouth), and these effects are critically determined by the circulating levels of testosterone.[30]

An intriguing question traces the source for the social-status-dependent alcohol effects in squirrel monkeys and in rats. At present, it is unclear at which developmental stage alcohol begins to engender aggression-heightening effects and whether these effects are a life-long characteristic. It is possible that dominant monkeys or resident rats acquire the sensitivity to the aggression-heightening effects of alcohol by repeated experiences with aggressive encounters and by repeated exposures to alcohol. If in fact distinctive experiential factors are critical for the aggression-heightening effects of alcohol, then it appears feasible to identify such decisive events in the natal group and in the postpubertal period.

2.2. Animal Models of Alcohol Self-Administration and Aggression

As illustrated in the preceding account, a major advantage of experimental research on the determinants of the link between alcohol and aggression is the control over the precise pharmacological conditions of alcohol. This is traditionally accomplished by administering alcohol at a specific dose and time. Of course, it is evident from the epidemiological statistics of violent and aggressive behavior that these acts are committed by alcohol-intoxicated individuals who have self-administered the drug; this route of administration needs to be implemented in laboratory studies in order to enhance the validity of experimental protocols. During the last decade, experimental preparations have been developed that achieve voluntary intake of alcohol at intoxicating doses, in both primate and rodent species (e.g., refs. 54,63,73,164). The application of these methodologies enables a detailed analysis of the conditions under which alcohol self-administration may lead to increased aggressive behavior and, vice versa, how situations of social confrontation influence alcohol self-administration.

Historically, the first approach to the study of social factors on alcohol self-administration has been to alter experimentally the housing conditions, comparing alcohol self-administration in singly housed versus pair- or group-housed animals. In general, individually housed rats have been shown to drink more than group-housed counterparts.[55–57] Yet, social factors have also been shown to increase alcohol self-administration. For example, Randall and Lester[58] speculated that "social facilitation" or "peer pressure" might explain why DBA mice, which usually avoid alcohol, consume significantly more of a 10% alcohol solution when housed with C57BL mice, which drink alcohol more readily. Similarly, cats drink more of a 10% alcohol–milk solution in the presence of a companion than when singly housed.[59] Unfortunately, often the past and present social behavior of alcohol-drinking group members is not assessed, rendering conclusions as to the impact of social housing and dominance status uncertain,[60–62] whereas the effect of alcohol directly on aggressive behavior was not studied at all.

Studies in primates are even more scarce, chiefly due to difficulties in implementing alcohol self-administration in primate colonies. For instance, Crowley and Andrews[63] investigated alcohol self-administration in macaques, but did not find a correlation between social status and alcohol consumption. In this valiant effort to induce alcoholiclike drinking, blood alcohol concentrations (BACs) in excess of 100 mg/dl were achieved only when food access was scheduled after alcohol availability. Curiously, no ill effects such as wounding or increased aggression were noted in alcohol drinking individuals. Interestingly, Ervin et al.[64] reported increased orientation to external stimuli, increased incidence of "stereotyped aggression," and decreased frequency of affiliative behaviors in stable social groups of vervet monkeys during periods of alcohol availability as compared to control periods. Stereotyped aggression was defined as aggressive overtures, including threats, slapping at, and physical displacement, which were neither responded to nor followed up by the instigator. Alcohol was presented in increasing concentrations from 7.5 to 20% in a 3% sucrose solution. It appeared that young animals drank more than older ones, whereas neither sexually mature males nor dominant females drank substantial quantities of alcohol. Unfortunately, no blood alcohol concentrations after self-administration were measured; however, 20–25% of alcohol-preferring animals were reported to drink occasionally to ataxia, while 5–8% drank to unconsciousness on at least one occasion. In another study, the effects of rearing conditions on alcohol self-administration in rhesus monkeys were established.[65] Monkeys that were reared among peers drank significantly more of an aspartame-sweetened 7% alcohol solution than monkeys reared with their mothers. Social isolation increased the level of alcohol consumption in mother-reared monkeys up to a similar level as peer-reared monkeys. Most monkeys were reported to drink alcohol in sufficient quantities to demonstrate signs of intoxication with ataxia, sway, and vomiting; BACs measured after intubation with a similar quantity as self-administered on the day of greatest intake ranged from about 40 to 380 mg/dl, with a mean BAC of about 275 mg/dl. In sum, these studies show that alcohol self-administration can be implemented in group-housed primate species; however, the effect of social housing and dominance status on self-administration or aggressive behavior remains unclear.

Other studies in rats tried to delineate a possible link between dominance status and alcohol self-administration. For instance, Ellison and co-workers[66] found that a larger proportion of individuals that had lived in large single-sex rat colonies under conditions of abundant and varied food consumed 10% alcohol in preference over water, as compared to single housed animals. Notably, these increases in alcohol self-administration were observed in a subpopulation of individuals, many of whom appeared to be less dominant within the colony.[67] In concordance with this observation, it was shown that subordinate group members in male–female rat colonies lapped at bottles containing 4 and 8% alcohol more often than dominant group members, and females did so more often than males.[68] Although both studies in rat colonies addressed the effect of dominance status on alcohol self-administration, they did not provide actual blood alcohol concentrations, which renders conclusions about individual alcohol intake somewhat tentative. Still, these observations suggest that lower-ranking individuals, who are often the recipients of aggression, are more likely to increase alcohol consumption than the individuals displaying aggressive behavior. However, the timing of self-administration with respect to the experience of "social stress" appears to be of crucial importance, as many studies have shown that exposure to stress (e.g., foot shock, restraint, or social stress) reduces alcohol self-administration during and immediately following stress, and increases in alcohol intake are only observed after termination of the stress period (e.g., refs. 69–71; van Erp *et al.*, submitted).

Recently, methodological advances have allowed a more systematic investigation of orally self-administered alcohol on aggressive behavior in animals[72] (van Erp *et al.*, submitted). The key developments are (1) the induction of concentration-dependent oral alcohol self-administration in laboratory rats under conditions that preserve the social structure and that avoid body weight reductions, and (2) the induction of aggressive behavior in laboratory rats that is very similar to the behavioral repertoire seen by the feral counterparts. Under the present conditions, male Long-Evans rats, each housed with a female, attacked a male intruder in their home cage during 5-min confrontations.[49] After establishing a baseline of reliable aggressive behavior toward intruders during repeated confrontations over the course of several weeks, "resident" rats were conditioned to drink a 10% alcohol solution during a daily 15-min access period in their home cage, using a sucrose substitution technique.[73] After ethanol intake stabilized for approximately 10 days, the resident rats confronted an intruder twice per week, 5 min after consuming alcohol. Behavioral data from confrontations that followed alcohol self-administration were grouped according to the BAC, as measured in samples that were taken immediately after the confrontation. The contemporary control level of aggressive behavior for a specific individual animal was assessed during confrontations with an intruder that were scheduled before or more than 3 hr after the ethanol access period, i.e., at a time when no BAC was detectable.

Under these conditions, resident rats drank up to 1.0 g/kg during the daily 15-min access period, resulting most often in BAC levels of 20–40 mg/dl with a range of 10–80 mg/dl. As discussed above, earlier studies had found aggression-heightening effects at lower acute ethanol doses, the focus was on the ascending limb of the ethanol dose–effect curve, and neither intoxication nor sedation were seen. As seen previously with experimenter-administered ethanol,[42] aggressive behavior increased after ethanol self-administration in certain individuals and remained unchanged in others (van Erp *et al.*, submitted). The magnitude of the increase in the frequency and duration of attacks and threats ranged from 40 to 90% above the control level (see Fig. 7). It is evident that individual differences in the effect of alcohol on aggressive behavior can be studied in rats, using limited-access self-administration and short-term aggressive confrontations. Although the overall group does not show an effect of alcohol on aggressive behavior, it appears that there is a subgroup of individuals that shows enhanced aggression after alcohol self-administration.

In sum, effects of alcohol on aggressive behavior have been studied in rodent and primate species using alcohol self-administration. Social factors under certain conditions may enhance alcohol self-administration and, vice versa, alcohol has been shown to enhance aggressive behavior in a sub-

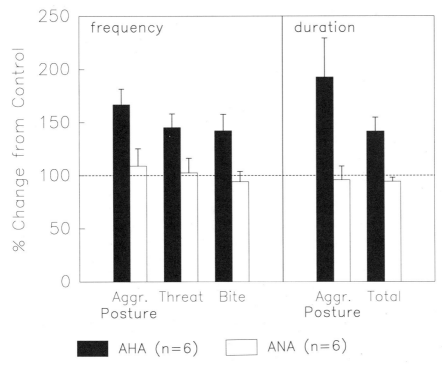

Figure 7.   Alcohol's effect on aggressive behavior in resident rats. Rats were assigned to the alcohol-enhanced aggression (AHA) group ($n = 6$) or the alcohol-nonenhanced aggression (ANA) group ($n = 6$), based on individual behavior during intruder confrontations with and without alcohol self-administration preceding the confrontation. Data are expressed as percentage change of control (confrontations without alcohol). The AHA group significantly differs from the ANA group for all the behaviors shown (frequency of aggressive posture/on top, sideways threat and bite; duration of aggressive posture/on top and total time spent on aggression). Data were analyzed with a one way analysis of variance ($P < 0.05$).

population of individuals. The most useful information derives from studies that establish self-administration in group-housed individuals, while monitoring individual alcohol intake and BACs. In addition, it is important to simultaneously assess social interactions between individuals in these groups and identify hierarchies and dominance status, in order to determine the effect of social factors on alcohol self-administration. Integrating these essential pharmacological and ethological features is bound to yield the most valid information on the interaction between aggression and alcohol self-administration. In identifying individuals who are more prone to increased alcohol intake and to increased aggression after alcohol intake, it is possible to assess pharmacological and neurochemical differences between these individuals and those that are not prone to those effects.

3. Pharmacological Evidence for Interactions between Alcohol and γ-Aminobutyric Acid-A Receptors and Aggression

3.1. Benzodiazepine Receptor

Several of alcohol's behavioral effects are linked to its action on subtypes of serotonin (5-HT), N-methyl-D-aspartate (NMDA), and γ-aminobutyric acid (GABA) receptors (e.g., refs. 74–76). Alcohol has been shown to potentiate behavioral, electrophysiological, and biochemical GABAergic responses.[77] Here, we focus on the GABA$_A$–benzodiazepine receptor complex as a site of action for alcohol in modulating aggressive behavior. Benzodiazepines, which are allosteric modulators of this complex, and alcohol share similar anxiolytic, amnesic, hypnotic, sedative, anticonvulsant, and ataxic effects. Further evidence linking ethanol and GABA$_A$ comes from studies showing that pharmacological blockade of the benzodiazepine site on the GABA$_A$–benzodiazepine receptor complex can antagonize several of ethanol's physiological, behavioral,[78–80] and neurochemical effects (e.g., refs. 81,82). In terms of aggression, mice that were selectively bred for high or low levels of aggressive behavior could be further differentiated by divergent GABA-dependent chloride uptake into cortical neurons, benzodiazepine receptor binding, and behavioral effects of chlordiazepoxide treatment.[83]

3.1.1. Effects of Alcohol on Aggression as Compared to Those of Benzodiazepine Agonists. A closely similar behavioral profile of effects by benzodiazepine receptor agonists and alcohol suggests, at least indirectly, potentially shared mechanisms for aggression-modulating effects (e.g., ref. 84). In the first decade of benzodiazepine research, alcohol and benzodiazepines were shown to reduce aggressive behavior, mostly due to their sedative and motor incoordinating properties at intermediate to higher doses in many animal species.[85–88] This evidence supported the characterization of benzodiazepines as antiaggressive drugs that could "tame" even feral animals.

Exploring a wider dose range, both chlordiazepoxide and diazepam, on the one hand, and alcohol on the other were found to share biphasic effects on aggressive behavior, with higher doses decreasing the frequency of threats and attacks and lower doses increasing these behaviors (e.g., refs. 19,21,89,90). For example, during confrontations between a resident and an intruder in rats and mice, the frequency of pursuits, attack bites, threatening acts, and postures was increased following administration of low acute alcohol doses ranging from 0.3 to 1.0 g/kg orally, while doses above 1.7 g/kg decreased these behaviors as well as prolonged inactivity (see Fig. 10).[21,53,91] Similarly, low doses of chlordiazepoxide (<10 mg/kg) and diazepam (0.3 mg/kg) increase the frequency of several behavioral elements of the aggressive repertoire, and higher doses have suppressive effects on these acts and postures as well as on all active elements of motor activity.[90,92]

However, not all benzodiazepine receptor agonists engender identical profiles of effects on aggressive, defensive, flight, and social behavior in rodents or primates, including humans. Alprazolam or oxazepam, two deschloro-phenyl derivatives, seem to be more selective in their reduction in defensive and escape activities and also in their antiaggressive effects in mice (e.g., ref. 92). This selective antiaggressive effect of alprazolam (>0.3 mg/kg, intraperitoneal) was confirmed in resident mice tested in an experimental protocol[93] that was designed to dissociate between effects on conditioned performance and aggressive behavior following the same drug treatment. Moreover, the same mice showed large increases in aggressive behavior after administration of low acute alcohol doses (e.g., 1.0 g/kg, orally).[43]

Recently, a comparison of the effects of chlordiazepoxide (0.3–10 mg/kg) and alcohol (0.1–1.0 g/kg) on vocalizations and threat displays during aggressive confrontations between rival dominant male squirrel monkeys showed a similar result. As illustrated in Fig. 8, threat peeps, the most prominent squirrel monkey call in social contexts, and aggressive displays such as genital threats, bipedal stances, and branch shakes were increased by low doses of alcohol and chlordiazepoxide.[10] Aggressive displays were in turn reduced by the moderate-to-high ataxic alcohol doses, but neither alcohol nor chlordiazepoxide reduced aggressive vocalizations in this behaviorally demanding situation.

These similar effects of alcohol and benzodiazepines on offensive-type aggressive behavior in different species may suggest shared mechanisms of action between these drugs. In order to test this possibility, it would be necessary to systematically investigate the interactions between alcohol and various types of benzodiazepine receptor agonists for their mutually potentiating effects on aggressive behavior. In male resident mice confronting an intruder, alcohol or chlordiazepoxide had no significant effects on aggressive behavior in nonsedative doses.[21] However, when attack rates were suppressed by conducting the agonistic confrontation in a neutral cage, a low dose of alcohol (0.3 g/kg orally) more than doubled the frequency of attacks and threats. In this latter condition, alcohol's proaggressive effect was further enhanced by chlordiazepoxide (5.0 mg/kg orally) pretreatment. These observations, if substantiated by systematic leftward shifts in the alcohol dose–effect curve, would in fact be consistent with the proposal of a common site of action for the aggression-heightening effects of alcohol and benzodiazepines.

3.1.2. Interactions with Benzodiazepine Receptor Antagonists.

More direct support for the GABA$_A$–benzodiazepine receptor complex as a site of action for alcohol's aggression-heightening effects can be accrued from studies with benzodiazepine receptor antagonists.[53] The rate of several aggressive acts and postures of dominant squirrel monkeys and resident male rats during the dyadic confrontations described above increases after administration of low

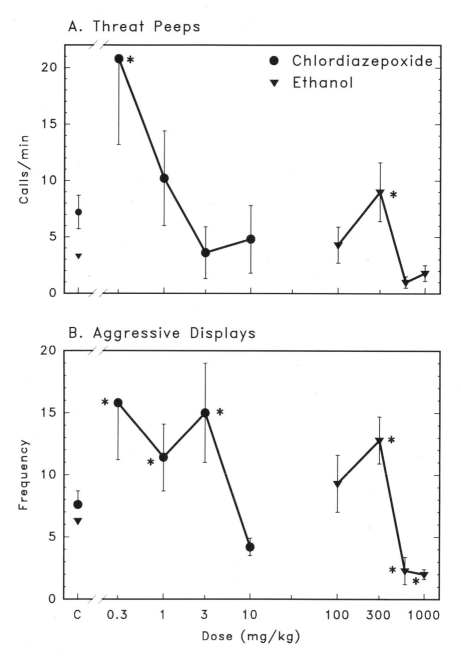

Figure 8. Effects of chlordiazepoxide and ethyl alcohol on (A) rate of threat peeps during the first minute of aggressive confrontations (B) frequency of aggressive behaviors. Asterisk indicate significant ($P < 0.05$) differences when compared to vehicle control. (Reprinted with permission from Weerts *et al.*[10])

acute alcohol doses (0.1–0.3 g/kg, orally). In a series of experiments, the alcohol dose–effect curves were redetermined after rats and monkeys were pretreated with one of two benzodiazepine receptor antagonists, ZK 93426 (3 mg/kg) or flumazenil (10 mg/kg). Figure 9 illustrates that both antagonists, the imidazobenzodiazepine as well as the β-carboline derivative, selectively prevented the aggression-heightening effects of lower alcohol doses, without having an effect on the aggression-decreasing and sedative effects of higher alcohol doses.

However, quantitative ethological analysis of the salient elements in the behavioral repertoire of socially housed squirrel monkeys revealed subtle differences in the way both benzodiazepine receptor antagonists modulated the sedative and motor-incoordinating effects of alcohol. Flumazenil, given before low alcohol doses (0.1–0.3 g/kg), actually decreased active locomotion and increased inactive postures to the low levels that are typically seen after higher alcohol doses (1.5 g/kg).[53] Flumazenil administration before high alcohol doses (1.5 g/kg) did not antagonize the characteristic motor incoordination, as measured by the incidence of staggering, but further intensified these effects. By contrast, ZK 93426 pretreatment prevented motor incoordination by higher alcohol doses. These data suggest a remarkably specific antagonism of alcohol's aggression-heightening effects, as distinct from other behavioral, i.e., sedative or motor-incoordinating effects, by the two benzodiazepine receptor antagonists.

The intrinsic effects of benzodiazepine receptor antagonists are of considerable interest in the interpretation of the interactive effects between alcohol and these substances. In a primate species such as squirrel monkeys that is particularly sensitive to the effects of GABA$_A$–benzodiazepine receptor manipulations, it is apparent that benzodiazepine receptor antagonists can engender readily behavioral effects such as increased food intake or decreased social interactions that have been interpreted to reflect either "anxiolytic" or "anxiogenic" properties.[94] Specific doses of ZK 93426 and flumazenil can decrease aggressive and social behavior in rats and in squirrel monkeys.[94–98] For example, higher doses of flumazenil (10 mg/kg) reduced isolation-induced aggression in mice, suggesting a partial benzodiazepine agonistlike activity of the compound.[99] Considering the continuously ongoing regulation of the GABA$_A$–benzodiazepine receptor complex by endogenous and exogenous factors, it may not be at all surprising that antagonist drugs can produce effects that are either similar to partial agonist or partial inverse agonist substances. These observations caution against any simple modulation of alcohol effects on aggressive behavior by benzodiazepine receptor antagonist.

3.1.3. Interactions with Partial Benzodiazepine Agonists. The benzodiazepine receptor partial inverse agonist Ro15-4513, introduced in the mid-1980s, has been studied for its prevention or reversal of physiological and behavioral alcohol effects.[100] Alcohol's sedative, ataxic, muscle relaxant, and hypnotic effects were demonstrated to be at least partially and transiently reduced by

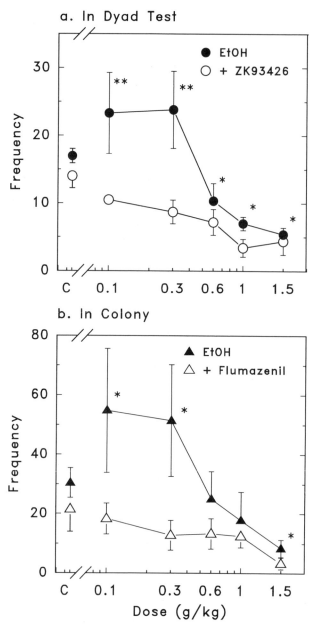

Figure 9. (A) Effects of alcohol (ETOH) and ZK 93426 (3 mg/kg) pretreatment on aggressive threats and displays in dominant male squirrel monkeys ($n = 6$) in dyadic confrontations. (B) Effects of ETOH and flumazenil (10 mg/kg) pretreatment on aggressive threats, grasps, and displays in dominant male squirrel monkeys ($n = 5$) directed toward untreated group members. * Represents $P < 0.05$ compared to vehicle control. ** Represents $P < 0.05$ compared to vehicle control and the same dose of ETOH alone. (Reprinted from Weerts et al.[53])

Ro15-4513.[78,80,101,102] Pretreatment with benzodiazepine receptor inverse agonists reduces the enhancing effects of alcohol on behavior that is suppressed by bright light[103,104] or electric shock.[103–106] Alcohol-induced reductions in exploratory motor behaviors[107,108] and social interactions between two familiar rats in a novel brightly lit arena[28] were prevented by inverse agonists. However, in attempts to antagonize the aggression-heightening effects of alcohol in squirrel monkeys, Ro15-4513 pretreatment produced tremors and seizures.[53,109] Similarly, Ro15-4513 also potentiates seizures in mice after alcohol withdrawal and leads to electrophysiological indices of seizurelike activity in rats.[110,111] The risk of inducing epileptogenic activity in a significant proportion of individuals renders benzodiazepine receptor partial inverse agonists such as Ro15-4513 unusable and the entire strategy as problematic for eventual clinical development.

In sum, there is evidence for the GABA$_A$–benzodiazepine receptor complex as a major site that differentiates highly aggressive animals from less aggressive individuals.[83] Additionally, there are data that suggest that this site is mainly involved in the potentiation or the reversal of alcohol's aggression-heightening effects by benzodiazepine agonists or antagonists, respectively.

A cautionary note is in order: the GABA$_A$–benzodiazepine receptor complex interacts with monoamines, steroids, and peptides, which in turn are influenced by many endogenous and exogenous factors. Considering the fact that alcohol does not act only at GABA$_A$ receptors, it remains to be determined if alcohol's interactions with the GABA$_A$–benzodiazepine receptor complex is the most important component of alcohol's proaggression effect.

3.2. Alcohol Interactions with Neurosteroids

3.2.1. Neurosteroids. Another class of compounds that can affect the GABA$_A$ receptor complex are certain C21 steroids. Although the genomic mechanism of steroid action mediated by intracellular receptors has been known for over 30 years,[112] recently it has been demonstrated that some steroids can act extracellularly at the GABA$_A$ receptor complex. Some of these GABA$_A$-active steroids have been found to be allosteric positive modulators of the GABA$_A$ receptor complex *in vitro*, while others are negative modulators. Among the most well documented of the positive modulators is the naturally occurring metabolite of progesterone, allopregnanolone (5α-pregnan-3α-ol-20-one). This steroid has been shown to competitively inhibit [^{35}S]t-butylbicy-clophosphorothionate (TBPS) from binding to the GABA$_A$ chloride ion channel in brain.[113–115] Additional research with rat cortical synaptoneurosomes has shown that allopregnanolone also increases the binding of the GABA$_A$ agonist [^{3}H]muscimol,[116] and nanomolar concentrations of the steroid potentiates the stimulatory effect of muscimol on ^{36}Cl$^-$ flux.[117] Moreover, this is a stereospecific effect, since its 3β isomer is inactive.[118] In addition to increasing muscimol binding, allopregnanolone enhances the binding of the benzodiazepine agonist flunitrazepam.[113,117] Another example of a steroid that positively modulates the $GABA_A$ complex is the synthetic steroid alphaxalone. This compound had been used for its anesthetic properties, but it was also one of the first steroids shown to acutely enhance [^{3}H]muscimol binding in rat brain membrane preparations.[119]

Behaviorally, steroids like allopregnanolone and alphaxalone have also been shown to share effects with other positive modulators of $GABA_A$ such as benzodiazepines, barbiturates, and ethanol. For example, they have anxiolytic,[120–124] anticonvulsant,[125] anesthetic,[126–128] and analgesic actions[129,130] when administered to rats. These effects have also been found to be quite potent. Allopregnanolone has anxiolytic effects in the elevated plus-maze[123,131] and on lick suppression,[124] at dosages of 10–20 mg/kg IP. The same dose range protects mice from pentylene tetrazole-induced seizures,[132] and loss of the righting reflex has been reported to have an ED_{50} of 1.05 mg/kg with intravenous administration.[133] The same effects are generally reduced by $GABA_A$ antagonists. For example, bicuculline reduces the analgesic effects of allopregnanolone.[134]

However, unlike with ethanol and benzodiazepines, there has been very little work on the effects of $GABA_A$-active steroids on aggression. The few papers that have appeared on this topic report effects that are consistent with the other $GABA_A$-active compounds. For example, we have found that acute administration of allopregnanolone to male mice has biphasic effects on aggression that are quite similar to those of ethanol.[135] As shown in Fig. 10, 10 mg/kg allopregnanolone was seen to increase the frequency of the salient components of male mouse aggressive behavior, while this effect disappeared at higher doses, and at 30 mg/kg, allopregnanolone reduced aggressive behavior. Such a biphasic dose–effect curve is also very similar in pattern to the behavioral responses to ethanol and to diazepam (Fig. 10). The close similarity in the dose–effect curves of these three drugs extends the proposal presented earlier in this chapter that their shared effects on the $GABA_A$ receptor complex underlies their actions on aggression.

Allopregnanolone is not the only neuroactive steroid with effects on aggression. Others have found that a negative modulator of $GABA_A$, dehydroepiandrosterone, inhibits aggression in either male or female mice toward lactating females.[136,137]

3.2.2. Interactions with Ethanol. Given that ethanol and these steroids have converging actions on the $GABA_A$–benzodiazepine receptor complex,[76] it should not be surprising that when administered jointly, the effects of either compound are altered. For example, Büküsoglu, Thalhammer, and Krieger[133] evaluated the role of the interactive effects of ethanol and allopregnanolone in a test for analgesic loss of the righting response (LRR). They found that when male albino mice were administered ethanol (0.5 and 1.1 g/kg) and allopregnanolone (0.3–3.0 mg/kg) intravenously, ethanol enhanced the steroid's analgesic effects in a dose-dependent manner. In addition, 5β-pregnan-3α-ol-20-one, another positive modulator of $GABA_A$, enhances the effects of ethanol on locomotion, body temperature, and sleep duration in mice.[138]

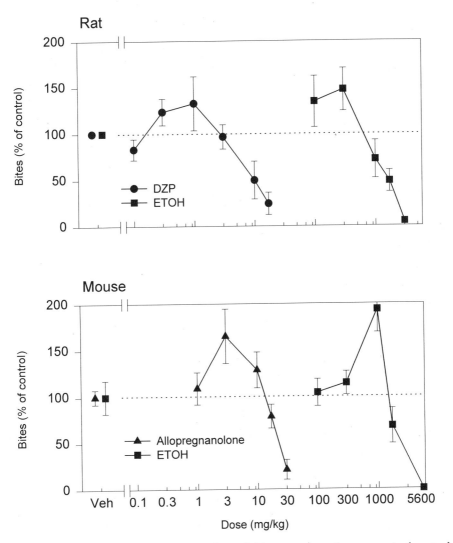

Figure 10. Changes in the frequency of attack bites, expressed as percent of control (100% = control, dashed horizontal line), as a function of dose diazepam (DZP) and ethanol (ETOH) in resident rats confronting an intruder (top), and of allopregnanolone and ethanol (ETOH) in resident mice confronting an intruder (bottom). Vertical lines in the data points indicate ± 1 SEM.

However, neuroactive steroids do not always interact with ethanol effects in ways that would be predicted based on the results of *in vitro* measures of their actions on the GABA$_A$ complex. Some of the steroids that act as negative modulators of GABA$_A$ in membrane preparations have not been found to reduce the effects of ethanol. For example, pregnenolone sulfate does not reduce the anticonvulsant or hypnotic effects of ethanol as would be predicted based on its ability to reduce the effects of GABA on Cl^- flux.[138] In fact, pregnenolone sulfate actually enhances ethanol-induced hypothermia. Another negative modulator of $GABA_A$, dehydroepiandrosterone sulfate, has also been reported to enhance ethanol-induced hypothermia.[139] Some of these unexpected effects may be due to *in vivo* metabolic conversion of the administered steroid into another steroid form with different activities. Rapid metabolism of neuroactive steroids to less active forms has also been used to explain the far greater analgesic potency of intraventricularly administered allopregnanolone in comparison to peripheral administration.[140] In addition, some of the steroids that are negative modulators of $GABA_A$ also interact with other neurotransmitter receptors. For example, pregnenolone sulfate has been shown to potentiate NMDA-mediated cellular responses *in vitro*[141,142] and to affect glycine receptors.[143] Ethanol can also alter these receptors in at least some neurons,[144] but it is less clear if these are the same neurons that are responsive to pregnenolone sulfate. These additional effects may complicate the behavioral outcome of modulating alcohol effects by neuroactive steroids.

4. Neurochemical Mechanisms for Alcohol–$GABA_A$ Interactions and Aggression

Ideally, evidence for a critical role of $GABA_A$ receptors in the aggression-heightening effects of alcohol should be derived from direct measurements of $GABA_A$ receptor functions in individuals who exhibit increased aggressive behavior while under the influence of alcohol. Unfortunately, such data are currently not available, and the role of $GABA_A$ receptors has to be inferred from studies that (1) demonstrate alcohol actions on these receptors at relevant doses, (2) implicate GABA in the regulation of relevant aggressive behavior patterns, and (3) correlate alcohol effects on aggressive behavior with those of the effects of modulators and direct agonists and antagonists at $GABA_A$ receptors.

An attractive and inviting reason for implicating $GABA_A$ receptors in the actions of alcohol is the evidence demonstrating chloride flux changes due to alcohol in cortical synaptosomes at nanomolar concentrations that may correspond to the oral doses that increase aggressive behavior.[78,145-147] So far, it is not clear whether or not individual differences in the *in vitro* chloride flux measurements at increasing alcohol concentrations actually exist and whether such differences would be relevant to the aggression-heightening effects. However, consistent with such reasoning is evidence from mice that were selected to be highly aggressive and that differ from those that were selected for a low level of aggressive behavior in several neurochemical systems,[148] most notably in muscimol-activated chloride flux in cortical tissue.[83]

As the two most apparent alternative possibilities, one can conceptualize the $GABA_A$ receptors as being either in parallel with several concurrently activated receptors or as the initiation site for a cascade of subsequent mechanisms that are required for the aggression-heightening effects of alcohol. Pharmacological strategies have been of limited use in deciding between GABA$_A$ receptors' place in sequential or parallel models, since blockade of many receptor types can modify alcohol's behavioral effects, including those on aggressive behavior. For example, in addition to the earlier-discussed benzodiazepine receptor antagonists, antagonists at opioid, serotonergic, dopaminergic, and noradrenergic receptors can block alcohol's behavioral effects (e.g., refs. 149–151). Yet, so far, only modulators of the GABA$_A$ receptor such as benzodiazepines, barbiturates, and neuroactive steroids mimic the biphasic dose–effect function of alcohol on aggressive behavior and actually can potentiate the effects of alcohol on these types of behavior.[152] To decide whether or not modulatory sites of a subpopulation of GABA$_A$ receptors are indeed one of the critical sites for intervention in reducing alcohol-heightened aggressive behavior has to await the development of more specific pharmacological tools.

An important characteristic of the GABA$_A$ receptor complex is its protein structure, most commonly being composed of two α, two β, and one γ subunit, but there is variety in the identity of each subunit in this mix. This heterogeneity in subunit composition has pharmacological implications. For example, the γ$_{2L}$ subunit has been reported to be required for ethanol sensitivity,[153] but the identity of the α and β subunits may also affect response.[144,154] In addition, subunit composition of the GABA$_A$ receptor not only can differentially affect sensitivity to different compounds, but subunit composition also varies across brain regions.[155–157] For example, the effect of ethanol on neural activity also varies across brain regions.[158] This may have implications for the effects of ethanol on aggression. Some brain regions have been specifically implicated in particular forms of aggressive behavior in laboratory animals.[159] It is possible that regional differences in GABA$_A$ subunit composition and in ethanol, benzodiazepine, and steroid sensitivity may provide a way to refine where alcohol acts in the brain to affect aggression.

There is some evidence tracing individual differences in physiological and behavioral alcohol effects to differences in GABA$_A$ receptor activation. For example, mice that have been selected to be resistant to alcohol withdrawal seizures differ from those who are prone to these seizures in terms of binding and functional characteristics of GABA$_A$ receptors.[160] Whether or not individual differences in increased aggressive behavior after alcohol can be linked to distinctive characteristics in subpopulations of GABA$_A$ receptors remains an experimental challenge.

One of the obvious problems in manipulating directly GABA$_A$ receptors in order to alter alcohol's aggression-heightening effects is the pervasive effects on many additional behavioral and physiological functions that range from convulsive to motor disorders.[161–163] Targeting modulatory sites on certain GABA$_A$ receptors with benzodiazepines, barbiturates, and neuroactive steroids may offer a wider range of tools to modify ethanol effects on aggressive behavior with fewer side effects than direct GABA receptor interventions.

ACKNOWLEDGMENTS. The experimental research from the authors' laboratory was supported by USPHS research grants AA 05122 and DA 02632. We are grateful to Dr. H. T. Barros and J. T. Sopko for their excellent assistance.

References

1. Reiss AJ Jr, Roth JA: *Understanding and Preventing Violence*. Washington, DC, National Academy Press, 1993.
2. Miczek KA, Haney M, Tidey J, *et al:* Neurochemistry and pharmacotherapeutic management of violence and aggression, in Reiss AJ, Miczek KA, Roth JA (eds): *Understanding and Preventing Violence: Biobehavioral Influences on Violence*. Washington, DC, National Academy Press, 1994, vol 2, pp 244–514.
3. Miczek KA: The psychopharmacology of aggression, in Iversen LL, Iversen SD, Snyder SH (eds): *Handbook of Psychopharmacology*. New York, Plenum, 1987, vol 19, pp 183–328.
4. Miczek KA, DeBold JF, Haney M, *et al:* Alcohol, drugs of abuse, aggression and violence, in Reiss AJ, Roth JA (eds): *Understanding and Preventing Violence: Social Influences on Violence*. Washington, DC, National Academy Press, 1994, vol 3, pp 377–570.
5. Cherek DR, Steinberg JL, Manno BR: Effects of alcohol on human aggressive behavior. *J Stud Alcohol* 46:321–328, 1985.
6. Shuntich RJ, Taylor SP: The effects of alcohol on human physical aggression. *J Exp Res Person* 6:34–38, 1972.
7. Zeichner A, Pihl RO: Effects of alcohol and behavior contingencies on human aggression. *J Abnorm Psychol* 88:153–160, 1978.
8. Huntingford FA, Turner AK: *Animal Conflict*. London, Chapman and Hall, 1987.
9. Pedigo NW, Yamamura HI, Nelson DL: Discrimination of multiple 3H-5-hydroxytrptamine binding sites by the neuroleptic spiperone in rat brain. *J Neurochem* 36:220–226, 1981.
10. Weerts EM, Miczek KA: Primate vocalizations during social separation and aggression: Effects of alcohol and benzodiazepines. *Psychopharmacology*, 127:255–264, 1996.
11. Miczek KA, Winslow JT, DeBold JF: Heightened aggressive behavior by animals interacting with alcohol-treated conspecifics: Studies with mice, rats and squirrel monkeys. *Pharmacol Biochem Behav* 20:349–353, 1984.
12. Huntingford FA: Some ethical issues raised by studies of predation and aggression. *Anim Behav* 32:210–215, 1984.
13. Berry MS, Smoothy R: A critical evaluation of claimed relationships between alcohol intake and aggression in infra-human animals, in Brain PF (ed): *Alcohol and Aggression*. London, Croom Helm, 1986, pp 84–137.
14. Bushman BJ, Cooper HM: Effects of alcohol on human aggression: Integrative research review. *Psychol B* 107:341–354, 1990.
15. Cherek DR, Steinberg JL: Effects of drugs on human aggressive behavior, in Burrows GD, Werry JS (eds): *Advances in Human Psychopharmacology*. Greenwich, CN, JAI Press, 1987, vol 4, pp 239–290.
16. Raynes AE, Ryback RS: Effect of alcohol and congeners on aggressive response in Betta splendens. *Q J Stud Alcohol* 5:130–135, 1970.
17. Ellman GL, Herz MJ, Peeke HVS: Ethanol in a cichlid fish: Blood levels and aggressive behavior. *Proc West Pharmacol Soc* 15:92–95, 1972.
18. Chance MRA, Mackintosh JH, Dixon AK: The effects of ethyl alcohol on social encounters between mice. *J Alcohol* 8:90–93, 1973.
19. Miczek KA, Barry H III: Effects of alcohol on attack and defensive–submissive reactions in rats. *Psychopharmacology* 52:231–237, 1977.

20. Pettijohn TF: The effects of alcohol on agonistic behavior in the Telomian dog. *Psychopharmacology* 60:295–301, 1979.
21. Miczek KA, O'Donnell JM: Alcohol and chlordiazepoxide increase suppressed aggression in mice. *Psychopharmacology* 69:39–44, 1980.
22. Peeke HVS, Cutler L, Ellman G, *et al*: Effects of alcohol, cogeners, and acetaldehyde of aggressive behavior of the convict cichlid. *Psychopharmacology* 75:245–247, 1981.
23. Yoshimura H: Pharmaco-ethological analysis of agonistic behavior between resident and intruder mice: Effects of ethyl alcohol. *Folia Pharmacol Japonica* 81:135–141, 1983.
24. DeBold JF, Miczek KA: Testosterone modulates the effects of ethanol on male mouse aggression. *Psychopharmacology* 86:286–290, 1985.
25. Blanchard RJ, Hori K, Flannelly K, Blanchard DC: The effects of ethanol on the offense and defensive behaviors of male and female rats during group formation. *Pharmacol Biochem Behav* 26:61–64, 1987.
26. Blanchard KJ, Flannelly KJ, Hori K, Blanchard DC: Ethanol effects on female aggression vary with opponent size and time within session. *Pharmacol Biochem Behav* 27:645–648, 1987.
27. Blanchard RJ, Hori K, Blanchard DC, Hall J: Ethanol effects on aggression of rats selected for different levels of aggressiveness. *Pharmacol Biochem Behav* 27:641–644, 1987.
28. Lister RG, Hilakivi LA: The effects of novelty, isolation, light and ethanol on the social behavior of mice. *Psychopharmacology* 96:181–187, 1988.
29. Winslow JT, Ellingboe J, Miczek KA: Effects of alcohol on aggressive behavior in squirrel monkeys: Influence of testosterone and social context. *Psychopharmacology* 95:356–363, 1988.
30. Winslow JT, Miczek KA: Androgen dependency of alcohol effects on aggressive behavior: A seasonal rhythm in high-ranking squirrel monkeys. *Psychopharmacology* 95:92–98, 1988.
31. Krsiak M, Borgesova M: Effect of alcohol on behaviour of pairs of rats. *Psychopharmacologia* 32:201–209, 1973.
32. Crowley TJ, Stynes AJ, Hydinger M, Kaufman IC: Ethanol, methamphetamine, pentobarbital, morphine, and monkey social behavior. *Arch Gen Psychiatry* 31:829–838, 1974.
33. Lagerspetz KMJ, Ekqvist K: Failure to induce aggression in inhibited and in genetically nonaggressive mice through injections of ethyl alcohol. *Aggressive Behav* 4:105–113, 1978.
34. Smoothy R, Bowden NJ, Berry MS: Ethanol and social behaviour in naive Swiss mice. *Aggressive Behav* 8:204–207, 1982.
35. Smoothy R, Berry MS: Effects of ethanol on behavior of aggressive mice from two different strains: A comparison of simple and complex behavioral assessments. *Pharmacol Biochem Behav* 19:645–653, 1983.
36. Smoothy R, Berry MS, Brain PF: Acute influences of ethanol on murine social aggression: Effects of dose, strain and fighting experience (Abstract). *Aggressive Behav* 9:119–120, 1983.
37. Benton D, Smoothy R: The relationship between blood alcohol levels and aggression in mice. *Physiol Behav* 33:757–760, 1984.
38. Smoothy R, Berry MS: Effects of ethanol on murine aggression assessed by biting of an inanimate target. *Psychopharmacology* 83:268–271, 1984.
39. Everill B, Berry MS: Effects of ethanol on aggression in three inbred strains of mice. *Physiol Behav* 39:45–51, 1987.
40. Berry MS: Ethanol-induced enhancement of defensive behavior in different models of murine aggression. *J Stud Alcohol* (Suppl 11):156–162, 1993.
41. Mos J, Olivier B: Differential effects of selected psychoactive drugs on dominant and subordinate male rats housed in a colony. *Neurosci Res Commun* 2:29–36, 1988.
42. Miczek KA, Weerts EM, Tornatzky W, *et al*: Alcohol and "bursts" of aggressive behavior: Ethological analysis of individual differences in rats. *Psychopharmacology* 107:551–563, 1992.
43. Wheatley MD: The hypothalamus and affective behavior in cats. *Arch Neurol Psychiatry* 52:296–316, 1944.
44. Barnett SA: *The Rat. A Study in Behavior*. Chicago, University of Chicago Press, 1975.
45. Crowcroft P: *Mice All Over*. London, Foulis, 1966.
46. Blanchard RJ, Blanchard CD: Aggressive behavior in the rat. *Behav Biol* 21:197–224, 1977.

47. Brain PF: Differentiating types of attack and defense in rodents, in Brain PF, Benton D (eds): *Multidisciplinary Approaches to Aggression Research*, Amsterdam, Elsevier, 1981, pp 53–78.

48. Miczek KA, O'Donnell JM: Intruder-evoked aggression in isolated and nonisolated mice: Effects of psychomotor stimulants and L-dopa. *Psychopharmacology* 57:47–55, 1978.

49. Miczek KA: A new test for aggression in rats without aversive stimulation: Differential effects of D-amphetamine and cocaine. *Psychopharmacology* 60:253–259, 1979.

50. Miczek KA, Thompson ML, Shuster L: Opioid-like analgesia in defeated mice. *Science* 215:1520–1522, 1982.

51. Miczek KA: Ethological analysis of drug action on aggression, defense and defeat, in Spiegelstein MY, Levy A (eds): *Behavioral Models and the Analysis of Drug Action*. Amsterdam, Elsevier, 1982, pp 225–239.

52. Winslow JT, Miczek KA: Social status as determinant of alcohol effects on aggressive behavior in squirrel monkeys (*Saimiri sciureus*). *Psychopharmacology* 85:167–172, 1985.

53. Weerts EM, Tornatzky W, Miczek KA: Prevention of the proaggressive effects of alcohol by benzodiazepine receptor antagonists in rats and in squirrel monkeys. *Psychopharmacology* 111:144–152, 1993.

54. Meisch RA, Carrol ME: *Establishment of Orally Delivered Drugs for Rhesus Monkeys: Some Relations to Human Drug Dependence*. Washington, DC, US Government Printing Office, 1981.

55. Deatherage G: Effect of housing density on alcohol intake in the rat. *Physiol Behav* 9:55–57, 1972.

56. Parker LF, Radow BL: Isolation stress and volitional ethanol consumption in the rat. *Physiol Behav* 12:1–3, 1974.

57. Wolffgramm J: Free choice ethanol intake of laboratory rats under different social conditions. *Psychopharmacology* 101:233–239, 1990.

58. Randall CL, Lester D: Social modification of alcohol consumption in inbred mice. *Science* 189:149–151, 1975.

59. Wyrwicka W, Long AM: The effect of companion on consumption of ethanol solution in cats. *Pavlovian J Biol Sci* 18:49–53, 1983.

60. Heminway DA, Furumoto L: Population density and alcohol consumption in the rat. *Q J Stud Alcohol* 33:794–799, 1972.

61. Kulkosky PJ, Zellner DA, Hyson RL, Riley AL: Ethanol consumption of rats in individual, group, and colonial housing conditions. *Physiol Psychol* 8:56–60, 1980.

62. Rockman GE, Gibson JEM: Effects of duration and timing of environmental enrichment on voluntary ethanol intake in rats. *Pharmacol Biochem Behav* 41:689–693, 1992.

63. Crowley TJ, Andrews AE: Alcoholic-like drinking in simian social groups. *Psychopharmacology* 92:196–205, 1987.

64. Ervin FR, Palmour RM, Young SN, et al: Voluntary consumption of beverage alcohol by vervet monkeys: Population screening, descriptive behavior and biochemical measures. *Pharmacol Biochem Behav* 36:367–373, 1990.

65. Higley JD, Hasert MF, Suomi SJ, Linnoila M: Nonhuman primate model of alcohol abuse– Effects of early experience, personality, and stress on alcohol consumption. *Proc Nat Acad Sci USA* 88:7261–7265, 1991.

66. Ellison G, Daniel F, Zoraster R: Delayed increases in alcohol consumption occur in rat colonies but not in isolated rats after injections of monoamine neurotoxins. *Exp Neurol* 65:608–615, 1979.

67. Ellison G: Stress and alcohol intake: The socio-pharmacological approach. *Physiol Behav* 40:387–392, 1987.

68. Blanchard RJ, Hori K, Tom P, Blanchard DC: Social structure and ethanol consumption in the laboratory rat. *Pharmacol Biochem Behav* 28:437–442, 1987.

69. Anisman H, Waller TG: Effects of inescapable shock and shock-produced conflict on self-selection of alcohol in rats. *Pharmacol Biochem Behav* 2:27–33, 1974.

70. Mills KC, Bean JW, Hutcheson JS: Shock-induced ethanol consumption in rats. *Pharmacol Biochem Behav* 6:107–115, 1977.

71. Rawleigh JM, Kushner MG, Fiszdon J, Carroll ME: The effects of restraint-stress on voluntary ethanol consumption in rats (submitted).
72. Van Erp AMM, Samson HH, Miczek KA: Alcohol self-administration, dopamine and aggression in rats. *Neurosci Abstr* 20:1614, 1994.
73. Samson HH: Initiation of ethanol reinforcement using a sucrose-substitution procedure in food- and water-sated rats. *Alcohol Clin Exp* 10:436–442, 1986.
74. Deitrich RA, Dunwiddie TV, Harris RA, Erwin VG: Mechanism of action of ethanol: Initial central nervous system actions. *Pharmacol Rev* 41:489–537, 1989.
75. Tabakoff B, Hoffman PL: Biochemical pharmacology of alcohol, in Meltzer HY (ed): *Psychopharmacology: The Third Generation of Progress*. New York, Raven Press, 1987, pp 1521–1526.
76. Lueddens H, Korpi ER: Biological function of GABA_A/benzodiazepine receptor heterogeneity. *J Psychiatr Res* 29:77–94, 1995.
77. Korpi ER: Role of GABA_A receptors in the actions of alcohol and in alcoholism: Recent advances. *Alcohol Alcoholism* 29:115–129, 1994.
78. Suzdak PD, Glowa JR, Crawley JN, *et al*: A selective imidazobenzodiazepine antagonist of ethanol in the rat. *Science* 234:1243–1247, 1986.
79. Deacon RMJ, Buddhram P, Thompson TA, Gardner CR: Differential interactions of Ro 15-4513 with benzodiazepines, ethanol and pentobarbital. *Eur J Pharmacol* 180:283–290, 1990.
80. Syapin PJ, Jones BL, Kobayashi LS, *et al*: Interactions between benzodiazepine antagonists, inverse agonists, and acute behavioral effects of ethanol in mice. *Brain Res B* 24:705–709, 1990.
81. Mehta AK, Ticku MK: Ethanol potentiation of GABAergic transmission in cultured spinal cord neurons involves gamma-aminobutyric acidA-gated chloride channels. *Journal of Pharmacology and Experimental Therapeutics* 246:558–564, 1988.
82. Harris RA, Allan AM, Daniell LC, Nixon C: Antagonism of ethanol and pentobarbital actions by benzodiazepine inverse agonists: Neurochemical studies. *Journal of Pharmacology and Experimental Therapeutics* 247:1012–1017, 1988.
83. Weerts EM, Miller LG, Hood KE, Miczek KA: Increased GABA_A-dependent chloride uptake in mice selectively bred for low aggressive behavior. *Psychopharmacology* 108:196–204, 1992.
84. Miczek KA, Krsiak M: Drug effects on agonistic behavior, in Thompson T, Dews PB (eds): *Advances in Behavioral Pharmacology*. New York, Academic Press, 1979, vol 2, pp 87–162.
85. Heise GA, Boff E: Taming action of chlordiazepoxide. *Fed Proc* 20:393, 1961.
86. Heuschele WP: Chlordiazepoxide for calming zoo animals. *J Am Vet Med Assoc* 139:996–998, 1961.
87. Christmas AJ, Maxwell DR: A comparison of the effects of some benzodiazepines and other drugs on aggressive and exploratory behaviour in mice and rats. *Neuropharmacology* 9:17–29, 1970.
88. Langfeldt T, Ursin H: Differential action of diazepam on flight and defense behavior in the cat. *Psychopharmacologia* 19:61–66, 1971.
89. Miczek KA: Intraspecies aggression in rats: Effects of D-amphetamine and chlordiazepoxide. *Psychopharmacologia* 39:275–301, 1974.
90. Olivier B, Mos J, Miczek KA: Ethopharmacological studies of anxiolytics and aggression. *Eur Neuropsychopharmacol* 1:97–100, 1991.
91. Krsiak M: Effect of ethanol on aggression and timidity in mice. *Psychopharmacology* 51:75–80, 1976.
92. Krsiak M, Sulcova A: Differential effects of six structurally related benzodiazepines on some ethological measures of timidity, aggression and locomotion in mice. *Psychopharmacology* 101:396–402, 1990.
93. Miczek KA, Haney M: Psychomotor stimulant effects of D-amphetamine, MDMA and PCP: Aggressive and schedule-controlled behavior in mice. *Psychopharmacology* 115:358–365, 1994.
94. Weerts EM, Tornatzky W, Miczek KA: "Anxiolytic" and "anxiogenic" benzodiazepines and beta-carbolines: Effects on aggressive and social behavior in rats and squirrel monkeys. *Psychopharmacology* 110:451–459, 1993.

95. Rodgers RJ, Waters AJ: Benzodiazepines and their antagonists: A pharmacoethological analysis with particular reference to effects on "aggression." *Neurosci B* 9:21–35, 1985.

96. File SE, Lister RG, Nutt DJ: The axiogenic action of benzodiazepine antagonists. *Neuropharmacology* 21:1033–1037, 1982.

97. File SE, Lister RG, Nutt DJ: Intrinsic actions of benzodiazepine antagonists. *Neurosci Lett* 32:165–168, 1982.

98. File SE, Pellow S: Intrinsic actions of the benzodiazepine receptor antagonist Ro 15-1788. *Psychopharmacology* 88:1–11, 1986.

99. Skolnick P, Reed GF, Paul SM: Benzodiazepine-receptor mediated inhibition of isolation-induced aggression in mice. *Pharmacol Biochem Behav* 23:17–20, 1985.

100. Lister RG, Nutt DJ: Alcohol antagonists—the continuing quest. *Alcohol Clin Exp Res,* 12:566–569, 1988.

101. Deacon RMJ, Guy AP, Gardner CR: Effects of selected imidazopyrimidine ligands for benzodiazepine receptors in rodent models of anxiety and behavioural impairment. *Drug Dev Res* 22:321–329, 1991.

102. Bonetti EP, Burkard WP, Gabl M, Mohler H: The partial inverse benzodiazepine agonist Ro 15-4513 antagonizes acute alcohol effects in mice and rats. *Br J Pharmacol* 86 (Suppl):463–467, 1985.

103. Belzung C, Misslin R, Vogel E: The benzodiazepine inverse agonists beta-CCM and RO 15-3505 both reverse the anxiolytic effects in mice. *Life Sci* 42:1765–1772, 1988.

104. Misslin R, Belzung C, Vogel E: Interaction of RO 15-4513 and ethanol on the behaviour of mice: Antagonistic or additive effects? *Psychopharmacology* 94:392–396, 1988.

105. Koob GF, Percy L, Britton KT: The effects of Ro 15-4513 on the behavioral actions of ethanol in an operant reaction time task and a conflict test. *Pharmacol Biochem Behav* 31:757–760, 1989.

106. Glowa JR, Crawley J, Suzdak PD, Paul SM: Ethanol and the GABA receptor complex: Studies with the partial inverse benzodiazepine receptor agonist Ro 15-4513. *Pharmacol Biochem Behav* 31:767–772, 1989.

107. Lister RG: Interactions of RO 15-4513 with diazepam, sodium pentobarbital and ethanol in a holeboard test. *Pharmacol Biochem Behav* 28:75–79, 1987.

108. Lister RG: The benzodiazepine receptor inverse agonists FG 7142 and RO 15-4513 both reverse some of the behavioral effects of ethanol in a holeboard test. *Life Sci* 41:1481–1489, 1987.

109. Bell R, Hobson H: 5-HT1a receptor influences on rodent social and agonistic behavior: A review and empirical study. *Neurosci B* 18:325–328, 1994.

110. Britton KT, Ehlers CL, Koob GF: Is ethanol antagonist Ro 15-4513 selective for ethanol? *Science* 239:648–649, 1988.

111. Lister RG, Karanian JW: RO 15-4513 induces seizures in DBA/2 mice undergoing alcohol withdrawal. *Alcohol* 4:409–411, 1987.

112. Jensen EV, Jacobsen HI: Basic guides to the mechanism of estrogen action. *Recent Prog Horm Res* 18:387–414, 1962.

113. Majewska MD, Harrison NL, Schwartz RD, et al: Steroid hormone metabolites are barbiturate-like modulators of the GABA receptor. *Science* 232:1004–1007, 1986.

114. Gee KW, Chang WC, Brinton RE, McEwen BS: GABA-dependent modulation of the Cl⁻ ionophore by steroids in rat brain. *Eur J Pharmacol* 136:419–423, 1987.

115. Gee KW, Bolger MB, Brinton RE, et al: Steroid modulation of the chloride ionophore in rat brain: Structure–activity requirements, regional difference and mechanism of action. *Journal of Pharmacology and Experimental Therapeutics* 246:803–812, 1988.

116. Lopez-Colome AM, McCarthy M, Beyer C: Enhancement of 3H-muscimol binding to brain synaptic membranes by progesterone and related pregnanes. *Eur J Pharmacol* 176:297–303, 1990.

117. Morrow AL, Suzdak PD, Paul SM: Steroid hormone metabolites potentiate GABA receptor-mediated chloride ion flux with nanomolar potency. *Eur J Pharmacol* 142:483–485, 1987.

118. Morrow AL, Pace JR, Purdy RH, Paul SM: Characterization of steroid interactions with

γ-aminobutyric acid receptor-gated chloride ion channels: Evidence for multiple steroid recognition sites. *Mol Pharmacol* 37:263–270, 1990.

119. Simmonds MA, Turner JP, Harrison NL: Interactions of steroids with the GABA-A receptor complex. *Neuropharmacology* 23:877–878, 1984.

120. Crawley JN, Glowa JR, Majewska MD, Paul SM: Anxiolytic activity of an endogenous adrenal stereoid. *Brain Res* 398:382–385, 1986.

121. Britton KT, Page M, Baldwin H, Koob GF: Anxiolytic activity of steroid anesthetic alphax-alone. *Journal of Pharmacology and Experimental Therapeutics* 258:124–129, 1991.

122. Norberg L, Wahlstrom G, Backstrom T: The anaesthetic potency of 3a-hydroxy-5a-preg-nan-20-one and 3a-hydroxy-5b-pregnan-20-one determined with an intravenous EEG-threshold method in male rats. *Pharmacol Toxicol* 61:42–47, 1987.

123. Bitran D, Hilvers RJ, Kellogg CK: Anxiolytic effects of 3a-hydroxy-5a β-pregnan-20-one: Endogenous metabolites of progesterone that are active at the GABA$_A$ receptor. *Brain Res* 561:157–161, 1991.

124. Wieland S, Lan NC, Mirasedeghi S, Gee KW: Anxiolytic activity of the progesterone metab-olite 5alpha-pregnan-3alpha-ol-20-one. *Brain Res* 565:263–268, 1991.

125. Belelli D, Gee KW: 5a-pregnan-3a,20a-diol behaves like a partial agonist in the modulation of GABA-stimulated chloride uptake by synaptoneurosomes. *Eur J Pharmacol* 167:173–176, 1989.

126. Gyermek L, Genther G, Fleming N: Some effects of progesterone and related steroids on the central nervous system. *Int J Neuropharmacol* 6:191–198, 1967.

127. Seeman P: The membrane actions of anesthetics and tranquilizers. *Pharmacol Rev* 24:583–655, 1972.

128. Kubli-Garfias C, Cervantes M, Beyer C: Changes in multiunit activity and EEG induced by the administration of natural progestins to flaxedil immobilized cats. *Brain Res* 114:71–81, 1976.

129. Mendelson WB, Martin JV, Perlis M, *et al*: Sleep induction by an adrenal steroid in the rat. *Psychopharmacology* 93:226–229, 1987.

130. Majewska MD: Actions of steroids on neuron: role in personality, mood, stress, and dis-ease. *Integr Psychol* 5:258–273, 1987.

131. Wieland S, Belluzzi JD, Stein L, Lan NC: Comparative behavioral characterization of the neuroactive steroids 3alpha-OH, 5alpha-pregnan-20-one and 3alpha-OH, 5beta-pregnan-20-one in rodents. *Psychopharmacology* 118:65–71, 1995.

132. Kokate TG, Svensson BE, Rogawski MA: Anticonvulsant activity of neurosteroids: Correla-tion with gamma-aminobutyric acid-evoked chloride current potentiation. *Journal of Phar-macology and Experimental Therapeutics* 270:1223–1229, 1994.

133. Büküsoglu C, Thalhammer JG, Krieger NR: Analgesia with anesthetic steroids and ethanol. *Anesth Analg* 77:27–31, 1993.

134. Kavaliers M, Wiebe JP: Analgesic effects of the progesterone metabolite, 3a-hydroxy-5a-pregnan-20-one and possible modes of action in mice. *Brain Res* 414:393–398, 1987.

135. DeBold JF, Barros H, So S, Miczek KA: The effects of allopregnanolone and alcohol on intramale aggression in mice. *Alcohol Clin Exp Res* 19:11A, 1995.

136. Haug M, Young J, Robel P, Baulieu EE: Neonatal testosterone administration potentiates the inhibitory effect of dehydroepiandrosterone on the display of aggression by spayed female mice towards lactating intruders. *C R Acad Sci III* 312:511–516, 1991.

137. Young J, Corpechot C, Haug M, *et al*: Suppressive effects of dehydroepiandrosterone and 3-b-methyl-androst-5-en-17-one on attack towards lactating female intruders by castrated male mice .2. Brain neurosteroids. *Biochem Biophys Res Commun* 174:892–897, 1991.

138. Melchior CL, Allen PM: Interaction of pregnanolone and pregnenolone sulfate with ethanol and pentobarbital. *Pharmacol Biochem Behav* 42:605–611, 1992.

139. Melchior CL, Ritzmann RF: Dehydroepiandrosterone enhances the hypnotic and hypother-mic effects of ethanol and pentobarbital. *Pharmacol Biochem Behav* 43:223–227, 1992.

140. Frye CA, Duncan JE: Progesterone metabolites, effective at the GABA(a) receptor complex, attenuate pain sensitivity in rats. *Brain Res* 643:194–203, 1994.

141. Wu FS, Gibbs TT, Farb DH: Pregnenolone sulfate: A positive allosteric modulator at the *n*-methyl-D-aspartate receptor. *Mol Pharmacol* 40:333–336, 1991.

142. Irwin RP, Lin S-Z, Rogawski MA, *et al:* Steroid potentiation and inhibition of N-methyl-D-aspartate receptor-mediated intracellular Ca^{++} responses: Structure-activity studies. *Journal of Pharmacology and Experimental Therapeutics* 271:677–682, 1994.

143. Farb DH, Gibbs TT, Wu FS, *et al:* Steroid modulation of amino acid neurotransmitter receptors, in Biggio G, Concas A, Costa E (eds): *GABAergic Synaptic Neurotransmission*. New York, Raven Press, 1992, pp 119–131.

144. Criswell HE, Simson PE, Duncan GE, *et al:* Molecular basis for regionally specific action of ethanol on gamma-aminobutyric acid-A receptors: Generalization to other ligand-gated ion channels. *Journal of Pharmacology and Experimental Therapeutics* 267:522–537, 1993.

145. Suzdak PD, Schwartz RD, Skolnick P, Paul SM: Ethanol stimulates gamma-aminobutyric acid receptor-mediated chloride transport in rat brain synaptoneurosomes. *Proc Natl Acad Sci USA* 83:4071–4075, 1986.

146. Allan AM, Harris RA: Gamma-aminobutyric acid and alcohol actions: Neurochemical studies of long sleep and short sleep mice. *Life Sci* 39:2005–2015, 1986.

147. Leidenheimer NJ, Harris RA: Acute effects of ethanol on GABA alpha receptor function: Molecular and physiological determinants, in Biggio G, Concas A, Costa E (eds): *GABAergic Synaptic Transmission*. New York, Raven Press, 1992, pp 269–279.

148. Lewis MH, Gariepy JL, Gendreau P, *et al:* Social reactivity and D1 dopamine receptors: Studies in mice selectively bred for high and low levels of aggression. *Neuropsychopharmacology* 10:115–122, 1994.

149. Grant KA: Emerging neurochemical concepts in the actions of ethanol at ligand-gated ion channels. *Behav Pharmacol* 5:383–404, 1994.

150. Hubbell CL, Marglin SH, Spitalnic SJ, *et al:* Opioidergic, serotonergic, and dopaminergic manipulations and rats' intake of a sweetened alcoholic beverage. *Alcohol* 8:355–367, 1991.

151. Nutt DJ, Peters TJ: Alcohol: The drug. *Br Med Bull* 50:5–17, 1994.

152. Miczek KA, DeBold JF, van Erp AMM: Neuropharmacological characteristics of individual differences in alcohol effects on aggression in rodents and primates. *Behav Pharmacol* 5:407–421, 1994.

153. Wafford KA, Burnett DM, Leidenheimer NJ, *et al:* Ethanol sensitivity of the GABA$_A$ receptor expressed in Xenopus oocytes requires 8 amino acids contained in the g2L subunit. *Neuron* 7:27–33, 1991.

154. Criswell HE, Simson PE, Knapp DJ, *et al:* Effect of zolpidem on gamma-aminobutyric acid (GABA)-induced inhibition predicts the interaction of ethanol with GABA on individual neurons in several rat brain regions. *Journal of Pharmacology and Experimental Therapeutics* 273:526–536, 1995.

155. Inglefield JR, Sieghart W, Kellogg CK: Immunohistochemical and neurochemical evidence for GABA(A) receptor heterogeneity between the hypothalamus and cortex. *J Chem Neuroanat* 7:243–252, 1994.

156. Wisden W, Laurie DJ, Monyer H, Seeburg PH: The distribution of 13-GABA$_A$ receptor subunit messenger RNAs in the rat brain 1. Telencephalon, diencephalon, mesencephalon. *J Neurosci* 12:1040–1062, 1992.

157. Zimprich F, Zezula J, Sieghart W, Lassmann H: Immunohistochemical localization of the alpha-1, alpha-2 and alpha-3 subunit of the GABA$_A$ receptor in the rat brain. *Neurosci Lett* 127:125–128, 1991.

158. Givens BS, Breese GR: Electrophysiological evidence that ethanol alters function of medial septal without affecting lateral septal function. *Journal of Pharmacology and Experimental Therapeutics* 254:528–538, 1990.

159. Siegel A, Mirsky AF: The neurobiology of violence and aggression, in Reiss AJ Jr, Miczek KA, Roth JA (eds): *Understanding and Preventing Violence. Biobehavioral Influences*. Washington, DC, National Academy Press, 1994, vol 2, pp 59–172.

160. Samson HH, Harris RA: Neurobiology of alcohol abuse. *Trends in Pharmacological Sciences* 13:206–211, 1992.

161. Mohler H: GABAergic synaptic transmission—Regulation by drugs. *Arzneim Forsch* 42(-1): 211–214, 1992.
162. Paredes RG, Agmo A: GABA and behavior: The role of receptor subtypes. *Neurosci B* 16:145–170, 1992.
163. Costa E: The allosteric modulation of GABA(a) receptors: Seventeen years of research. *Neuropsychopharmacology* 4:225–235, 1991.
164. Samson HH, Tolliver GA, Lumeng L, Li TK: Ethanol reinforcement in the alcohol non-preferring rat: Initiation using behavioral techniques without food restriction. *Alcohol Clin Exp Res* 13:378–385, 1989.

8

Serotonin in Early-Onset Alcoholism

Matti Virkkunen and Markku Linnoila

Abstract. This chapter examines current, common schemes to subgroup alcoholics to arrive at relatively homogeneous groups of patients to facilitate psychobiological and molecular genetic studies. Early-onset, male-limited alcoholism is commonly associated with antisocial personality disorder or antisocial behavioral traits. It is often preceded by early-onset aggressiveness, which is followed by conduct disorder. Early-onset alcoholism among men is associated with low central serotonin turnover rate. The data concerning platelet MAO activity and serotonin uptake to platelets among early-onset alcoholics are conflicting. Recent molecular genetic and brain imaging studies on early-onset alcoholics are preliminary but appear very promising.

Alcoholism is the most common mental disorder among men in the United States. Its prevalence is highest among the 24 to 40 age group.[1] Like many mental disorders, alcoholism is a heterogeneous condition.

1. Subgrouping Alcoholics

Various classification schemes have been developed to obtain relatively homogeneous subgroups of alcoholics to facilitate scientific research. A generally accepted classification of alcoholics takes advantage of the common comorbidity of many mental disorders with alcoholism among treatment-seeking patient samples. Patients whose alcoholism started before the symptoms of other mental disorders appeared or who have only alcoholism are classified as primary alcoholics. In secondary alcoholics, the onset of another mental disorder precedes the onset of alcoholism.[2]

Matti Virkkunen • Department of Psychiatry, Helsinki University Central Hospital, Helsinki 00180, Finland.   **Markku Linnoila** • Laboratory of Clinical Studies, Division of Intramural Clinical and Biological Research, National Institute on Alcohol Abuse and Alcoholism, Bethesda, Maryland 20892-1256.

Recent Developments in Alcoholism, Volume 13: Alcoholism and Violence, edited by Marc Galanter. Plenum Press, New York, 1997.

The Achilles heel of this classification system lies in the possibility that an age-appropriate expression of genetic vulnerability toward alcoholism, which precedes the onset of alcoholism, is different from alcoholism. This may be the case for a subgroup of boys with attention deficit disorder,[3] conduct disorder, or excessive early-onset aggressiveness.[4] Thus, the above classification scheme may be of limited utility for genetic studies on subtypes of alcoholism.

An innovative, large-scale, adoption study based on a general population sample in Sweden, conducted by Cloninger et al.,[5] has been of great heuristic value for the field. This study defined two relatively homogenous subgroups of alcoholics called type 1 and type 2. This subgrouping scheme has been successfully utilized in a number of studies on personality, biochemistry, and genetics of alcoholics. A significant problem with this classification scheme, however, is the lack of validated and agreed upon diagnostic criteria for the subgroups applicable to samples of treatment-seeking alcoholics.[6]

2. Type 2 Alcoholism and Early-Onset Alcoholism

Cloninger et al.,[5] in a large-scale Swedish adoption study of 862 men and 913 women, defined male-limited, type 2 alcoholism. It is characterized by high heritability from fathers to sons, early onset, and is related to antisocial, often violent behavioral traits. Twenty-five percent of alcoholic men in the sample of Cloninger et al.[5] were deemed to have type 2 alcoholism. Seventy-five percent of men and all women in this cohort fulfilled criteria for type 1 alcoholism. These patients were characterized by a relatively late age of onset of excessive drinking, anxious personality traits, and adverse environmental conditions during development. A recent, separate adoption study conducted in Sweden by Sigrardsson et al.[7] included 577 men and 660 women. The findings confirmed all of the previously reported distinctions between these two subtypes of alcoholism in terms of age of onset, patterns of inheritance, and differences in gender distribution and personality traits. Cloninger[8] has repeatedly emphasized that type 2 alcoholism is not only associated with teenage onset of alcohol abuse, but also with recurrent criminal and often violent behaviors.

There have been several attempts to apply the findings of Cloninger and colleagues[5,7,8] to treatment-seeking alcoholics. Babor et al.[9] proposed the terminology of types A and B to subgroups of treatment-seeking alcoholics with characteristics similar to Cloninger and co-workers'[5] subgroups, but without taking into account family history. von Knorring et al.[10] operationalized a two-group classification scheme based primarily on age of onset criteria and secondarily on complications thought to be consequences of antisocial behavioral traits. Even though von Knorring et al.[10] did not use paternal family history as a criterion, early-onset alcoholics were labeled as type 2 and late-onset alcoholics as type 1. In clinical samples, Irwin et al.[11] and Lamparski et *al.*[6] were only partially successful in applying the findings of Cloninger *et al.*[5] Thus, there is no consensus about the exact criteria for type 2 alcoholism to be used in subgrouping clinical samples of alcoholics.

Gilligan *et al.*[12] and Sullivan *et al.*[13] have developed sets of clinical criteria for the type 1 and type 2 subgrouping. Anthenelli *et al.*[14] found that type 1 and 2 subgroups classified according to the criteria of Sullivan *et al.*[13] significantly overlap the subgroups diagnosed according to the primary–secondary alcoholism scheme. There was a 73% concordance between the type 2 subgroup and the subgroup with primary antisocial personality disorder and secondary alcoholism in the Anthenelli *et al.*[14] study.

Most researchers are of the opinion that, among male inpatients, early onset of alcoholism is the central feature of the type 2 criteria.[10–15] Furthermore, there seems to be a reasonable consensus that this form of alcoholism is common among the paternal male relatives, and the fathers often have an antisocial personality disorder or marked antisocial behavioral traits.

Hill[16] has proposed a third type of alcoholism that affects primarily men and is characterized by early onset, alcoholic fathers free of an antisocial personality disorder, and brothers with repeated episodes of fighting while intoxicated. Furthermore, Hill[16] found no evidence that these fathers would have explosive behavioral traits without satisfying criteria of antisocial personality disorder, different from the findings of Virkkunen *et al.*[17,18] Turner *et al.*[19] used a pattern analysis of inheritance of alcoholism to demonstrate that both father and mother may contribute equally to early age of onset of alcoholism in the offspring. Although the mother may or may not be an alcoholic, her brothers and father often are. This finding is consistent with X-linked transmission of vulnerability to alcoholism,[20] but differs from models proposed by Cloninger *et al.*[5,21] Consistent with both models, Linnoila *et al.*[22] found that a majority of early-onset, impulsive violent male alcoholics had impulsive alcoholic fathers. However, a minority had a mother who herself was not an alcoholic but had an alcoholic father and brothers.

Type 2 alcoholics have been reported to be prone to violence during intoxication.[8,10,17,21,23,24] According to Moss *et al.*,[25] the strongest correlate of aggressivity in the son is the father's negative affectivity in the Multidimensional Personality Questionnaire, which correlates positively with the propensity of the father for physical aggression. This is consistent with a large proportion of this subgroup of alcoholics actually having antisocial personality disorder.[11] The propensity for violent behavior among a subgroup of type 2 alcoholics is highlighted by the finding that among all perpetrators of recidivist homicides in Finland, 85% had type 2 alcoholism and antisocial personality disorder.[24]

3. Antisocial Personality Disorder and Early-Onset Alcoholism

There is a consensus on antisocial personality disorder being very common among men with early-onset alcoholism. Alcoholics with antisocial personality disorder are younger at the onset of alcohol-related problems and they experience more adverse social consequences of drinking, especially while under the influence of alcohol. They are also younger at first treatment and have a generally worse outcome than alcoholics who do not meet criteria for antisocial personality disorder at the time of or before the onset of alcoholism.[26–30]

According to Schuckit et al.,[31] it is difficult to identify any other reliable personality profile than antisocial personality disorder that is associated with an individual's risk of alcoholism. Hesselbrock[32] found that, in the United States, 60 to 80% of patients with antisocial personality disorder have concomitant alcohol and/or other substance dependence. Antisocial personality disorder and type 2 alcoholism clearly overlap in many population samples, and some of the clinical relevance of the type 1/type 2 classification is lost if individuals with antisocial personality disorder are excluded.[33] There are, however, a number of early-onset alcoholics, both men and women, who do not fulfill the diagnostic criteria of antisocial personality disorder.[34,35]

The same personality features, high novelty seeking, low harm avoidance, and low reward dependence on the Tridimensional Personality Questionnaire,[8,21] are characteristic of both type 2 alcoholism and antisocial personality disorder. Hesselbrock and Hesselbrock[36] found men with antisocial personality disorder to be higher than men without antisocial personality disorder on measures of impulsivity, sensation seeking, and monotony avoidance but not on harm avoidance and reward dependence. As young adults, individuals characterized by these personality traits are at high risk to commit violent crimes[37] and to receive the psychiatric diagnosis of antisocial personality disorder.[38] Furthermore, they have recently been found to have a prominent character trait termed *uncooperativeness*, which is defined as a lack of empathy, social tolerance, compassion, and moral principles.[39]

Cadoret et al.[40,41] have published adoption studies that point to high heritability of antisocial personality disorder (i.e., a biological parent with antisocial traits is at high risk to produce an adoptee with antisocial personality disorder). The antisocial personality disorder is hypothesized to be conducive to the development of alcoholism. The conclusion concerning the direction of the effect is based on the fact that, in most patients, antisocial personality disorder manifests itself in childhood and adolescence as conduct disorder. This diagnosis precedes the characteristically early onset of substance abuse in these individuals.

4. Is Early-Onset Aggressivity Specifically Conducive to the Development of Early-Onset Alcohol Abuse?

In a prospective study on precursors to problem drinking among young adults in Finland, Pulkkinen and Pitkanen[4] found that early aggression measured at the age of 8 contributed specifically but indirectly to adult problem drinking. A high rating of early aggression preceded the development of a full-blown conduct disorder at the age of 14 when the youngsters were investigated the second time. An alcoholism screening test, the CAGE questionnaire,[42] was administered and peer and teacher ratings were collected at both ages among the original sample that was drawn in 1968 from 369 second-grade students. They were followed until adulthood. Criminal records were investigated at the ages of 20 and 26. Problem drinking was defined by the CAGE questionnaire and arrests for alcohol abuse and disorderly or criminal conduct while intoxicated. A factor analysis confirmed the existence of a factor "problem drinking," which differed clearly from "social drinking" and "controlled drinking." Among women, the score on the scale for problem drinking was unrelated to aggression, but it correlated positively with anxiety. Among males, it correlated positively with aggression at the 8-, 14-, and 26-year interviews and negatively with the scores of social anxiety and prosociality. Thus, among men, early aggressiveness preceded conduct disorder, which preceded antisocial personality disorder and alcoholism. These prospective findings are compatible with the Cloninger et al.[5] findings on type 2, male-limited alcoholism.

5. Psychobiology of Early-Onset Alcoholism

There are a number of studies that support the idea that a child's early behavioral characteristics, especially aggression and conduct problems among boys, predict problem drinking.[43–49] According to Pulkkinen,[50] poor impulse control is the primary cause of early-onset aggressivity. Because low brain serotonin turnover rate, as indicated by a low cerebrospinal fluid (CSF) 5-hydroxyindoleacetic acid (5-HIAA) concentration, prospectively predicts habitual violence and impaired impulse control among rhesus monkeys,[51] young alcoholic violent men,[17,52] and adolescent males with disruptive behavioral disorders,[53] it may be a biochemical risk marker for both early-onset aggressiveness and early-onset alcohol abuse.

In addition to low CSF 5-HIAA concentration, low CSF ACTH,[54] low urinary 24-hr cortisol secretion,[55] and high CSF free testosterone[54] are common among habitually violent offenders who have antisocial personality disorder and early-onset alcoholism. Additionally, Bergman and Brismar[56] have found that abusive and suicidal behaviors among von Knorring's type 2 alcoholics are often associated with high testosterone and low cortisol outputs among the violent subgroup but not among the suicidal subgroup free of interpersonally violent behavior. Low CSF ACTH and 24-hr urinary cortisol may be features associated with low trait anxiety, which is one of the personality features characteristic of early-onset male problem drinkers.

King et al.[57] also found that young substance abusers, most of whom had alcohol problems, had low plasma cortisol levels when measured at 8:00 AM after an overnight fast. Moreover, they observed that low plasma cortisol levels were associated with impulsivity among normal controls. Thus, they speculated that impulsivity per se might influence plasma cortisol concentrations. Future psychobiological studies on early-onset alcoholism should include indicators of hypothalamic–pituitary–gonadal and hypothalamic–pituitary–adrenal axes activities.

6. Early-Onset Alcoholism and Antisocial Personality Disorder Are Associated with Reduced Brain Serotonin Turnover Rate and Transmission

6.1. Serotonin Turnover Rate (CSF 5-HIAA)

There is an increasing body of evidence that reduced central serotonin turnover rate is associated with early-onset alcoholism and antisocial personality traits.[8] We have found among alcoholics that a majority of the violent type 2 patients are characterized by a low CSF 5-HIAA concentration.[23,52,58,59]

In prospective follow-up studies, low CSF 5-HIAA and low blood glucose nadir after a glucose challenge were predictive of recidivist violent crimes under the influence of alcohol among early-onset male alcoholic violent offenders.[17] Low CSF 5-HIAA was particularly associated with a family history positive for paternal alcoholism and violence[22] compatible with Cloninger's findings.[5]

In our most recent follow-up study, alcoholic recidivists who committed new violent crimes after release from prison had significantly lower CSF 5-HIAA, and 3-methoxy-4-hydroxyphenylglycol (MHPG) (main central metabolite of norepinephrine concentrations.[52] Low CSF 5-HIAA concentrations were associated with family histories positive for both paternal violence and alcoholism but not with family histories positive for paternal alcoholism but negative for paternal violence. Again, these findings are compatible with family histories characteristic of type 2 alcoholism as defined by Cloninger *et al.*[5] In a prospective follow-up study among American children and adolescents with disruptive behavioral disorders (mainly conduct disorder), Kruesi *et al.*[53] also found low CSF 5-HIAA and HVA to be predictive of future violent behavior.

Among the impulsive alcoholic violent offenders, high novelty seeking, low monotony avoidance, high irritability, and low socialization scores on the Karolinska Scales of Personality are associated with low CSF 5-HIAA concentrations.[18] However, Cloninger[8] postulates that although a central serotonergic deficit is consistently correlated with antisocial character traits, it is only indirectly and inconsistently associated with personality traits such as high novelty seeking,[60] low harm avoidance,[60] other measures of impulsivity,[18] or history of aggressiveness.[18]

In addition to alcoholic violent patients with antisocial personality disorder, alcoholic violent patients with impulsive personality disorders other than antisocial personality disorder, who repeatedly exhibit explosive behaviors under the influence of alcohol, also have extremely low CSF 5-HIAA concentrations. Typically, these patients have not, however, fulfilled all the diagnostic criteria for attention deficit or conduct disorders during childhood or early adolescence, and their problems do not become manifest until after puberty. Usually, by 20 years of age, they have developed alcoholism. Biologically, many of these patients are characterized by a profound disturbance of day and night activity rhythm.[54] These differences between patients with antisocial personality and intermittent explosive disorder emphasize the important role early impulsive aggressivity can play in the very early onset of alcohol abuse among patients with antisocial personality disorder.

Even among alcoholics without personality disorders, those with an early onset ($\leq$ 25 years) have a lower mean CSF 5-HIAA concentration than late-onset (> 25 years) alcoholics.[35] It is important to note, however, that the mean CSF 5-HIAA concentration among these American patients with early-onset alcoholism was much higher (85.6 ± 34.7 nmole/liter) than the mean CSF 5-HIAA concentration among the violent antisocial and explosive criminal alcoholics (58.8 ± 25.2 nmole/liter) in Finland who often also had a history positive for suicide attempts.[54] A history positive for suicide attempts has been repeatedly associated with extremely low CSF 5-HIAA concentration among the alcoholic violent Finns.[17,52,54,61] This finding was not, however, replicated in our two recent American studies on nonviolent alcoholics, most of whom did not have personality disorders.[35,58] Among late-onset alcoholics in the American study,[35] the mean CSF 5-HIAA concentration was 103.6 ± 38.9 nmole/liter.

Also, our earlier American study[58] reported a lower mean CSF 5-HIAA concentration among early- as compared to late-onset alcoholics, but the finding was not statistically significant. The major differences between the two studies were the larger sample size and the elimination of between-assay variability in the Fils-Aime et al.[35] study and a different age of onset criterion. The age of onset criterion in the Fils-Aime et al.[35] study was selected to directly test the postulates of Cloninger et al.[5] and Irwin et al.[11]

Many other investigators have reported reduced CSF 5-HIAA concentrations in abstinent alcoholics, but they have not addressed the issue of subgrouping. Ballenger et al.[62] studied abstinent, young male alcoholics and reported one of the largest differences in CSF 5-HIAA between alcoholics and controls. The demographics of their sample made it very likely that a large proportion of their patients were early-onset alcoholics. Banki[63] found low CSF 5-HIAA in both recently abstinent alcoholic men and women, and Takahashi et al.[64] found low CSF 5-HIAA concentrations only in alcoholics who had experienced severe withdrawals.

6.2. Serotonin Receptor Challenges in Early- versus Late-Onset Male Alcoholics

Recent pharmacological challenge studies[65–67] suggest that serotonergic dysregulation may be more prominent among von Knorring's type 2 than among type 1 alcoholics and healthy subjects. Meta-chlorophenylpiperazine (mCPP), a primary serotonin (5-HT$_{2c}$) receptor agonist, has been found to produce blunted prolactin and cortisol responses in alcoholics compared to healthy volunteers but to elicit alcohol-like cues mainly among von Knorring's type 2 alcoholics.[65–67] In addition to the 5-HT$_{2c}$ receptor, mCPP may also affect 5-HT$_{1a}$, 5-HT$_{1d}$, 5-HT$_{2a}$, 5-HT$_3$, and 5-HT$_7$ receptors.[66] Blunted hormonal responses to mCPP have also been observed in patients with antisocial personality disorder and substance abuse.[68]

6.3. Abnormal Tryptophan–Large Neutral Amino Acid Ratio in Plasma

Fernström and Wurtman[69,70] reported in the early 1970s that tryptophan–large neutral amino acid (LNAA) ratio in plasma regulates the availability of tryptophan to the brain among laboratory rodents. They suggested that the rate of entry of tryptophan regulated the rate of serotonin synthesis in the brain. The physiological importance of this system under steady-state conditions, however, has not been extensively elucidated in humans.

Buydens-Branchey et al.[71] observed that among alcoholics who had started to abuse alcohol before 20 years of age there was an association between a low tryptophan–LNAA ratio in plasma and depressive and aggressive behaviors. The ratio was measured 1 day after cessation of drinking and the ratio increased progressively for at least 2 to 3 weeks after detoxification. Many of the subjects who had exhibited early-onset alcohol-seeking behavior had also committed crimes of violence and had a history of paternal alcoholism.

Branchey et al.[72] also found that the tendency to experience blackouts, i.e., to lose one's memory under the influence of alcohol, was associated with a low plasma tryptophan concentration quantified after 2 weeks abstinence. On the other hand, Buydens-Branchey et al.[71] and Virkkunen and Narvanen[73] found an elevated tryptophan–LNAA ratio among violent male alcoholics.

Interestingly, Fils-Aime et al.[35] found a nonsignificant negative correlation between CSF 5-HIAA and tryptophan concentrations among early-onset alcoholics. According to these data, under steady-state conditions in humans, tryptophan crossing the blood–brain barrier may not be the rate-limiting step for serotonin synthesis.[70] These findings are in accordance with our recent postulate that in humans, under steady-state conditions, the activity of tryptophan hydroxylase rather than the availability of tryptophan may be rate-limiting for the turnover rate of central serotonin.[74]

6.4. Platelet Monoamine Oxidase

Monoamine oxidase (MAO) is the major enzyme that metabolizes biogenic monoamine neurotransmitters, including serotonin, by oxidative deamination. Two forms of MAO, A and B, are widely distributed in the human body, with high activity of the B form in blood platelets.[75,76] There is a relatively large number of published studies correlating behavioral characteristics with platelet MAO activity. A lack of correlation between platelet and brain MAO activities renders the meaning of platelet MAO findings uncertain for CNS disorders.[77] Clinical and experimental findings support, however, the hypothesis that platelet MAO activity may be a marker of the functional capacity of the central serotonin system.[78,79]

Many authors have reported that platelet MAO activity is lower among alcoholics than healthy volunteers.[80-88] von Knorring et al.[10,89,90] and Sullivan et al.[13] both found that early-onset male alcoholics had low mean platelet MAO activity compared to late-onset alcoholics and healthy volunteers, who did not differ from each other. In these studies, type 2 alcoholics were characterized by early onset of alcoholism, alcoholism in first-degree relatives, and a high prevalence of drug abuse and social complications. Similar to these findings, low platelet MAO activity has also been reported in patients with antisocial personality and borderline personality disorders.[91,92] Yates et al.[85] and Anthenelli et al.,[86] however, did not find platelet MAO activity differences between type 1 and 2 alcoholics.

Platelet MAO activity has been found to be negatively correlated with the personality traits of impulsivity and sensation seeking,[93] which are among the traits associated with early-onset alcohol abuse among men, as reviewed above. These are also traits that, according to genetic studies, have high heritability and characterize many children with conduct disorder who have often been exposed to family discord and disruption.[94] As reviewed above, impaired impulse control has been repeatedly associated with reduced brain serotonin turnover rate.

Moreover, symptoms of conduct disorder commonly precede early alcohol problems and the illness often progresses to an antisocial personality disorder. Therefore, it is surprising that platelet MAO activity has been reported to be higher in sons of substance-abusing fathers who have conduct disorder than in sons of substance-abusing fathers who do not have conduct disorder or among sons of nonsubstance-abusing fathers who have conduct disorder.[95] Furthermore, Stoff et al.[96] found that impulsivity, which is often an important clinical feature of conduct disorder, was positively correlated with platelet MAO activity. Shekim et al.,[97] on the other hand, found that both low and high platelet MAO activities were associated with impulsivity among healthy children. Bowden et al.[98] found lower platelet MAO activity among youths with conduct and attention deficit disorder than among youths with only attention deficit disorder.

Interestingly, among adults with personality disorders, prolactin response to dl-fenfluramine has been found to be inversely correlated with measures of aggression, motor impulsivity, assaultiveness, and irritability.[99] In a study by Halperin et al.,[100] the prolactin response to a dl-fenfluramine challenge among youth with attention deficit disorder and a history of exhibiting aggressive behaviors was positively correlated with aggressiveness. The subjects in the study were too young to have developed alcohol abuse.

The cause of the differences between the findings among the adults and children and adolescents is unclear.[101] It is possible that physiological changes associated with puberty or increasing alcohol and other substance abuse reverse the relationships between the platelet MAO activity, prolactin responsiveness to fenfluramine, and behavior. Also, it is possible that although by definition symptoms of conduct disorder always precede antisocial personality disorder,[102] boys with conduct disorder and high platelet MAO activity may differ from boys with conduct disorder who are more likely to become alcoholics with antisocial personality disorder with increasing age. This suggestion is compatible with the finding of Gabel et al.[101] that only a very small proportion of the youths in their study had positive histories for substance abuse at the mean age of 12.3 ± 2.0 years.

6.5. Uptake of Serotonin to Platelets

Many peripheral indicators of serotonin metabolism are currently being investigated among alcoholics and especially among early-onset alcoholics.[33] Blood platelets have been thought to be a representative peripheral model for central serotonergic neuronal function because the kinetics of serotonin in platelets resemble the kinetics of serotonin in synaptosomes.[103] Thus far, preliminary findings suggest that family-history-positive and family-history-negative young men may have different platelet serotonin uptake rates. Family history positives had higher maximum velocity (V_{max}) of the uptake of serotonin than family history negatives.[104] Furthermore, Ernouf et al.[105] found that descendants of alcoholics of both genders had a higher V_{max} for serotonin uptake than healthy age-matched offspring of nonalcoholics. Studies on alcoholics have also reported increased serotonin uptake by platelets of alcoholics compared to controls.[106,107] Only the directly quantified serotonin uptake rate was higher among alcoholics than healthy volunteers, whereas no differences between alcoholics and healthy volunteers were found for platelet paroxetine-binding variables.[107] Neiman et al.,[108] however, found an elevated affinity constant (K_m) for serotonin in alcoholics only during withdrawal but a normal rate of uptake in alcoholics during continued abstinence. Furthermore, Kent et al.[109] found platelet serotonin uptake to be reduced by 18% on the average in male alcoholics who had been abstinent for 2 weeks as compared to healthy volunteers.

At this time, there are no studies available specifically investigating serotonin uptake among patients with early-onset alcoholism, type 2 alcoholism or alcoholism and antisocial personality disorder. Platelet serotonin uptake, however, was found to be reduced among habitually violent impulsive offenders,[110] but this preliminary study contains no information concerning alcohol use among the subjects.

Despite the conflicting reports, higher V_{max} values among alcoholics and their descendants as compared to healthy volunteers, if confirmed in future studies, are particularly interesting because platelet serotonin uptake in major depression has been reported to have a reduced V_{max} in about 75% of the studies.[103] However, the issue of whether platelet uptake reflects serotonin uptake in the brain remains unresolved.

6.6. Molecular Genetic Findings Associated with Early-Onset Alcoholism

Molecular genetic findings concerning early-onset or type 2 alcoholism are preliminary, but several groups are pursuing this line of investigation. Our approach, with Dr. David Goldman at the National Institute on Alcohol Abuse and Alcoholism has been to directly scan the coding sequences of serotonergic candidate genes for structural variants.

We have reported polymorphisms of several serotonin receptor genes[111–113] and the tryptophan hydroxylase (TPH) gene[114] among violent alcoholics. However, the only common amino acid substitution producing polymorphism (5-HT$_{cys23-ser23}$) is in the 5-HT$_{2c}$ receptor gene. The rarer variant has an allelic frequency of about 13% among Caucasians.[112] Among Finns, 5-HT$_{2c-ser23}$ showed a negative association in alcoholics as compared to healthy volunteers matched for age, sex, and socioeconomic class, but it was not associated with antisocial personality disorder or CSF 5-HIAA concentrations.[115] Thus, the only abundant structural variant discovered so far does not seem to play a role in the vulnerability toward early-onset or type 2 alcoholism.[115]

An intronic polymorphism was identified in the TPH gene that may influence serotonergic activity, and it has been genotyped as a single-strand conformational polymorphism. Our preliminary data suggest an association between the TPH "L" allele, severity of impulsivity, relatively low CSF 5-HIAA, and a history positive for suicide attempts among impulsive, violent Finnish alcoholics.[74] Because of the association between low CSF 5-HIAA and the "L" allele, this polymorphism may be associated with type 2 and early-onset alcoholism. Further mechanistic studies, however, are needed to elucidate the meaning, if any, of these associations because the polymorphism is intronic. Analysis of the TPH promoter has identified several regions required for tissue-specific and basal expression. Furthermore, Nielsen et al.[114] have discovered a novel transcription factor, which is being cloned and sequenced, that regulates negatively TPH gene expression.

Vanyukov et al.[116] have found an association between the vulnerability toward early-onset alcoholism and substance abuse and a recently discovered dinucleotide repeat-length polymorphism of the MAOA gene. A significant correlation between the presence or absence off early-onset alcoholism and substance abuse and the length of the MAOCA-1 repeat was found among men but not among women. "Long" alleles (repeat length above 115 base pairs) were associated with an early age of onset of substance abuse. At the present time, these findings are difficult to interpret. This is because it is low-platelet MAO activity that has been found to be associated with early-onset alcoholism,[10,13,89,90] and the MAO in platelets is MAOB, which is coded by a different gene. The molecular genetic data on early-onset or type 2 alcoholism are still very preliminary but promising.

6.7. Brain Neuroimaging Findings in Alcoholism

Using single-photon emission computed tomography (SPECT), Tiihonen et al.[117] found that patients with the most abundant type of alcoholism, which in their study clinically resembles type 1 alcoholism as described by Cloninger et al.,[5,21] can be distinguished from violent patients with early-onset alcoholism and from healthy volunteers by increased density of dopamine transporters in the caudate putamen. Cloninger[8] regards this finding as the first identification of a specific neuroregulatory deficit in type 1 alcoholics. Among early-onset alcoholics who had committed very severe violent crimes under the influence of alcohol, the striatal density of the dopamine uptake sites was only slightly higher than among controls. At this time, there are no brain-imaging findings that have been identified to be characteristic of early-onset or type 2 alcoholism.

7. Conclusion

Alcoholism is a common, heterogeneous disorder that, according to Cloninger et al.,[5] can be usefully divided into two relatively homogeneous subgroups. The subgroup that consists of 25% of alcoholic men and is characterized by early onset, antisocial personality traits, and a high degree of heritability from fathers to sons may have a reduced central serotonin turnover rate. This disorder may share the same genetic background as antisocial personality disorder. Early aggressiveness among boys, which is conducive to the development of conduct disorder, may predispose these individuals to the development of early-onset alcoholism and other substance abuse. Because of the high heritability and relative homogeneity of this disorder, it is a prime target for molecular genetic investigations.

ACKNOWLEDGMENTS. The authors are grateful to David Goldman, MD and Michael Eckardt, PhD for their thoughtful review and constructive comments and to Ms. Andrea Hobbs for typing and editorial assistance.

References

1. Robins LN, Helzer JE, Weissman MM, et al: Lifetime prevalence of specific psychiatric disorders in three sites. Arch Gen Psychiatry 41:948–958, 1984.
2. Schuckit M, Pitts FN, Reich T, et al: Alcoholism I: Two types of alcoholism in women. Arch Gen Psychiatry 20:301–306, 1969.
3. Tarter RE, McBride H, Buonpane N, Schneider DU: Differentiation of alcoholics. Arch Gen Psychiatry 34:761–768, 1977.

4. Pulkkinen L, Pitkanen T: A prospective study of the precursors to problem drinking in young adulthood. *J Stud Alcohol* 55:578–587, 1994.
5. Cloninger CR, Bohman M, Sigvardsson S: Inheritance of alcohol abuse: Cross-fostering analysis of adopted men. *Arch Gen Psychiatry* 38:861–868, 1981.
6. Lamparski DM, Roy A, Nutt DJ, Linnoila M: The criteria of Cloninger *et al* and von Knorring *et al* for subgrouping alcoholics: A comparison in a clinical population. *Acta Psychiatr Scand* 84:497–502, 1991.
7. Sigrardsson S, Bohman M, Cloninger CR: Replication of the Stockholm adoption study of alcoholism: Confirmatory cross-fostering analysis. *Arch Gen Psychiatry* 53:681–687, 1996.
8. Cloninger CR: The psychobiological regulation of social cooperation. *Nature Med* 7:623–625, 1995.
9. Babor TF, Hofmann M, DelBoca FK, *et al:* Types of alcoholics. I. Evidence for an empirically derived typology based on indicators of vulnerability and severity. *Arch Gen Psychiatry* 49:599–608, 1992.
10. von Knorring AL, Bohman M, von Knorring L, Oreland L: Platelet MAO activity as a biological marker in subgroups of alcoholism. *Acta Psychiatr Scand* 72:51–58, 1985.
11. Irwin M, Schuckit MA, Smith TL: Clinical importance of age at onset in type 1 and 2 primary alcoholics. *Arch Gen Psychiatry* 47:320–324, 1990.
12. Gilligan SB, Reich T, Cloninger CR: Alcohol-related symptoms in heterogenous families of hospitalized alcoholics. *Alcohol Clin Exp Res* 12:671–678, 1988.
13. Sullivan JL, Baenziger JC, Wagner DL, *et al:* : Platelet MAO in subtypes of alcoholism. *Biol Psychiatry* 27:911–922, 1990.
14. Anthenelli RM, Smith TL, Irwin MR, Schuckit MA; A comparative study of criteria for subgrouping alcoholics: The primary/secondary diagnostic scheme versus variations of the type 1/type 2 criteria. *Am J Psychiatry* 151:1468–1474, 1994.
15. Penick EC, Powell BJ, Nickel EJ, *et al:* Examination of Cloninger's type 1 and 2 alcoholism with a sample of men alcoholics in treatment. *Alcohol Clin Exp Res* 14:623–629, 1990.
16. Hill SY: Absence of paternal sociopathy in the etiology of severe alcoholism: Is there a type 3 alcoholism? *J Stud Alcohol* 53:161–169, 1992.
17. Virkkunen M, DeJong J, Bartko J, *et al:* Relationship of psychobiological variables to recidivism in violent offenders and impulsive fire setters: A follow-up study. *Arch Gen Psychiatry* 46:600–603, 1989.
18. Virkkunen M, Kallio E, Rawlings R, *et al:* Personality profiles and state aggressiveness in Finnish alcoholic violent offenders, fire setters and healthy volunteers. *Arch Gen Psychiatry* 51:28–33, 1994.
19. Turner WM, Cutter HSG, Worobec TG, *et al:* Family history models of alcoholism: Age of onset, consequences and dependence. *J Stud Alcohol* 54:164–171, 1993.
20. Kaij L, Dock J: Grandsons of alcoholics: A test of sex-linked transmission of alcohol abuse. *Arch Gen Psychiatry* 39:1379–1381, 1975.
21. Cloninger CR: Neurogenetic adaptive mechanisms in alcoholism. *Science* 236:410–416, 1987.
22. Linnoila M, DeJong J, Virkkunen M: Family history of alcoholism in violent offenders and impulsive fire setters. *Arch Gen Psychiatry* 46:613–616, 1989.
23. Virkkunen M, Linnoila M: Brain serotonin, type 2 alcoholism and impulsive violence. *J Stud Alcohol* 11:163–169, 1993.
24. Tiihonen J, Hakola P: Psychiatric disorders and homicide recidivism. *Am J Psychiatry* 151:436–438, 1994.
25. Moss HB, Mezzich A, Yao JK, *et al:* Aggressivity among sons of substance-abusing fathers: Association with psychiatric disorder in the father and son, paternal personality, pubertal development and socioeconomic status. *Am J Drug Alcohol Abuse* 21:195–208, 1995.
26. Virkkunen M: Alcoholism and antisocial personality. *Acta Psychiatr Scand* 59:493–501, 1979.
27. Cadoret RJ, Troughton E, Widmer R: Clinical differences between antisocial and primary alcoholics. *Compr Psychiatry* 25:1–8, 1984.
28. Hesselbrock VM, Hesselbrock MN, Stabenau JR: Alcoholism in men patients subtyped by family history and antisocial personality. *J Stud Alcohol* 46:59–64, 1985.

29. Schuckit MA: The clinical implications of primary diagnostic groups among alcoholics. *Arch Gen Psychiatry* 42:1043–1049, 1985.

30. Liskow B, Powell BJ, Nickel E, Penick E: Antisocial alcoholics: Are there clinically significant diagnostic subgroups? *J Stud Alcohol* 52:62–69, 1991.

31. Schuckit MA, Klein J, Twitchell G, Smith T: Personality test scores as predictors of alcoholism almost a decade later. *Am J Psychiatry* 151:1038–1042, 1994.

32. Hesselbrock MN: Gender comparison of antisocial personality disorder and depression in alcoholism. *J Subst Abuse* 3:205–219, 1991.

33. Schuckit MA: A clinical model of genetic influences in alcohol dependence. *J Stud Alcohol* 55:5–17, 1994.

34. Helmi S, Penick EG, Nickel EJ, et al: Early onset male alcoholics with and without antisocial personality disorder, in *148th Annual Meeting Proceedings of the American Psychiatric Association*. Miami, APA Press, 1995, p. 91.

35. Fils-Aime M-L, Eckardt MJ, George DT, et al: Early-onset alcoholics have lower cerebrospinal fluid 5-hydroxyindoleacetic acid levels than late-onset alcoholics. *Arch Gen Psychiatry* 53:211–216, 1996.

36. Hesselbrock MN, Hesselbrock VM: Relationships of family history, antisocial personality disorder and personality traits in young men at risk for alcoholism. *J Stud Alcohol* 53:619–625, 1992.

37. Cloninger CR, Przybeck TR, Svrakic DM, Wetzel R: *The Temperament and Character Inventory: A Guide to Its Development and Use*. St. Louis, Washington University Center for Psychobiology and Personality, 1994.

38. Svrakic DM, Whitehead C, Przybeck TR, Cloninger CR: Differential diagnosis of personality disorders by the seven-factor model of temperament and character. *Arch Gen Psychiatry* 50:991–999, 1993.

39. Svrakic N, Svrakic DM, Cloninger CR: A general quantitative model of personality development: Fundamentals of a self-organizing psychobiological complex. *Dev Psychopathol*, in press.

40. Cadoret RJ, O'Gorman TW, Troughton E, Heywood E: Alcoholism and antisocial personality: Interrelationships, genetic and environmental factors. *Arch Gen Psychiatry* 42:161–167, 1985.

41. Cadoret RJ, Troughton E, O'Gorman TW: Genetic and environmental factors in alcohol abuse and antisocial personality. *J Stud Alcohol* 48:1–8, 1987.

42. Mayfield D, McLeod G, Hall P: The CAGE questionnaire: Validation of a new alcoholism screening instrument. *Am J Psychiatry* 131:1121–1123, 1974.

43. McCord W, McCord J: *Origins of Alcoholism*. Stanford, CA, Stanford University Press, 1960.

44. Donovan JE, Jessor R, Jessor L: Problem drinking in adolescence and young adulthood: A follow-up study. *J Stud Alcohol* 44:109–137, 1983.

45. Barnes GM, Welte JW: Patterns and predictors of alcohol use among 7–12th grade students in New York State. *J Stud Alcohol* 47:53–62, 1986.

46. Andersson T, Bergman LR, Magnusson D: Patterns of adjustment problems and alcohol abuse in early adulthood: A prospective longitudinal study. *Dev Psychopathol* 1:119–131, 1989.

47. Robins LN, McEvoy L: Conduct problems as predictors of substance abuse, in Robins LN, Rutter M (eds): *Straight and Devious Pathways from Childhood to Adulthood*. New York, Cambridge University Press, 1990, pp 182–204.

48. van Kammen WB, Loeber R, Stouthammer-Loeber M: Substance use and its relationship to conduct problems and delinquency in young boys. *J Youth Adolesc* 20:399–413, 1991.

49. Boyle MH, Offord DR, Racine YA, et al: Predicting substance use in late adolescence: Results from the Ontario Child Health Study follow-up. *Am J Psychiatry* 149:761–767, 1992.

50. Pulkkinen L: Self-control and continuity from childhood to late adolescence, in Baltes PB, Brim OG Jr (eds): *Life-span Development and Behavior*. San Diego, Academic Press, 1982, vol 4, pp 63–105.

51. Mehlman P, Higley J, Faucher J, et al: Low 5-HIAA concentrations and severe aggression and impaired impulse control in nonhuman primates. *Am J Psychiatry* 151:1485–1491, 1994.

52. Virkkunen M, Eggert M, Rawlings R, Linnoila M: A prospective follow-up study of alcoholic violent offenders and fire setters. *Arch Gen Psychiatry* 53:523–529, 1996.

53. Kruesi MJP, Hibbs ED, Zahn TP, *et al:* A 2-year prospective follow-up study of children and adolescents with disruptive behavior disorders: Prediction by cerebrospinal fluid 5-hydroxyindoleacetic acid, homovanillic acid and autonomic measures? *Arch Gen Psychiatry* 49:429–435, 1992.

54. Virkkunen M, Rawlings R, Tokola R, *et al:* CSF biochemistries, glucose metabolism, and diurnal activity rhythms in violent offenders, impulsive fire setters, and healthy volunteers. *Arch Gen Psychiatry* 51:20–27, 1994.

55. Virkkunen M: Urinary free cortisol secretion in habitually violent offenders. *Acta Psychiatr Scand* 72:40–44, 1985.

56. Bergman B, Brismar B: Hormone levels and personality traits in abusive and suicidal male alcoholics. *Alcohol Clin Exp Res* 18:311–316, 1994.

57. King RJ, Scheuer JW, Curtis D, Zarkone VP: Plasma cortisol correlates of impulsivity and substance abuse. *Person Individ Diff* 3:287–291, 1990.

58. Roy A, DeJong J, Lamparski D, *et al:* Mental disorders among alcoholics: Relationship to age of onset and cerebrospinal fluid neuropeptides. *Arch Gen Psychiatry* 48:423–427, 1991.

59. Virkkunen M, Linnoila M: Serotonin in early onset, male alcoholics with violent behavior. *Ann Med* 22:327–331, 1990.

60. Limson R, Goldman D, Roy A, *et al:* Personality and cerebrospinal fluid monoamine metabolites in alcoholics and controls. *Arch Gen Psychiatry* 48:437–441, 1991.

61. Linnoila M, Virkkunen M, Scheinin M, *et al:* Low CSF 5-HIAA concentration differentiates impulsive from nonimpulsive violent behavior. *Life Sci* 33:2609–2614, 1983.

62. Ballenger J, Goodwin F, Major L, Brown G: Alcohol and central serotonin metabolism in man. *Arch Gen Psychiatry* 36:224–227, 1979.

63. Banki C: Factors influencing monoamine metabolites and tryptophan in patients with alcohol dependence. *J Neural Transm* 50:98–101, 1981.

64. Takahashi S, Yamane H, Kondo H, Tani M: CRF monoamine metabolites in alcoholism, a comparative study with depression. *Folia Psychiat Neurol Japan* 28:347–354, 1974.

65. Benkelfat C, Murphy DL, Hill JL, *et al:* Ethanollike properties of the serotonergic partial agonist m-chlorophenylpiperazine in chronic alcoholic patients. *Arch Gen Psychiatry* 48:383, 1991.

66. Krystal JH, Webb E, Cooney N, *et al:* Specificity of ethanollike effects elicited by serotonergic and noradrenergic mechanisms. *Arch Gen Psychiatry* 51:898–911, 1994.

67. George DT, Benkelfat C, Hill JL, *et al:* A comparison of behavioral and biochemical responses to mCPP in subtypes of alcoholics. *Am J Psychiatry,* 1996, in press.

68. Moss HB, Yao JK, Panzak GL: Serotonergic responsivity and behavioral dimensions in antisocial personality disorder with substance abuse. *Biol Psychiatry* 28:325–328, 1990.

69. Fernstrom JD, Wurtman RJ: Brain serotonin content: Increase following ingestion of carbohydrate diet. *Science* 174:1023–1025, 1971.

70. Fernstrom JD, Wurtman RJ: Brain serotonin content: Physiological regulation by plasma neural amino acids. *Science* 178:414–416, 1972.

71. Buydens-Branchey L, Branchey MH, Noumair D, Lieber CS: Age of alcoholism onset: Relationship to susceptibility to serotonin precursor availability. *Arch Gen Psychiatry* 46:231–236, 1989.

72. Branchey L, Branchey M, Zucker D, *et al:* Association between low plasma tryptophan and blackouts in male alcoholic patients. *Alcohol Clin Exp Res* 9:393–395, 1985.

73. Virkkunen M, Narvanen S: Plasma insulin, tryptophan and serotonin levels during the glucose tolerance test among habitually violent and impulsive offenders. *Neuropsychobiology* 17:19–23, 1987.

74. Nielsen DA, Goldman D, Virkkunen M, *et al:* Suicidality and 5-hydroxyindoleacetic acid concentration associated with a tryptophan hydroxylase polymorphism. *Arch Gen Psychiatry* 51:34–38, 1994.

75. Fowler CJ, Oreland L: Human platelet monoamine oxidase: Some biochemical findings, in

Kamijo K, Usdin K, Nagatsu T (eds): *Monoamine Oxidase: Basic and Clinical Frontiers*. Amsterdam, Excerpta Medica, 1981, pp 28–39.

76. Fowler CJ, Tipton KF, MacKay AVP, Youdim MBH: Human platelet monoamine oxidase: A useful enzyme in the study of psychiatric disorders. *Neuroscience* 7:1577–1594, 1982.
77. Young WF, Laws ER, Sharbrough PW, Weinshilboum RM: Human monoamine oxidase: Lack of brain and platelet correlation. *Arch Gen Psychiatry* 43:604–609, 1986.
78. Oreland L: The activity of human brain and thrombocyte monoamine oxidase (MAO) in relation to various psychiatric disorders: I. MAO activity in some disease states, in Singer T, von Korff R, Murphy D (eds): *Monoamine Oxidase: Structure, Function and Altered Functions*. New York, Academic Press, 1979, pp 379–387.
79. Oreland L, Shaskan EG: Monoamine oxidase activity as a biological marker. *Trends Pharmacol Sci* 4:339–341, 1983.
80. Wiberg A, Gottfries CG, Oreland L: Low platelet MAO activity in human alcoholics. *Med Biol* 55:181–186, 1977.
81. Faraj BA, Lenton JD, Kutner M, *et al*: Prevalence of low monoamine oxidase function in alcoholism. *Alcohol Clin Exp Res* 11:464–467, 1987.
82. Faraj BA, Davis DC, Camp VM, *et al*: Platelet monoamine oxidase activity in alcoholics, alcoholics with drug dependence, and cocaine addicts. *Alcohol Clin Exp Res* 18:1114–1120, 1994.
83. Pandey GN, Fawcett J, Gibbons R, *et al*: Platelet monoamine oxidase in alcoholism. *Biol Psychiatry* 24:15–24, 1988.
84. Mukassa H, Nakamura J, Yamada S, *et al*: Platelet monoamine oxidase activity and personality traits in alcoholics and metamphetamine dependents. *Drug Alcohol Depend* 26:251–254, 1990.
85. Yates WR, Wilcox J, Knudson R, *et al*: The effect of gender and subtype of platelet MAO in alcoholism. *J Stud Alcohol* 51:463–467, 1990.
86. Anthenelli RM, Smith TL, Craig CE, *et al*: Platelet monoamine oxidase levels in subgroups of alcoholics: Diagnostic, temporal and clinical correlates. *Biol Psychiatry* 38:361–368, 1995.
87. Sherf F, Hallman J, Oreland L: Low platelet gamma-aminobutyrate aminotransferase and monoamine oxidase activities in chronic alcoholic patients. *Alcohol Clin Exp Res* 16:1014–1020, 1992.
88. Devor EJ, Cloninger CR, Kwan SW, Abell CW: A genetic familial study of monoamine oxidase B activity and concentration in alcoholics. *Alcohol Clin Exp Res* 17:263–267, 1993.
89. von Knorring L, Oreland L, von Knorring AL: Personality traits and platelet MAO activity in alcoholic and drug abusing teenage boys. *Acta Psychiatr Scand* 75:307–314, 1987.
90. von Knorring AL, Hallman J, von Knorring L, Oreland L: Platelet MAO oxidase activity in type 1 and 2 alcoholism. *Alcohol Alcohol* 26:409–416, 1991.
91. Lidberg L, Modin I, Oreland L, *et al*: Low platelet monoamine oxidase activity and psychopathy. *Psychiatr Res* 16:339–343, 1985.
92. Yehuda R, Southwick SM, Edell WS, Giller EL Jr: Low platelet monoamine oxidase activity in borderline personality disorder. *Psychiatry Res* 30:265–273, 1989.
93. von Knorring L, Oreland L, Winblad B: Personality traits related to monoamine oxidase (MAO) in platelets. *Psychiatry Res* 12:11–26, 1984.
94. Rutter M: Concluding remarks in Rutter M (ed): *Genetics of Criminal and Antisocial Behavior*. Chichester, Wiley, 1996, 265–271.
95. Gabel S, Stadler J, Bjorn J, *et al*: Homovanillic acid and monoamine oxidase in sons of substance-abusing fathers: Relationships to conduct disorder. *J Stud Alcohol* 56:135–139, 1995.
96. Stoff DM, Friedman E, Pollock L, *et al*: Elevated platelet MAO is related to impulsivity in disruptive behavior disorders. *J Am Acad Child Adolesc Psychiatry* 28:754–760, 1989.
97. Shekim WO, Hodges K, Horwitz E, *et al*: Psychoeducational and impulsivity correlates of platelet MAO in normal children. *Psychiatry Res* 11:99–106, 1984.
98. Bowden CL, Deutsch CK, Swanson JM: Plasma dopamine beta-hydroxylase and platelet

monoamine oxidase in attention deficit disorder and conduct disorder. *J Am Acad Child Adolesc Psychiatry* 27:171–174, 1988.

99. Coccaro EF, Siever LJ, Klar H, *et al:* Serotonergic studies of personality disorder: Correlates with behavioral aggression and impulsivity. *Arch Gen Psychiatry* 46:587–589, 1989.

100. Halperin JM, Sharma V, Siever LJ, *et al:* Serotonergic function in aggressive and nonaggressive boys with attention deficit hyperactive disorder. *Am J Psychiatry* 151:243–248, 1994.

101. Gabel S, Stadler J, Bjorn J, *et al:* Monoamine oxidase and homovanillic acid in male youth with predisposition to substance abuse. *Alcohol Clin Exp Res* 18:1137–1142, 1994.

102. American Psychiatric Association, Committee on Nomenclature and Statistics: *Diagnostic and Statistical Manual of Mental Disorders,* 4th ed. Washington, DC, American Psychiatric Press, 1994.

103. Meltzer HY, Arora RC: Platelet serotonin studies in affective disorders: Evidence for a serotonergic abnormality? in Sandler M, Coppen A, Harnett S (eds): *5-Hydroxytryptamine in Psychiatry: A Spectrum of Ideas.* New York, Oxford University Press, 1991, pp 50–89.

104. Rausch JL, Monteiro MG, Schuckit MA: Platelet serotonin uptake in men with family histories of alcoholism. *Neuropsychopharmacology* 4:83–86, 1991.

105. Ernouf D, Compagnon P, Lothion P, *et al:* Platelet 3H 5HT uptake in descendants from alcoholic patients: A potential risk factor for alcohol dependence? *Life Sci* 52:989–995, 1993.

106. Boismare F, Lhuintre JP, Daoust M, *et al:* Platelet affinity for serotonin is increased in alcoholics and former alcoholics. *Alcohol Alcohol* 22:155–159, 1987.

107. Daoust M, Lhuintre JP, Ernouf D, *et al:* Ethanol intake and 3H-serotonin uptake. II: A study in alcoholic patients using platelets 3H-paroxetine binding. *Life Sci* 48:1977–1983, 1991.

108. Neiman J, Bewing H, Malmgren R: Platelet uptake of serotonin (5HT) during ethanol withdrawal in male alcoholics. *Thromb Res* 46:803–809, 1987.

109. Kent TA, Campbell JL, Pazdernik TL, *et al:* Blood platelet uptake of serotonin in men alcoholics. *J Stud Alcohol* 46:357–359, 1985.

110. Brown CS, Kent TA, Bryant SG, *et al:* Blood platelet uptake of serotonin in episodic aggression. *Psychiatry Res* 27:5–12, 1989.

111. Lappalainen J, Dean M, Charbonneau L, *et al:* Mapping of the serotonin 5-HT$_{1DB}$ autoreceptor gene on chromosome 6 using a coding region polymorphism. *Am J Med Genet* 60:157–161, 1995.

112. Lappalainen J, Zhang L, Dean M, *et al:* Identification, expression and pharmacology of a cys23-ser23 substitution in the human 5HT$_{2c}$ receptor gene. *Genomics* 27:274–279, 1995.

113. Ozaki N, Lappalainen J, Dean M, *et al:* Mapping of the serotonin 5HT$_{1Da}$ autoreceptor gene (5HTR$_{1D}$) on chromosome 1 using a silent polymorphism in the coding region. *Am Med Genet* 60:162–164, 1995.

114. Nielsen D, Nakhai B, Schuebel K, *et al:* Tryptophan hydroxylase and the 5HT$_{1a}$ receptor: Behavioral and gene expression studies, in *Proceedings of the 33rd Annual Meeting of the American College of Neuropsychopharmacology.* San Juan, ACNP, 1994, p. 28.

115. Lappalainen J, Virkkunen M, Dean M, *et al:* Identification of a cys23-ser23 substitution in the 5HT$_{2c}$ receptor gene and allelic association to violent behavior and alcoholism. Manuscript in preparation.

116. Vanyukov MM, Moss HB, Yu LM, *et al:* Preliminary evidence for an association of dinucleotide repeat polymorphism at the MAOA gene with early onset alcoholism/substance abuse. *Am J Med Genet* 60:122–126, 1995.

117. Tiihonen J, Kuikka J, Bergstrom K, *et al:* Altered striatal dopamine reuptake site densities in habitually violent and nonviolent alcoholics. *Nature Med* 7:664–657, 1995.

9

A Nonhuman Primate Model of Excessive Alcohol Intake

Personality and Neurobiological Parallels of Type I- and Type II-Like Alcoholism

J. Dee Higley and Markku Linnoila

Abstract. Developmental, biochemical, and behavioral concomitants of voluntary excessive alcohol consumption were investigated using a nonhuman primate model. Studies were designed to investigate potential neurobiological and behavioral parallels of Cloninger's subtypes of type I and type II alcoholism in nonhuman primates. The studies have shown that a subpopulation of primates chronically consume intoxicating amounts of alcohol. Subjects that chronically consume intoxicating amounts of alcohol often exhibit neurobiological and behavioral features that were predicted by Cloninger's model for subtypes of alcoholism among humans. Investigations showed that behavior patterns and biological indices that characterize high anxiety, whether constitutionally or stress induced, were correlated with high rates of alcohol consumption, consistent with predictions for type I alcoholism. Early untoward rearing experiences that increased anxiety increased the probability that subjects would chronically drink alcohol to intoxication. Investigations of type II-like alcohol consumption patterns focused on subjects with low central nervous system (CNS) serotonin functioning [as measured by reduced cerebrospinal fluid (CSF) concentrations of the serotonin metabolite 5-hydroxyindoleacetic acid (5-HIAA)]. CSF 5-HIAA in infancy was shown to be a relatively stable neurobiological trait across development into adulthood. An individual CSF 5-HIAA concentration in infancy was shown to be a consequence of paternal and maternal genetic influences. Early parental neglect reduced CSF 5-HIAA concentrations. Low CSF 5-HIAA and CNS norepinephrine functioning were shown to predict excessive alcohol consumption in adolescence. Behaviorally, subjects with low CSF 5-HIAA demonstrated

J. Dee Higley • Laboratory of Clinical Studies, Primate Unit, National Institute on Alcohol Abuse and Alcoholism, Poolesville, Maryland 20837.   **Markku Linnoila** • Laboratory of Clinical Studies, Division of Intramural Clinical and Biological Research, National Institute on Alcohol Abuse and Alcoholism, Bethesda, Maryland 20892-1256.

Recent Developments in Alcoholism, Volume 13: Alcoholism and Violence, edited by Marc Galanter. Plenum Press, New York, 1997

impaired impulse control, which resulted in excessive and inappropriate aggression, infrequent and inept social behaviors, low social status, social isolation and expulsion from social groups at an early age, and high rates of early mortality. With some exceptions, these findings were consistent with predictions from Cloninger's type II model of excessive alcohol consumption among men who exhibit impaired impulse control and violent and antisocial behaviors.

> *The time has come for a study of inebriety from a medical stand-point, and when it is treated as a special disease its curability will be found equal to any other disease.*
> —Franklin D. Clum, MD, 1892

1. Introduction

During the past two decades, remarkable progress has been made in the study of alcohol abuse and alcoholism. As the field has become increasingly refined, more accurate classification and typology of patients have become possible. With the advances of classification, there has been the recognition that alcohol abuse and alcoholism are heterogeneous conditions with multiple etiological components.[1–3] Biological and psychological research has identified relatively homogeneous subgroups of alcohol-abusing and dependent patients, with each group exhibiting somewhat different psychobiological traits. Cloninger's neurogenetic, tridimensional theory of personality structure is among the most influential of the current psychobiological models.[4]

Cloninger identified two subtypes of alcoholism. The first, labeled type I, is characterized by high levels of traitlike anticipatory anxiety. Individuals with type I alcoholism are postulated to consume alcohol primarily for its antianxiety properties.[4,5] Excessive anxiety and the resulting increased alcohol consumption patterns are hypothesized to result from an interaction between untoward rearing experiences and genetic background. Type II alcoholism, on the other hand, is distinguished by impaired impulse control resulting in excessive alcohol consumption. Initial consumption is thought to be primarily motivated by the euphorogenic effects of alcohol, followed by high rates of alcohol consumption that result from loss of control once alcohol consumption begins. A cluster of behaviors related to impaired impulse control characterizes individuals with type II alcoholism. Essentially, Cloninger portrays the behaviors of type II alcoholics as physically aggressive, risk taking, and having difficulties functioning socially[4,6] (see ref. 7, for example). Each of the two types of alcoholism is proposed to have a different neurogenetic background, with anxiety-mediated type I alcoholism based primarily on a CNS norepinephrine excess, and impulse-mediated type II alcoholism based primarily on a CNS serotonin deficit.[4]

Because the systematic study of alcoholism is a relatively new discipline, until recently our understanding of the syndrome has been somewhat sparse. Animal models of human diseases are limited by the current understanding of the pathophysiology of the disease in question. To model a disease, its symptoms, causal, and precipitating factors must be defined in humans with such precision that they can be reproduced in another species.[8–10] An animal model is only useful to the extent that the essential features of the disease to be modeled are clearly defined and potential causal mechanisms are delineated. This is particularly difficult for syndromes, which typically have numerous symptoms along with multiple potential causal and precipitating factors. Advances in defining the necessary criteria and symptomatology for alcohol abuse and alcoholism have allowed researchers to develop animal models of the syndromes and to investigate the basic mechanisms of their components.[11–15]

2. Why Study Nonhuman Primates?

Recently, nonhuman primates have been used to model some features of alcohol abuse and alcoholism.[16–20] Nonhuman primates are our closest phylogenetic relatives, and as a result share a large percentage of their DNA with humans. These similarities in DNA makeup yield physiological, neuroanatomical, and behavioral similarities, if not actual homologies, that allow researchers to extrapolate their results to the human condition more readily than with results obtained from less closely related animal species. Many of the precursors and consequences of alcohol problems are social in nature. Like humans, the typical primate is a social being, living in a complex society with multiple social stressors and social responsibilities. Because of these similarities, nonhuman primates are particularly suited as research subjects for modeling the antecedents and concomitants of human alcohol problems.

3. Difficulties Producing a Nonhuman Primate Model of Alcohol Abuse

Given these advantages for using nonhuman primates to study alcohol abuse and alcoholism, it is surprising that the use of nonhuman primates to model alcohol abuse and dependence is a relatively new phenomenon. There are indications that this is a result of both theoretical and practical problems. For alcohol abuse and alcoholism, only recently have the descriptive data and our understanding of the pathophysiology achieved an adequate level of sophistication to allow the development of standardized diagnostic systems.[21–24] With these recent advances, nonhuman primate models relevant to alcohol abuse have begun to be developed.[8,18,25]

An independent limiting factor that has impeded the development of nonhuman primate models of alcohol abuse has been the difficulty in producing high levels of voluntary consumption of alcohol among normal nonhuman primates. Until recently, it was widely believed that nonhuman primates would not consume alcohol (e.g., refs. 16, 26, 27). Recent studies have shown, however, that at least for some species of nonhuman primates, when the alcohol solution is palatable and freely available, some (but not all) subjects will readily consume it in quantities that produce pharmacological effects. In many cases individual subjects will consume sufficient quantities of alcohol to produce blood levels exceeding the limits of legal intoxication for most states of the United States, resulting in stupor and at times unconsciousness.[18,28] Such recent observations have prompted investigators to use nonhuman primates in research on alcohol abuse and alcoholism.

4. Human and Nonhuman Primate Parallels in Alcohol Use

There are a number of demographic and epidemiological descriptions of alcohol consumption patterns in human society. Most humans find the initial taste of alcohol aversive, and, as a result, in human society alcohol is rarely consumed in its pure state. Instead, alcohol is consumed in solutions with low concentrations and often the taste is disguised using colas, fruit juices, and other flavorings. Despite its aversive taste properties, most people who try alcohol persist either because of expectations concerning its effects, social pressure, or because they find they enjoy its pharmacological effects.[29–31] Eventually, most individuals develop a pattern of modest consumption, with minimal alcohol-related problems.[32,33] Similarly, in at least some species of nonhuman primates, when the solution is palatable and the concentration of alcohol is under 15–20%, most subjects will consume alcohol at rates producing pharmacological effects, but only about 10–20% of normally reared subjects will freely consume palatable alcohol solutions at rates that consistently produce blood alcohol levels greater than the legal level of intoxication for most states.[19,25,28] Because only a few individual subjects consume alcohol at high rates, a problem that researchers face when using nonhuman primates is that they must have access to a large population of monkeys to identify a pool of subjects to study excessive alcohol consumption.

5. Methodology

Over the course of the past 4 years, more than 70 rhesus monkeys from our laboratory have been allowed to consume alcohol while living socially in their home cages. To perform this research, the monkeys are provided unfettered access to a palatable water–alcohol solution (8.5% v/v, flavored to taste with aspartame and colored with food coloring) for 1 hr each day while they are in their home environment. To precipitate initial consumption of alcohol at rates that produce pharmacological effects, subjects are first trained to drink a colored aspartame-water vehicle by hanging a bottle or a burette on the side of the cage and connecting it to a drinking spout. When all of the subjects are drinking the sweetened solution, the color is changed, and sufficient alcohol is added to make an 8.5% v/v alcohol solution. Over a 30- to 10-day period, most subjects consume alcohol at rates that produce pharmacological effects. Over an additional 5–15 days, individual response rates are established and the data collection phase of the experiment begins.

Subjects are not food- or water-deprived throughout their exposure, and they have alcohol available 5 days a week for 1 hr each day. To assure that the subjects are not drinking the alcohol solution just for its sweetened taste, subjects are provided simultaneous access to the sweetened vehicle, tap water, and the alcohol solution. In all of our studies to date, the first 10 days of the experimental paradigms have served as baseline periods and are identical in methodology except for the social arrangement of the home cage where the subjects have access to alcohol. The subjects are provided alcohol in their home cages, which include housing in pairs (both single and mixed gender pairs), social group housing in a pen containing 7 to 10 other monkeys, and occasionally in single cages. Those subjects living in social groups are maintained under stable social conditions, having lived in their social groups for at least a year prior to the beginning of the study. Because rhesus monkeys maintain a social dominance hierarchy that probably affects free access to the alcohol solution,[18,28,34] social groups receiving alcohol are subdivided according to relative dominance rankings. The cage is physically divided into smaller subsections, and subjects receiving alcohol are alternatively placed into high or low social dominance portions of the cage. Multiple drinking spouts are present in each subdivision of the cage. When subjects are tested in pairs, an alcohol dispenser is provided for each monkey: typically, one in the front and one in the back of the cage. Our paradigm has been designed to provide all subjects with sufficient time and opportunity to drink alcohol during each session; indeed, during the majority of the second half-hour-long alcohol session, the drinking spouts are not occupied.

6. Biological and Behavioral Measures

All behavioral and biochemical observations are obtained when the subjects are alcohol-free. In our studies, repeated cisternal CSF samples are collected from each of the subjects to measure CNS monoamine functioning. Simultaneous blood samples are drawn to quantify stress hormones. Behavioral observations are recorded during home-cage baseline conditions and during a stressful period such as social separation by trained observers who are blind to the subjects' monoamine status and specific hypotheses of the study. All cisternal CSF and blood samples are obtained between 1300 and 1500. All behavioral data are collected in the morning between 0900 and 1130, before alcohol is dispensed, using a standardized behavior scoring system described in detail in the original articles.[35]

7. Studies of Interindividual Differences

Studies by us and others have shown that although the rates of consumption vary between individual monkeys, once rates of consumption stabilize, average interindividual differences in alcohol consumption are markedly stable over time,[18] showing that the underlying motivation to consume alcohol may be traitlike. This suggests the possibility that within nonhuman primate societies, the 10–20% of individual nonhuman primates that consume alcohol at high rates may be homologous to the 10–20% of humans who at some period of their life abuse alcohol.[36] Researchers studying alcohol consumption in nonhuman primates have made significant progress in developing a nonhuman primate model of alcohol abuse by focusing on those subjects that show high rates of alcohol consumption.

8. Studies Investigating Features of Type I Alcoholism

> *The tranquilizer of greatest value since the early history of man, and which may never become outdated, is alcohol, when administered in moderation.*
>
> —Nathan Masor[37]

Nonhuman primates have been used with increasing frequency to investigate features of type I, or anxiety-related alcoholism. Some of the first researchers to investigate alcohol consumption in nonhuman primates indicated that under certain conditions stress may increase alcohol consumption.[16,38,39] Subsequent systematic studies using adolescent rhesus macaques have shown that social stress increases alcohol consumption, and that during nonstressful periods interindividual rates of alcohol consumption are positively correlated with interindividual traitlike anxiety and fearfulness.[18] For example, in these studies, interindividual differences in alcohol consumption were positive correlated with anxietylike behaviors such as self-directed orality and clasping of the body. Moreover, biological measures of stress and anxiety such as plasma corticotropin are also positively correlated with alcohol consumption.[18]

Research has further delineated the conditions and the underlying psychobiology related to stress-induced excessive alcohol consumption. This research has shown that alcohol consumption may attenuate the response to a stressful event. One measure that is quite sensitive to stress is social play. It typically declines following a number of different stressors.[40–43] In one study, social play declined to an almost nonexistent level following the exposure to a stressor. However, when a moderate dose of alcohol was given to the stressed monkeys, social play increased to and even exceeded the baseline levels.[44] Others have also found that a modest-to-moderate dosage of alcohol reduces adverse consequences of stress, resulting in increased social play and other positive social behaviors.[45] As levels of intoxication increase, however, play decreases below baseline levels.[38]

Play is not the only behavior reduced by stress that returns to baseline levels following alcohol consumption. Ervin and colleagues[28] found that in vervet monkeys there was not a uniform increase in play following the consumption of alcohol; rather, the idiosyncratic behavioral patterns of individual subjects that were suppressed by stress were the same behaviors that increased following alcohol consumption. Further evidence of alcohol's stress-reducing properties was seen when subjects underwent the stress of a social separation. During periods of social separation, rates of despair and anxiety-like behaviors were attenuated by low doses of alcohol.[44] This finding is consistent with a body of literature from rodent studies showing the similarities between benzodiazepines and alcohol in attenuating anxiety,[46] and suggests that at low to moderate doses, alcohol possesses anxiolytic effects. It is noteworthy, however, that while small doses of alcohol may attenuate stress, high doses of alcohol were more likely to exacerbate anxiety and depressionlike behaviors.[44] Interestingly, while it is widely held that alcohol use is related to or may exacerbate depressive symptoms in humans, in their relatively exhaustive review of laboratory studies that assessed the activating and depressing effects of alcohol, Tucker and colleagues[47] noted that at blood levels below 10%, alcohol typically acts as an antidepressant. While high doses are seldom used in the laboratory, the few studies that have shown increased depressive symptoms following alcohol consumption have utilized high doses.[47] This again suggests the utility of the primate model to investigate alcohol effects, particularly in cases where ethical concerns, such as administering high doses of alcohol to volunteers, make human studies impossible to perform.

Probably because alcohol has stress-reducing properties, nonhuman primates typically consume more alcohol in stressful settings than in otherwise identical but less stressful settings.[18,19,38] Such stress-induced alcohol consumption may be substantial. For example, following a social separation stressor, adolescent subjects reared in normal settings double their rates of alcohol consumption, often to levels that produce blood alcohol concentrations in excess of 100 mg/dl, the limit of legal intoxication in most of the United States.[18,19] Nevertheless, some subjects' rates of alcohol consumption seem relatively unaffected by increased stress; still others seem particularly prone to increase their consumption during even minimal stress. Studies of nonhuman primates indicate that these differences in how stress affects alcohol consumption may be, at least in part, due to early experiences that serve to decrease the threshold for experiencing anxiety. One of the best illustrations of this comes from studies of rhesus macaques reared under what is termed a peer-only or peer-rearing condition. These subjects are reared from birth with constant access to other same-aged peers but without mothers or any adults. In the absence of adult guidance, these peer-reared monkeys develop trait-like, chronic anxiety.[35,48,49] From infancy and into adolescence, they exhibit chronic activation of the hypothalamic–pituitary–adrenal axis.[18,50–52] They are more likely to show fearfulness and anxietylike behavior in the face of a challenge than mother-reared controls.[35,48,49] While other factors probably play a role, at least in part as a result of this predisposition to anxiety and fear,

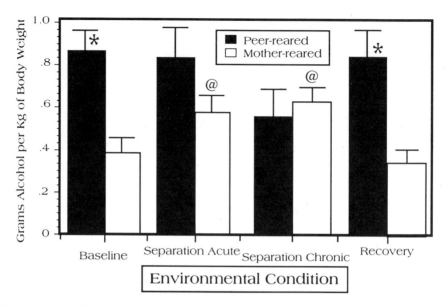

Figure 1.   An illustration of the effects of early rearing experiences and social separation on alcohol consumption ($n = 22$, $F(3.60) = 5.02$, $P = 0.007$). Each bar represents the average and SD of alcohol consumption in grams per kilogram of body weight for each group over experimental conditions. Solid bar represents peer-reared and open bar represents mother-reared subjects. The preseparation baseline period is the average of 10 days of home-cage consumption. The average consumption of the four separations is divided into an overall acute phase (mean of first day of each of the four separations) and an overall chronic phase (mean of remaining 3 days of each separation). The postseparation recovery phase is the average of 10 days of alcohol consumption following the social separations. A significant difference between the peer-reared subjects and the mother-reared subjects within the same period, with the peer-reared subjects showing an increased consumption ($P < 0.05$). @, A significant increase in alcohol consumption for the mother-reared subjects during social separation relative to home-cage consumption ($P < 0.05$). The apparent reduction in alcohol consumption by the peer-reared monkeys during the chronic phase of the social separations is not statistically significant ($T = 1.56$, $P > 0.10$). (From Higley et al.[18])

peer-reared subjects are more likely than mother-reared controls to consume alcohol at rates that produce intoxication when alcohol is freely available in the home cage.[18] On the other hand, when a stressor such as a social separation is applied, the mother-reared subjects, who normally consume only limited amounts of alcohol, increase their levels of consumption to levels that equal those of the peer-reared monkeys[18] (see Fig. 1).

Interestingly, within each of the rearing groups there are wide interindividual differences in alcohol consumption rates. A few of the mother-reared subjects consume alcohol at rates similar to the peer-reared subjects; on the other hand, some of the peer-reared subjects seem relatively unaffected by the early rearing experience and consume alcohol at rates similar to the mother-reared subjects. These within-group interindividual differences in alcohol consumption are maintained across settings and time.[18] Clues suggesting the possible genesis of these within-group individual differences come from measuring the anxietylike behaviors and biological markers indicative of stress responsiveness and anxiety prior to alcohol exposure. Interindividual differences in both anxietylike behaviors and biological markers of anxiety correlate positively with interindividual differences in alcohol consumption. For example, there is a positive correlation between individual alcohol consumption rate and the severity of prestress anxietylike behaviors. These anxietylike behaviors are also positively correlated with plasma cortisol.[18] As might be predicted, plasma cortisol is positively correlated with alcohol consumption rate.[18] These findings suggest that the intrinsic predisposition to experience anxiety when stressed may be related to differences in alcohol consumption rates. Kraemer *et al.*[20] also found evidence for Cloninger's prediction of high CNS norepinephrine functioning among rhesus monkeys exhibiting type I-like excessive alcohol consumption. According to these authors, nonhuman primates that show large increases in CSF norepinephrine concentrations following an alcohol bolus are more likely to show a high rate of stress-induced alcohol consumption relative to those that exhibit only minimal CSF norepinephrine increases.[20] These results suggest possible reasons why under apparently identical stressful conditions some subjects increase their alcohol consumption, while others appear to be relatively invulnerable to the same stressor.

These findings indicate that early experiences that result in increased levels of anxietylike behaviors can have a major impact on alcohol consumption. Studies of human alcoholics have shown that for type I alcoholism early developmental experiences are important factors in determining alcohol abuse patterns.[4] The results suggest that early rearing experiences, which predispose monkeys to increased fear-related behaviors, produce excessive alcohol consumption under normal living conditions. Furthermore, a major stressful challenge such as social separation increases alcohol consumption to levels producing intoxication even in monkeys not particularly vulnerable to stress.

9. Serotonin and Type II Alcoholism

> At the moment, serotonin is the hottest item (in this author's opinion) in the search for a biochemical explanation for what appears to be a genetically determined transmission of alcoholism.
> —Donald W. Goodwin[53]

Recently, nonhuman primates have been used to model features of type II alcoholism. These studies used group-living adolescent and adult rhesus monkeys to investigate high alcohol consumption in subjects with reduced

CNS serotonin functioning.[54-57] As noted earlier, a distinguishing neurobiological feature of type II alcoholism is impaired impulse control, which is believed to result in part from impaired CNS serotonin functioning.[7] The underlying theory of Cloninger's model of type II alcoholism postulates that initial alcohol consumption among individuals with the vulnerability is primarily motivated by the euphorogenic effects of alcohol; but because these individuals are unable to curb their impulses, once consumption begins, loss of controlled drinking results. In his original formulation and other publications, Cloninger discusses an overall behavioral style that characterizes individuals with type II alcohol problems as having a pattern of behaviors that are related to impaired impulse control, such as physically aggressive behaviors, antisocial traits, excessive risk taking, and difficulties in social relationships.[4,6] Unlike the risk for expressing type I alcoholism, the risk for expressing type II alcoholism appears to be primarily genetically transmitted and relatively unaffected by early experiences.

10. Reduced CNS Serotonin Functioning as a Long-Term Enduring Trait

A principal neurobiological feature of type II alcoholism is a CNS serotonin deficit.[4] This is typically measured by assaying CSF for concentrations of the major serotonin metabolite, 5-hydroxyindoleacetic acid (5-HIAA). Several nonhuman primate studies have suggested that interindividual differences in CSF 5-HIAA concentrations are traitlike (i.e., highly stable across time and experimental settings). For example, when 14 CSF samples were obtained over a 1-year period from the same adult female subjects, interindividual stability was high, with the average correlation coefficient in excess of $r = .51$.[58] When Raleigh and colleagues obtained repeated CSF samples from adult males of a closely related species of an Old World primate, they also found a high degree of intraindividual stability in CSF 5-HIAA concentrations among adult males.[59,60] This high degree of intraindividual stability is not limited to the laboratory setting, where environmental changes are closely controlled. When adolescent male macaques that live in a free-ranging forest were trapped once in 1991 and again in 1992, and a CSF sample was obtained during each of the two captures, the between-year average correlation in CSF 5-HIAA was $r = 0.54$.[61]

Although absolute concentrations of CSF 5-HIAA vary with age and situations,[52,62] interindividual differences stabilize starting early in life, during infancy. For example, in one recently completed study, CSF 5-HIAA concentrations obtained from infant monkeys on day 14 correlated with samples obtained on days 30, 60, 90, 120, and 150.[62] This interindividual stability is also present across situations and settings. In another study of 6-month-old infant rhesus monkeys, home-cage baseline CSF 5-HIAA concentrations were strongly correlated with CSF 5-HIAA concentrations obtained under conditions of social separation, when samples were taken 2 and 4 weeks apart.[52,63] Kraemer *et al.*[64] also found traitlike stability in infant rhesus monkey across repeated sampling during the first year of life, particularly among infants reared by their mothers. These early interindividual differences that stabilize in infancy also appear to be stable across longer periods, with the mean of CSF monoamine samples taken in infancy (6 months of age) predicting mean concentrations in middle childhood, a year later.[52] A recent study of these same subjects showed this traitlike response of the serotonin system may endure into adulthood. CSF 5-HIAA samples obtained when the subjects were 6 months old were positively correlated with CSF 5-HIAA samples obtained 5 years later, when the subjects were adults.[56]

11. Impaired CNS Serotonin Functioning and High Alcohol Consumption

Numerous studies have shown that men with low CSF 5-HIAA concentrations exhibit evidence of impaired impulse control such as increased fire setting[65] and increased violent criminal recidivism.[66] A large number of animal studies show excessive or high rates of alcohol consumption among animals with reduced central serotonin functioning (e.g., see ref. 67 for a recent review). Among humans, clinical studies show evidence of reduced central serotonin functioning in subjects at risk for or who exhibit alcohol abuse and alcoholism (e.g., see ref. 68 for a recent review). For example, when they are compared to healthy volunteers, young alcoholic men and women have low CSF 5-HIAA concentrations, even during periods of abstinence.[69–71] Depressed patients with first-degree alcoholic relatives have significantly lower CSF 5-HIAA and 3-methoxy-4-hydroxyphenylglycol (MHPG) concentrations than depressed patients without alcoholic relatives.[72] Like humans, nonhuman primates with low CSF 5-HIAA concentrations are more likely to exhibit behaviors characteristic of impaired impulse control such as spontaneous, long leaps at dangerous heights and repeated jumping into baited traps where they are captured.[61,73]

Because they are impaired in controlling their impulses, we postulated that subjects with low CSF 5-HIAA would exhibit high rates of alcohol consumption. This hypothesis is consistent with one of the postulates of Cloninger's tridimensional model of alcoholism that type II alcoholism is mediated by central serotonin and norepinephrine deficits.[4,74] In what is to our knowledge the first study of this hypothesis in nonhuman primates, we found that alcohol consumption was related to reduced CNS serotonergic and noradrenergic functioning.[18,56] High rates of alcohol consumption during the stressful conditions of a social separation were correlated with low CSF 5-HIAA[56] and MHPG[18,56] concentrations obtained during the social separation stress. MHPG obtained during social separation was also negatively correlated with alcohol consumption during nonstress conditions.[56] To the degree that nonhuman primate findings can be extrapolated to the human condition, our findings suggest that serotonin-deficit-associated excessive alcohol consumption may be particularly associated with stressful conditions; reduced norepinephrine, on the other hand, was correlated with high alcohol consumption under both stressful and nonstressful conditions. This suggests that the level of stress should be taken under consideration when obtaining CSF 5-HIAA to use as a biological marker to predict alcohol consumption.

Additional evidence that serotonin is involved in excessive alcohol consumption comes from investigations that use serotonin-function-enhancing drugs to treat alcohol consumption. While primarily norepinephrine-affecting antidepressant treatments have met with little success in treating alcohol abuse, some recent studies using the antidepressants that are highly selective for serotonin have shown promise as adjunctive pharmacological treatments for maintenance of abstinence (see, for example, ref. 68). In a recent, unpublished study using rhesus monkeys, we investigated treatment of excessive alcohol consumption with the serotonin reuptake inhibitor sertraline. Baseline alcohol consumption patterns were established in adolescent monkeys. They were then treated for alcohol consumption with the serotonin reuptake inhibitor sertraline. Subjects who were modest alcohol consumers, who typically consumed alcohol at rates that would not produce intoxicating blood alcohol levels, were unaffected by the treatment. On the other hand, subjects that consumed alcohol on a daily basis to the point of visible intoxication (i.e., acquired blood alcohol levels in excess of 100 mg/dl) reduced their rates of consumption to match the modest alcohol consumers. This reduction in alcohol consumption occurred only after chronic but not acute sertraline treatment. The treatment effect was not a result of a loss of appetite, since food consumption was unaltered by the sertraline treatment.[75] It is also of note that our findings are consistent with a large number of animal studies showing high rates of alcohol consumption and an increased alcohol preference in subjects with reduced CNS serotonin functioning.[67]

12. Serotonin and Violence

> The trait nature of the serotonin dysfunction could be
> an advantage for the potential detection of a
> propensity for impulsive violent behavior and perhaps
> for the prediction of dangerousness.
>
> —Jan Volavka[76]

A number of studies have suggested that impaired CNS serotonin functioning underlies excessive, unprovoked aggression. For example, many men with low CSF 5-HIAA concentrations exhibit increased unplanned aggression and violence.[65,77–86] Paralleling studies in humans, recent studies using nonhuman primates have demonstrated that low CSF 5-HIAA concentrations are correlated with increased rates of wounding, unprovoked and unrestrained

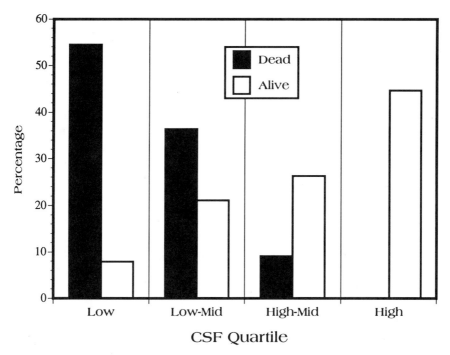

Figure 2. The percentage of subjects dead or alive 4 years after a CSF sample was obtained to quantify CSF 5-HIAA concentrations. Subjects are grouped in quartiles according to CSF 5-HIAA concentrations. Units of 5-HIAA concentrations are in picomoles per milliliter. The figure shows a monotonic increase in death rates with lower quartiles of CSF 5-HIAA. None of the subjects from the highest quartile of CSF 5-HIAA died over the course of the study. (From Higley et al.[135])

violence, and inappropriate aggression.[25,58,61,73,87,88] This relationship between impaired CNS serotonin functioning and violence appears to be particularly strong in nonhuman primate subjects with less competent social skills, characterized by low social ranking.[60]

The data suggest, however, that low CSF 5-HIAA is not correlated with overall levels of aggression; rather, it is only spontaneous, impulsive aggression that tends to escalate to physically damaging conflicts that shows a negative correlation with CSF 5-HIAA concentrations.[60,73,88] An illustration of this comes from a study that investigated the separate roles that central testosterone and serotonin functioning play in controlling aggression and impulsivity.[61] CSF testosterone and 5-HIAA and aggressive behaviors were measured twice in the same free-ranging adolescent male nonhuman primates with the samples taken 1 year apart. CSF free testosterone concentrations were positively correlated with aggressiveness and with behaviors indicative of high social dominance but not with behaviors indicative of impulsivity.

CSF 5-HIAA concentrations were negatively correlated with impulsive leaps and with violent aggression that escalated into assaults, wounds, and prolonged chase sequences (escalated aggression), but CSF 5-HIAA was not correlated with overall rates of aggression. Dimensional analyses showed that subjects with low CSF 5-HIAA exhibited high rates of most forms of aggression; nevertheless, rates of aggression were augmented even further if a subject with low CSF 5-HIAA also had a high CSF testosterone concentration (see Fig. 2). Measures of social dominance were highest among males with both high CSF testosterone and high CSF 5-HIAA concentrations.[61]

13. Reduced CNS Serotonin Functioning and Antisociallike Behavior

In humans, type II alcoholism is associated with various antisocial traits and other problems of impaired social functioning, such as reduced social affiliation and less competent social skills.[74] Indeed, some of the most frequent correlates of type II alcoholism are antisocial personality traits.[6,89,90] For example, there is evidence that impaired social functioning beginning early in life is predictive of excessive alcohol use in adolescence.[90] Adolescents who rate themselves as socially isolated are more likely to abuse alcohol.[91] Young and elderly men with few friends are more likely to abuse alcohol,[92] and adult children of alcoholics rate themselves as more socially isolated and with few friends.[93] Indeed, in one study the best predictor of successful alcoholism treatment outcome for type II alcoholics was the degree of impaired social functioning, with less social impairment predicting a better outcome.[94]

Nonhuman primates are close to ideal subjects to investigate the relationship between CNS serotonin responses and social functioning. They are inherently social, living in complex settings with numerous partners and fluid social interchanges. As in human society, the rules for such interchanges are orderly, structured by status and emotional and physical needs. Like humans, individual primates vary in their sociality, with some subjects highly gregarious and others solitary. Chamove, Eysenck, and Harlow[95] identified sociality as one of three personality traits in rhesus monkeys. Sociality in monkeys is a trait that is similar to the personality trait extroversion, that Eysenck's identified in humans.[96] Sociality is an enduring trait in monkeys[97,98] as well as in humans.[99] Several studies among nonhuman primates have demonstrated that sociality is positively correlated with CNS serotonin function. For example, across repeated studies of captive vervet monkeys (*Cercopithecus aethiops*, a highly social Old World primate species that is closely related to macaques), Raleigh and colleagues[100-103] found that enhancing serotonin functioning by administering the serotonin precursor tryptophan, the uptake inhibitor fluoxetine, or the serotonin agonist quipazine increased positive social behaviors such as approaching and grooming other monkeys. When investigators reduced serotonin functioning by administering the tryptophan hydroxylase inhibitor para-chlorophenylananine (PCPA) to the monkeys, it produced opposite effects. Instead, the monkeys withdrew from and avoided social proximity and affiliative social interactions.[101,103,104]

More recently, research with our collaborators demonstrated that naturally occurring reduced serotonin functioning is correlated with reduced sociality. For example, in a sample of free-ranging adolescent male monkeys, subjects with low CSF 5-HIAA concentrations exhibited reduced levels of four measures of sociality: time spent grooming other monkeys (a measure of affection in nonhuman primates); time spent in close proximity to other group members; time spent in general affiliative social behaviors; and mean number of companions within a 5-m radius (<5 m).[88] Low rates of positive social interactions are also associated with low CSF 5-HIAA concentrations among juveniles of both sexes and adult females.[58]

Several studies have also shown that diminished central serotonin activity is correlated with diminished social competence. For example, Kruesi and colleagues[105] found that in behaviorally disturbed and obsessive–compulsive children, independent of psychiatric classification, reduced social competence was correlated with low CSF 5-HIAA concentrations. Similarly, studies of both aggressive humans[78] and nonhuman primates[98,106,107] have shown that individuals high in social deviancy, or who are rated as low in competent social behaviors,[106] have relatively low CSF 5-HIAA concentrations.

Type II alcoholism in humans is closely linked to antisocial behavior. Given that nonhuman primates with infrequent and less competent social interactions often possess low CSF 5-HIAA concentrations, one might predict that reduced sociality would be related to high rates of alcohol consumption. These postulates were tested by measuring the rate and complexity of social behaviors prior to alcohol exposure and correlating them with alcohol consumption. The complexity of social behaviors used during interchanges varies positively with the degree of social competence. For example, infants engage in frequent ventral clinging with caregivers, a behavior seldom seen between adults. With increasing social complexity these infantlike affiliative social behaviors change, and by adulthood, when subjects spend time in close proximity to each other, they groom and huddle together[105,108] but seldom if ever cling ventrally to each other. We predicted that ostracized subjects, as indexed by minimal time in social affiliation, would consume more alcohol than subjects spending a lot of time in social affiliation. Moreover, immature, less competent social behaviors would correlate positively with high rates of alcohol consumption. Consistent with our predictions, infrequent social interactions were predictive of high alcohol consumption; and when the subjects that consumed high volumes of alcohol interacted socially, they used less mature social behaviors such as infantlike ventral clinging, a behavior that is characteristic of infants and seldom seen between adults.[56]

One measure of social competence among nonhuman primates is social dominance ranking. Social dominance among nonhuman primates is generally measured by observing who has primary access to prized or limited resources. As male monkeys' tenure in their new troops is prolonged, competence in forming and maintaining social relationships increases social dominance. Because size and weight play little role in acquiring social dominance,[109,110] it is clear that physical prowess alone is not sufficient to gain success in social competition. Indeed, rarely is the highest-ranking male of a troop the most aggressive.[110,111] Instead, social dominance is acquired and maintained through the formation of affiliative bonds with other troop members who then support the dominant male in hostile and challenging social encounters.[110–113] Building coalitions and maintaining social support is crucial to acquire and maintain a high social dominance rank.[114–118] One of the most replicated findings among nonhuman primates with low CSF 5-HIAA[56,58,60,102,105] or pharmacologically lowered CNS serotonin functioning[60,102,118,119] is low social dominance ranking.

14. Low CSF 5-HIAA as a Risk Factor for Social Ostracism and Early Mortality

Nonhuman primates that exhibit excessive aggressiveness in a naturalistic environment are typically ostracized and often forcibly expelled from their social group.[110,120] Given these findings, it is not surprising that there is a strong association between the length of a male's tenure in a troop and the number of relationships the male is able to form and maintain, especially with the adult females of the troop, and the social dominance ranking he attains.[121] These findings appear to have important consequences for the adolescent male macaques migrating between social groups.

One of the most critical life-history events among feral-living male macaques is emigration from the natal group. This is a universal event for male macaques that the species utilize to prevent inbreeding. Migration to a new troop is a dangerous and highly stressful event for young males. Wounding and death is not uncommon.[122–129] With the exception of human encroachment, for a number of different primates the most frequent cause of adolescent and young adult male death is aggression by other monkeys or intraspecies resources competition.[130–133] While some males migrate early in adolescence, when their growth acceleration is just beginning,[88] other subjects are able to delay migration until they are fully mature and more socially sophisticated.[134] An additional benefit of delaying migration is that older brothers and other familiar conspecifics may have migrated to nearly troops, facilitating an immigrant's integration into a new social group.[121,135] While males with high CSF 5-HIAA concentrations remain in their troops of origin until they are older than this normative age of migration,[134] males with low CSF 5-HIAA typically migrate from their social group of origin when they are younger and often not fully mature.[88]

Based on the above observations, we hypothesized that subjects with low CSF 5-HIAA concentrations would show disproportionally high rates of mortality during the period that most males migrate from their social groups of origin. When CSF 5-HIAA samples were obtained from 49 free-ranging, 2-year-old prepubertal male rhesus monkeys, low CSF 5-HIAA concentrations were predictive of which subjects died, with 46% of the subjects with low CSF 5-HIAA concentrations dead or presumed dead 4 years later.[136] Indeed, 91% of the dead subjects came from the two lowest quartiles of CSF 5-HIAA concentrations. Direct observations of aggressive behavior showed that subjects that were dead or missing initiated escalated aggression, a measure of unrestrained aggression that has a high probability of trauma or injury, at a higher rate than subjects that were known to be alive.[136] The cause of death could be ascertained for 6 of the 11 dead subjects. The four subjects that were known to die as a consequence of violence all came from the lowest quartile of CSF 5-HIAA concentrations and had been rated as more aggressive during their initial capture.[136] None of the subjects from the highest CSF 5-HIAA concentration quartile were dead or missing.

15. CSF 5-HIAA, Frontal Cortex Serotonin Functioning, and Impulsive Behaviors

While it is clear that CNS serotonin has crucial effects on impulse control, aggression, overall social functioning, and ultimately on the rate of early mortality, it is less clear which areas of the brain are involved in these behaviors and what the measurement of CSF 5-HIAA concentrations represents. In primates but not in rodents, the dorsal raphe nucleus is the origin of the major ascending serotonin pathway from the brain stem (the major source of CNS serotonin) to the frontal and prefrontal cortices.[137] Moreover, the dorsal prefrontal cortex may be the only cortical area that projects directly back to the dorsal raphe nucleus.[138] Stanley et al.[139] found a high positive correlation between frontal cortex tissue and lumbar CSF 5-HIAA concentrations postmortem in humans. Other human studies have also found strong positive correlations between frontal cortex 5-HIAA and cisternal CSF 5-HIAA concentrations.[140,141] In a PET study on nonhuman primates, designed to measure the relationship between CSF 5-HIAA concentrations and regional glucose utilization, the strongest correlation between CSF 5-HIAA concentrations and glucose utilization was with the orbitofrontal cortex region.[142] Moreover, ratings for aggressivity were correlated with both CSF 5-HIAA concentrations and glucose utilization in the orbitofrontal cortex.[142] Two recent exhaustive reviews of serotonin receptor functioning in suicide victims concluded that most studies show low serotonin-2 receptor density in frontal cortex of suicide victims.[143,144] Furthermore, individuals with frontal brain injury exhibit deficits in impulse control,[145,146] increased episodes of violence,[147] and low CSF 5-HIAA concentrations.[148] These and other systematic studies of nonhuman primates and humans with frontal lobe injury show the importance of the frontal and prefrontal cortices for the regulation of impulses and maintenance of goal-oriented behavior.[149,150] Taken together, these studies suggest that cisternal CSF 5-HIAA concentrations correlate with frontal cortex functioning and the possible importance of frontal cortex serotonin in impulse control.

16. Etiology of Low CSF 5-HIAA

16.1. Genetic Influences

The nonhuman primate model has made important contributions toward understanding genetic contributions to serotonin functioning. Despite the potential importance for understanding mechanisms underlying differences in behavior and mental disorders, only one study of humans utilizing a small number of monozygotic and dizygotic twins has investigated genetic contributions to CSF monoamine metabolite concentrations. In that study, CSF 5-HIAA concentrations were not found to be heritable.[151] Environmental and genetic contributions to CSF monoamine metabolite concentrations were investigated in a number of nonhuman primate infants with different rearing backgrounds. To study genetic contributions to CSF monoamine concentrations, 55 young rhesus monkeys were reared apart from their 10 fathers to perform a paternal half-sibling analysis. To study maternal genetic contributions, 23 infants were reared with their mothers, 23 infants were removed from their mothers at birth and fostered to unrelated lactating females, and 24 infants were removed from their mothers at birth and reared in peer-only groups. When the monkeys reached 6 months of age, CSF was obtained via cisternal puncture prior to and during a series of social separations. When the results were statistically pooled according to the biological father, CSF 5-HIAA showed significant heritable effects ($h^2 > 0.5$) for both sons and daughters. In addition, there were substantial maternal genetic influences on the young offsprings' 5-HIAA ($h^2 > 0.5$). Although they did not study maternal contributions, the finding of a paternal genetic contribution to CSF 5-HIAA concentrations has recently been replicated in a study by Clarke and colleagues.[152] These findings suggest that a significant portion of the variance in the turnover rate of CNS serotonin is determined by genetic mechanisms. While somewhat speculative, these findings may suggest the mode of genetic transmission of type II alcoholism. It predicts that low serotonin functioning is genetically transmitted, which leads to deficits of impulse control and ultimately to increased risk for excessive alcohol consumption once alcohol consumption begins. This pattern, however, does not fit Cloninger's predictions and findings replicating his original research, since those studies have shown that type II is transmitted from fathers to sons[153] and our studies show that low serotonin functioning is genetically transmitted by both mothers and fathers.

16.2. Environmental Influences

Primate societies are explicitly structured to assure that the infant acquires and practices its social skills in a relatively safe, protected environment. Among most Old World monkey societies, neonate monkeys initially develop their social skills within the watchful tutelage of their biological mother. Mothers are especially important social agents through which infant and juvenile monkeys develop the capacity to properly inhibit and express emotions, including aggression.[49,108,154–156] Infants and young monkeys deprived of opportunities to interact with their mothers are likely as adolescents and adults to show diminished affiliative social behaviors necessary for maintaining social bonds and relationships,[157] and in initial interactions with peers show less frequent and less skilled aggression to maintain social dominance.[158] Later in development, as young monkeys' motor and cognitive capacities mature, peers become central in developing and practicing social skills. Through social play, interactions with peers have a crucial role for acquiring knowledge regarding the proper settings and intensity for exhibiting aggression. Monkeys deprived of adult role models and opportunities to practice social behaviors with peers are likely to express aggression at inappropriate targets or settings and to demonstrate deviant social responses and social relationships.[159–162]

Adults not only affect the acquisition and development of observed behavior, they play a crucial role in the organization and proper development of the CNS. For example, a number of studies using nonhuman primates have shown that prior experiences affect serotonin functioning during infancy and childhood.[52,63,64] These studies have shown that adult influences, particularly maternal input, is critical to govern the development of the CNS serotonin system. In the absence of adult influence, serotonin functioning is impaired. For example, one rearing condition that has been widely studied in monkeys is peer-rearing. These subjects are removed from their mothers at birth and reared with other age-matched infants. When CSF 5-HIAA was obtained from neonatal peer- and mother-reared monkeys on days 14 and 30, 60, 90, 120, and 150, parentally neglected peer-reared subjects exhibited lower CSF 5-HIAA than mother-reared subjects.[62] One study with a limited sample size suggested that the effect of early rearing experiences on CSF 5-HIAA may disappear by adolescence.[51] In a study with a larger sample size, in which peer- and mother-reared subjects were longitudinally studied from infancy into adulthood, peer-reared subjects exhibited lower CSF 5-HIAA concentrations than mother-reared subjects both in infancy and adulthood.[56]

Behaviorally, peer-reared subjects exhibit a number of deficits. Even in the absence of threatening stimuli, juvenile-aged peer-reared monkeys are highly fearful, and in the face of a prolonged stressor such as social separation they are more likely to exhibit behaviors characteristic of despair.[108] There is evidence that these behavioral differences persist into early adulthood. In a recent study, we investigated 22 young peer- and mother-reared adult rhesus monkeys. The peer-reared monkeys were more likely than the mother-reared subjects to show regressive, infantlike behaviors such as self-orality and self-clasping. In addition, they had higher blood plasma concentrations of adrenocorticotropin and cortisol.[18]

Paralleling the findings of peer-rearing in nonhuman primates, prospective and retrospective studies show that a rearing history of parental neglect is very frequent during early development among aggressive children diagnosed as having conduct disorder[163,164] and among delinquent adolescents and adults with personality disorders.[90,165–169] It is also common among children who have poor relations with their peers and who exhibit excessive aggression.[90,170,171] Other studies show that children neglected by their parents are likely to use and abuse tobacco, alcohol, and other drugs.[90,172–174] Peer-rearing in nonhuman primates has been described as a model of parental neglect.[105,116] As we noted earlier, the peer-reared monkeys were also more likely to abuse alcohol than the mother-reared monkeys.[18]

The behaviors of peer-reared subjects parallel the behaviors of normally reared subjects with low CSF 5-HIAA concentrations. They exhibit inappropriate and excessive aggression.[105,116] For example, as adolescents, they were placed in a room with an infant and required to "baby-sit." All of the mother-reared monkeys demonstrated high levels of caregiving to the infant. The peer-reared monkeys, on the other hand, avoided contact with the infant and were more likely to threaten and show aggression to the infant.[105] Aggression to an infant is a behavior that is virtually never seen in normally reared subjects. This inappropriate aggression extended to other settings as well. While severe aggression hardly ever occurs in rhesus monkeys that have lived together for prolonged periods, peer-reared subjects were more likely to exhibit severe aggression to their cage-mates with whom they had lived for most of their lives.[105]

There are indications that these differences in aggressiveness between peer- and mother-reared monkeys persist beyond adolescence. In a colony-wide assessment of inappropriate maternal behavior, adult female monkeys who were peer-reared were more likely than adult female mother-reared monkeys to neglect and abuse their own infants.[175] In addition, we have recently acquired new evidence regarding long-term effects of early peer rearing. Although in our colony adult mother-reared monkeys outnumber peer-reared monkeys by 3 to 1, over a 2-year period, of 12 adult males producing injuries to a female requiring veterinary treatment, 10 were peer-reared (statistically significant at $P < 0.05$ using a Chi-square test). Of the seven females who had to be removed from stable social groups because of fight wounds or self-aggression requiring veterinary treatment, six were peer-reared (statistically significant at $P < 0.05$ using a Chi-square test).[105] This finding was recently replicated with a new cohort.[176]

Like the subjects with naturally occurring low CSF 5-HIAA concentrations, peer-reared subjects are socially inept. They are more likely as juveniles and young adolescents to achieve low social dominance ranking.[176] They are less likely to exhibit adultlike social huddling and more likely to engage in infantlike ventral clinging, even as adults.[61,136] One of the most important findings from these studies is that early parental absence has long-term effects on central serotonin and perhaps norepinephrine functions, which in turn are associated with excessive alcohol consumption, impaired social functioning, and disruptive social behaviors. The effects of rearing on alcohol consumption and neurophysiological functioning parallel the interindividual negative correlation between CSF 5-HIAA concentrations and alcohol consumption, with the high-alcohol-consuming peer-reared subjects[18] exhibiting low CSF 5-HIAA concentrations. This effect of early experience on type II-like behaviors and alcohol abuse is not consistent with Cloninger's predictions of no effect of developmental environment on type II alcoholism. It is consistent with recent studies showing that early experiences shape and account for antisocial behavior among adolescents and young adults, however.[177] It is also noteworthy that the peer-reared subjects exhibit high levels of fear and anxietylike behaviors, which is predicted by type I alcoholism. This suggests that, at least in this monkey model, the psychobiology of the two types of alcoholism may overlap in some subjects.

17. Summary and Conclusions

Within the general rhesus monkey population, a phenotype for high rates of alcohol consumption exists. Subjects with this phenotype chronically consume alcohol at rates producing intoxication. Our findings show that underlying etiological mechanisms and biobehavioral correlates parallel many of the predictions of Cloninger's neurogenetic model of alcoholism. Behavior patterns and biological indices that characterize high anxiety, whether constitutionally or stress induced, were correlated with high rates of alcohol consumption, consistent with predictions of type I alcoholism. Reduced CNS serotonin functioning early in life, as measured by low CSF 5-HIAA concentration, is a risk factor for low serotonin functioning later in life. Subjects with low CSF 5-HIAA concentrations have impaired impulse control, resulting in frequent violence, infrequent and less competent social behaviors, and low social status. They are shunned as companions and forced to leave their social groups at an early age and are likely to suffer from early mortality, often as an adjunct consequence to violent behavior. CSF 5-HIAA concentrations are genetically influenced, and parental neglect during early childhood may contribute to reduced central serotonin functioning during adolescence and early adulthood. Reduced central serotonin and norepinephrine functioning, decreased social affiliation, and less competent social functioning are risk factors that may contribute to excessive alcohol consumption in adulthood. Early rearing experiences that reduce serotonin functioning appear to exaggerate an inherited predisposition for alcohol consumption. These findings suggest the potential utility of this nonhuman primate model for understanding the neurobiology of controlled alcohol consumption and competent social functioning on one hand and excessive alcohol consumption, disruptive social behaviors, and excessive aggression on the other hand.

ACKNOWLEDGMENTS. The authors would like to thank Alan Dodson, Maribeth Champoux, Mariken Hasert, Sue Higley, Ted King, Karen Lucas, Patrick Mehlman, Stephen Suomi, and Kristin Zajicek, who assisted in various aspects of the studies.

References

1. Cloninger CR: Etiologic factors in substance abuse: An adoption study perspective. *NIDA Res Monogr* 89:52–72, 1988.
2. Gilligan SB, Reich T, Cloninger CR: Etiologic heterogeneity in alcoholism. *Genet Epidemiol* 4:395–414, 1987.
3. Nurnberger JI, Gershon ES: Genetics of affective disorders, in Post RM, Ballenger JC (eds): *Neurobiology of Mood Disorders*. Baltimore, Williams & Wilkins, 1984, pp 76–101.
4. Cloninger CR: Neurogenetic adaptive mechanisms in alcoholism. *Science* 236:410–416, 1987.
5. Cloninger CR: Anxiety and theories of emotion, in Noyes R Jr, Roth M, Burrows GD (eds): *Handbook of Anxiety, vol. 2: Classification, Etiological Factors and Associated Disturbances*. New York, Elsevier Science Publishers, 1988, pp 1–29.
6. Cloninger CR: A unified biosocial theory of personality and its role in the development of anxiety states. *Psychiatr Dev* 3:167–226, 1986.
7. Linnoila M, Virkkunen M, George T, *et al:* Serotonin, violent behavior and alcohol. *Experientia* 71:155–163, 1994.
8. McKinney WT: *Models of Mental Disorders: A New Comparative Psychiatry*. New York, Plenum Medical, 1988.
9. McClearn GE: Animal models in alcohol research. *Alcohol Clin Exp Res* 12:537–576, 1988.
10. Samson HH, Li T-K: Models of ethanol self-administration: Introduction. *Alcohol Clin Exp Res* 12:571–572, 1988.
11. Cicero TJ: Animal models of alcoholism? in Eriksson K, Sinclair JD, Kiianmaa K (eds): *Animal Models in Alcohol Research*. New York, Academic Press, 1980, pp 99–117.
12. Crabbe JC, Belknap JK, Buck KJ: Genetic animal models of alcohol and drug abuse. *Science* 264:1715–1723, 1994.
13. Li T-K, Lumeng L, Doolittle DP: Selective breeding for alcohol preference and associated responses. *Behav Genet* 23:163–170, 1993.
14. Rogers AE, Fox JG, Whitney K, *et al:* Acute and chronic effects of ethanol in nonhuman primates, in Hayes KC (ed): *Primates in Nutritional Research*. New York, Academic Press, 1979, pp 249–289.
15. Winger G: Animal models for understanding alcohol as a reinforcer, in Cox WM (ed): *Why People Drink*. New York, Gardner Press, 1990, pp 9–36.
16. Crowley TJ, Weisbard C, Hydinger-MacDonald MJ: Progress toward initiating and maintaining high-dose alcohol drinking in monkey social groups. *J Stud Alcohol* 44:569–590, 1983.
17. Crowley TJ, Andrews AE: Alcoholic-like drinking in simian social groups. *Psychopharmacology* 92:196–205, 1987.
18. Higley JD, Hasert MF, Suomi SJ, Linnoila M: Nonhuman primate model of alcohol abuse: Effects of early experience, personality, and stress on alcohol consumption. *Proc Nat Acad Sci USA* 88:7261–7265, 1991.
19. Kraemer GW, McKinney WT: Social separation increases alcohol consumption in rhesus monkeys. *Psychopharmacology* 86:182–189, 1985.
20. Kraemer GW, Lake CR, Ebert MH, McKinney WT: Effect of alcohol on cerebrospinal fluid norepinephrine in rhesus monkeys. *Psychopharmacology* 85:444–448, 1985.
21. Alcoholism NIAAA: *Diagnosis and Assessment of Alcohol Use Disorders*. Seventh Special Report to the US Congress on Alcohol and Health. 1990, pp 181–208. Rockville, MD, US Department of Health and Human Services.
22. Association AP: American Psychiatric Association. Washington, DC, American Psychiatric Association, 1987.

23. American Psychiatric Association: *Diagnostic and Statistical Manual of Mental Disorders*, 4th ed. Washington, DC, Author, 1994.

24. Cottler LB: Comparing DSM-III-R and ICD-10 substance use disorders. *Addiction* 88:689–696, 1993.

25. Higley JD, Suomi SJ, Linnoila M: Progress toward developing a nonhuman primate model of alcohol abuse and alcoholism. *Soc Sci Med* in press.

26. Mello NK, Mendelson JH: The effects of drinking to avoid shock on alcohol intake in primates, in Roach MK, McIsaac WM, Creaven PJ (eds): *Biological Aspects of Alcohol*. Austin, University of Texas Press, 1971, pp 313–332.

27. Meisch RA, Henningfield JE, Thompson T: Establishment of ethanol as a reinforcer for rhesus monkeys via the oral route: Initial results. *Adv Exp Med Biol* 59:323–342, 1975.

28. Ervin FR, Palmour RM, Young SN, *et al:* Voluntary consumption of beverage alcohol by vervet monkeys: Population screening, descriptive behavior and biochemical measures. *Pharmacol Biochem Behav* 36:367–373, 1990.

29. Gustafson R: Is the strength and the desirability of alcohol-related expectancies positively related? A test with an adult Swedish sample. *Drug Alcohol Depend* 28:145–150, 1991.

30. Gustafson R: The development of alcohol-related expectancies from the age of 12 to the age of 15 for two Swedish adolescent samples. *Alcohol Clin Exp Res* 16:700–704, 1992.

31. Gustafson R: Alcohol-related expected effects and the desirability of these effects for Swedish college students measured with the Alcohol Expectancy Questionnaire (AEQ). *Alcohol Alcohol* 28:469–475, 1993.

32. Andersson T, Magnusson D: Drinking habits and alcohol abuse among young men: A prospective longitudinal study. *J Stud Alcohol* 49:245–252, 1988.

33. Grant BF, Harford TC, Grigson B: Stability of alcohol consumption among youth: A national longitudinal survey. *J Stud Alcohol* 49:253–260, 1988.

34. Jones RJ, Bowden DM: Social factors influencing alcohol consumption: A primate model, in Eriksson K, Sinclair JD, Kiianmaa K (eds): *Animal Models in Alcohol Research*. New York, Academic Press, 1980, pp 185–189.

35. Higley JD, Hopkins WD, Thompson WW, *et al:* Peers as primary attachment sources in yearling rhesus monkeys (*Macaca mulatta*). *Dev Psychol* 28:1163–1171, 1992.

36. Robins, LN: Lifetime prevalence of specific psychiatric disorders in three sites. *Arch Gen Psychiatry* 41:949–58, 1984.

37. Gerald MC: Alcohol and alcoholism, in Gerald MC (ed): *Pharmacology: An Introduction to Drugs*. Englewood Cliffs, NJ, Prentice-Hall, 1981, p 221.

38. Cadell TE, Cressman R: Group social tension as a determinant of alcohol consumption in *Macaca mulatta*, in Goldsmith EI, Moor-Jankowski J (eds): *Medical Primatology*. New York, S. Karger, 1972, pp 250–259.

39. Mello NK, Mendelson JH: Factors affecting alcohol consumption in primates. *Psychosom Med* 28:529–550, 1966.

40. Higley JD: *Continuity of Social Separation Behaviors in Rhesus Monkeys from Infancy to Adolescence*. Unpublished doctoral dissertation, University of Wisconsin, Madison, 1985.

41. Smith PK: Does play matter? Functional and evolutionary aspects of animal and human play. *Behav Brain Sci* 5:139–184, 1982.

42. Suomi SJ: Peers, play and primary prevention in primates, in Kent M, Rolf J (eds): *Primary Prevention of Psychopathology: Social Competence in Children*. Hanover, NH, Press of New England, 1979, pp 127–149.

43. Zimmerman RR, Strobe DA, Steere P, Geist CR: Behavior and malnutrition in the rhesus monkey, in Rosenblum LA (ed): *Primate Behavior*. New York, Academic Press, 1975, pp 241–265.

44. Kraemer GW, Daria HL, Moran EC, McKinney WT: Effects of alcohol on the despair to peer separation in rhesus monkeys. *Psychopharmacology* 73:307–310, 1981.

45. Crowley TJ: Substance abuse research in monkey social groups. *Prog Clin Biol Res* 131:255–275, 1983.

46. Gray JA: *The Psychology of Fear and Stress*. New York, Cambridge University Press, 1987.

47. Tucker JA, Vuchinich RE, Sobell MB: Alcohol's effects on human emotions: A review of the stimulation/depression hypothesis. *Int J Addict* 17:155–180, 1982.

48. Chamove AS, Rosenblum LA, Harlow HF: Monkeys (*Macaca mulatta*) raised with only peers. A pilot study. *Anim Behav* 21:316–325, 1973.

49. Harlow HF: Age-mate or peer affectional system. *Adv Study Behav* 2:333–383, 1969.

50. Champoux M, Coe CL, Schanberg S, *et al:* Hormonal effects of early rearing conditions in the infant rhesus monkey. *Am J Primatol* 19:111–117, 1989.

51. Higley JD, Suomi SJ, Linnoila M: CSF monoamine metabolite concentrations vary according to age, rearing, and sex, and are influenced by the stressor of social separation in rhesus monkeys. *Psychopharmacology* 103:551–556, 1991.

52. Higley JD, Suomi SJ, Linnoila M: A longitudinal assessment of CSF monoamine metabolite and plasma cortisol concentrations in young rhesus monkeys. *Biol Psychiatry* 32:127–145, 1992.

53. Goodwin DW: *Alcoholism: The Facts.* New York, Oxford University Press, 1994.

54. Higley JD, Hasert MF, Dodson A, *et al:* Diminished central nervous system serotonin functioning as a predictor of excessive alcohol consumption: The role of early experiences. *Am J Primatol* 33:214, 1994.

55. King ST, Higley JD, Dodson A, *et al:* Alcohol consumption in rhesus monkeys: Effects of genetics, gender, early rearing experience, and social setting. *Am J Primatol* 30:323, 1993.

56. Higley JD, Suomi SJ, Linnoila M: A nonhuman primate model of Type II excessive alcohol consumption? (Part 1): Low CSF 5-HIAA concentrations and diminished social competence correlate with excessive alcohol consumption. *Alcohol Clin Exp Res* 20:629–642, 1996.

57. Higley JD, Suomi SJ, Linnoila M: A nonhuman primate model of Type II excessive alcohol consumption? (Part 2): Diminished social competence and excessive aggression correlates with low CSF 5-HIAA concentrations. *Alcohol Clin Exp Res* 20:643–650, 1996.

58. Higley JD, King ST, Hasert MF, *et al:* Stability of interindividual differences in serotonin function and its relationship to aggressive wounding and competent social behavior in rhesus macaque females. *Neuropsychopharmacology* 14:67–76, 1996.

59. Raleigh MJ, Brammer GL, McGuire MT, *et al:* Individual differences in basal cisternal cerebrospinal fluid 5-HIAA and HVA in monkeys. The effects of gender, age, physical characteristics, and matrilineal influences. *Neuropsychopharmacology* 7:295–304, 1992.

60. Raleigh MJ, McGuire MT: Serotonin, aggression, and violence in vervet monkeys, in Masters RD, McGuire MT (eds): *The Neurotransmitter Revolution.* Carbondale, Southern Illinois University Press, 1994, pp 129–145.

61. Higley JD, Mehlman PT, Poland RE, *et al:* A nonhuman primate model of violence and assertiveness: CSF 5-HIAA and CSF testosterone correlate with different types of aggressive behaviors. *Biol Psychiatry,* in press.

62. Shannon C, Champoux M, Higley JD, *et al:* Interindividual differences in neonatal serotonin functioning: Stability of interindividual differences and behavioral correlates. *Am J Primatol* 36:155, 1995.

63. Higley JD, Thompson WT, Champoux M, *et al:* Paternal and maternal genetic and environmental contributions to CSF monoamine metabolite concentrations in rhesus monkeys (*Macaca mulatta*). *Arch Gen Psychiatry* 50:615–623, 1993.

64. Kraemer GW, Ebert MH, Schmidt DE, McKinney WT: A longitudinal study of the effect of different social rearing conditions on cerebrospinal fluid norepinephrine and biogenic amine metabolites in rhesus monkeys. *Neuropsychopharmacology* 2:175–189, 1989.

65. Virkkunen M, Nuutila A, Goodwin FK, Linnoila M: Cerebrospinal fluid monoamine metabolite levels in male arsonists. *Arch Gen Psychiatry* 44:241–217, 1987.

66. Virkkunen M, De Jong J, Bartko J, *et al:* Relationship of psychobiological variables to recidivism in violent offenders and impulsive fire setters. A follow-up study. *Arch Gen Psychiatry* 46:600–603, 1989.

67. LeMarquand D, Pihl RO, Benkelfat C: Serotonin and alcohol intake, abuse, and dependence: Findings of animal studies. *Biol Psychiatry* 36:395–421, 1994.

68. LeMarquand D, Pihl RO, Benkelfat C: Serotonin and alcohol intake, abuse, and dependence: Clinical evidence. *Biol Psychiatry* 36:326–337, 1994.
69. Ballenger JC, Goodwin FK, Major LF, Brown GL: Alcohol and central serotonin metabolism in man. *Arch Gen Psychiatry* 36:224–227, 1979.
70. Banki CM: Factors influencing monoamine metabolites and tryptophan in patients with alcohol dependence. *J Neural Transm* 50:89–101, 1981.
71. Borg S, Kvande H, Liljeberg P, *et al*: 5-Hydroxyindoleacetic acid in cerebrospinal fluid in alcoholic patients under different clinical conditions. *Alcohol* 2:415–418, 1985.
72. Rosenthal NE, Davenport Y, Cowdry RW, *et al*: Monoamine metabolites in cerebrospinal fluid of depressive subgroups. *Psychiatry Res* 2:113–119, 1980.
73. Mehlman PT, Higley JD, Faucher I, *et al*: Low CSF 5-HIAA concentrations and severe aggression and impaired impulse control in nonhuman primates. *Am J Psychiatry* 151:1485–1491, 1994.
74. Cloninger CR: A unified biosocial theory of personality and its role in the development of anxiety states: A reply to commentaries. *Psychiatr Dev* 6:83–120, 1988.
75. Higley JD, Hasert MF, Dodson A, *et al*: Treatment of excessive alcohol consumption using the serotonin reuptake inhibitor sertraline using a nonhuman primate model of alcohol abuse. Paper presented at Research Society on Alcoholism, San Diego, CA, June 13–18, 1992.
76. Volavka J: *Neurobiology of Violence*. Washington, DC, American Psychiatric Press, 1995.
77. Brown GL, Goodwin FK, Ballenger JC, *et al*: Aggression in humans correlates with cerebrospinal fluid amine metabolites. *Psychiatry Res* 1:131–139, 1979.
78. Brown GL, Ebert MH, Goyer PF, *et al*: Aggression, suicide, and serotonin: Relationships to CSF amine metabolites. *Am J Psychiatry* 139:741–746, 1982.
79. Lidberg L, Tuck JR, Åsberg M, *et al*: Homicide, suicide and CSF 5-HIAA. *Acta Psychiatr Scand* 71:230–236, 1985.
80. Limson R, Goldman D, Roy A, *et al*: Personality and cerebrospinal fluid monoamine metabolites in alcoholics and controls. *Arch Gen Psychiatry* 48:437–441, 1991.
81. Linnoila M, Virkkunen M, Scheinin M, *et al*: Low cerebrospinal fluid 5-hydroxyindoleacetic acid concentration differentiates impulsive from nonimpulsive violent behavior. *Life Sci* 33:2609–2614, 1983.
82. Linnoila M, DeJong J, Virkkunen M: Family history of alcoholism in violent offenders and impulsive fire setters. *Arch Gen Psychiatry* 46:613–616, 1989.
83. Linnoila M: Monoamines, glucose metabolism, and impulse control, in van Praag HM, Plutchik R, Apter A (eds): *Violence and Suicidality: Perspectives in Clinical and Psychobiological Research*. New York, Brunner/Mazel, 1990, pp 218–244.
84. Roy A, Adinoff B, Linnoila M: Acting out hostility in normal volunteers: Negative correlation with levels of 5HIAA in cerebrospinal fluid. *Psychiatry Res* 24:187–194, 1988.
85. Virkkunen M, Rawlings R, Tokola R, *et al*: CSF biochemistries, glucose metabolism, and diurnal activity rhythms in alcoholic, violent offenders, fire setters, and healthy volunteers. *Arch Gen Psychiatry* 51:20–27, 1994.
86. Virkkunen M, Kallio E, Rawlings R, *et al*: Personality profiles and state aggressiveness in Finnish alcoholic, violent offenders, fire setters, and healthy volunteers. *Arch Gen Psychiatry* 51:28–33, 1994.
87. Higley JD, Mehlman P, Taub D, *et al*: Cerebrospinal fluid monoamine and adrenal correlates of aggression in free-ranging rhesus monkeys. *Arch Gen Psychiatry* 49:436–441, 1992.
88. Mehlman P, Higley JD, Faucher I, *et al*: Correlation of CSF 5-HIAA concentrations with sociality and the timing of emigration in free-ranging primates. *Am J Psychiatry* 152:907–913, 1995.
89. Helzer JE, Pryzbeck TR: The co-occurrence of alcoholism with other psychiatric disorders in the general population and its impact on treatment. *J Stud Alcohol* 49:219–224, 1988.
90. Windle M: A longitudinal study of antisocial behaviors in early adolescence as predictors of late adolescent substance use: Gender and ethnic group differences. *J Abnorm Psychol* 99:86–91, 1990.

91. Andersson T, Magnusson D: Patterns of adjustment problems and alcohol abuse in early childhood: A prospective longitudinal study. *Dev Psychopathol* 1:119–131, 1989.

92. Windle M, Miller-Tutzauer C, Barnes GM, Welte J: Adolescent perceptions of help-seeking resources for substance abuse. *Child Dev* 62:179–89, 1991.

93. Meyers AR, Hingson R, Mucatel M, Goldman E: Social and psychologic correlates of problem drinking in old age. *J Am Geriatr Soc* 30:452–456, 1982.

94. Domenico D, Windle M: Intrapersonal and interpersonal functioning among middle-aged female adult children of alcoholics. *J Consult Clin Psychol* 61:659–666, 1993.

95. Litt MD, Babor TF, DelBoca FK, *et al:* Types of alcoholics, II. Application of an empirically derived typology to treatment matching. *Arch Gen Psychiatry* 49:609–614, 1992.

96. Chamove AS, Eysenck HJ, Harlow HF: Personality in monkeys: Factor analysis of rhesus social behavior. *Q J Exp Psychol* 24:496–504, 1972.

97. Eysenck SB, Eysenck HJ: A comparative study of criminals and matched controls on three dimensions of personality. *Br J Soc Clin Psychol* 10:362–366, 1971.

98. McGuire MT, Raleigh MJ, Pollack DB: Personality factors in vervet monkeys: The effects of sex, age, social status, and group composition. *Am J Primatol* 33:1–13, 1994.

99. Stevenson-Hinde J, Simpson MJA: Subjective assessment of rhesus monkeys over four successive years. *Primates* 21:66–82, 1980.

100. Buss AH, Plomin R: *Temperament: Early Developing Personality Traits.* Hillsdale, NJ, Erlbaum, 1984.

101. Raleigh MJ, Brammer GL, Yuwiler A, *et al:* Serotonergic influences on the social behavior of vervet monkeys (*Cercopithecus aethiops sabaeus*). *Exp Neurol* 68:322–334, 1980.

102. Raleigh MJ, Brammer GL, McGuire MT: Male dominance, serotonergic systems, and the behavioral and physiological effects of drugs in vervet monkeys (*Cercopithecus aethiops sabaeus*), in Miczek KA (ed): *Ethopharmacology: Primate Models of Neuropsychiatric Disorders.* New York, Alan R. Liss, 1983, pp 185–197.

103. Raleigh MJ, Brammer GL, McGuire MT, Yuwiler A: Dominant social status facilitates the behavioral effects of serotonergic agonists. *Brain Res* 348:274–282, 1985.

104. Raleigh MJ, McGuire MT: Social influences on endocrine function in male vervet monkeys, in Ziegler TE, Bercovitch FB (eds): *Socioendocrinology of Primate Reproduction.* New York, Wiley-Liss, 1990, pp 95–111.

105. Higley JD, Linnoila M, Suomi SJ: Ethological contributions: Experiential and genetic contributions to the expression and inhibition of aggression in primates, in Hersen M, Ammerman RT, Sisson L (eds): *Handbook of Aggressive and Destructive Behavior in Psychiatric Patients.* New York, Plenum Press, 1994, pp 17–32.

106. Kruesi MJ, Rapoport JL, Hamburger S, *et al:* Cerebrospinal fluid monoamine metabolites, aggression, and impulsivity in disruptive behavior disorders of children and adolescents. *Arch Gen Psychiatry* 47:419–426, 1990.

107. Raleigh MJ, McGuire MT, Brammer GL: Subjective assessment of behavioral style: Links to overt behavior and physiology in vervet monkeys. *Am J Primatol* 18:161–162, 1989.

108. Higley JD, Suomi SJ: Temperamental reactivity in non-human primates, in Kohnstamm GA, Bates JE, Rothbart MK (eds): *Temperament in Childhood.* New York, John Wiley & Sons, 1989, pp 153–167.

109. McGuire MT, Raleigh MJ: Serotonin–behavior interactions in vervet monkeys. *Psychopharmacol Bull* 21:458–463, 1985.

110. Smuts BB: Gender, aggression and influence, in Smuts BB, Cheney DL, Seyfarth RM, *et al* (eds): *Primate Societies.* Chicago, University of Chicago Press, 1987, pp 400–412.

111. Raleigh MJ, Steklis HD: Effect of orbitofrontal and temporal neocortical lesion on the affiliative behavior of vervet monkeys (*Cercopithecus aethiops sabaeus*). *Exp Neurol* 73:378–379, 1981.

112. Packer C, Pusey AE: Female aggression and male membership in troops of Japanese macaques and olive baboons. *Folia Primatol* 31:212–218, 1979.

113. Walters JR, Seyfarth RM: Conflict and cooperation, in Smuts BB, Cheney DL, Seyfarth RM, *et al* (eds): *Primate Societies.* Chicago, University of Chicago Press, 1987, pp 306–317.

114. Chapais B: Why do male and female rhesus monkeys affiliate during the birth season? in Rawlins RG, Kessler M (eds): *The Cayo Santiago Macaques*. Chicago, SUNY Press, 1986, pp 173–200.

115. Chapais B: Rank maintenance in female Japanese macaques: Experimental evidence for social dependency. *Behaviour* 102:41–59, 1988.

116. Higley JD, Suomi SJ: Reactivity and social competence affect individual differences to severe stress in children: Investigations using nonhuman primates, in Pfeffer CR (ed): *Intense Stress and Mental Disturbance in Children*. Washington, DC, American Psychiatric Press, 1996, pp 1–69.

117. Raleigh MJ, McGuire MT: Animal analogues of ostracism: Biological mechanisms and social consequences. *Ethol Sociobiol* 7:53–66, 1986.

118. Raleigh MJ, McGuire MT, Brammer GL: Serotonergic mechanisms promote dominance acquisition in adult male vervet monkeys. *Brain Res* 559:181–190, 1991.

119. Raleigh MJ, Brammer GL, Ritvo ER: Effects of chronic fenfluramine on blood serotonin, cerebrospinal fluid metabolites, and behavior in monkeys. *Psychopharmacology* 90:503–508, 1986.

120. Smuts BB: *Sex and Friendship in Baboons*. New York, Aldine, 1985.

121. Drickamer LC, Vessey SH: Group changing in free-ranging male rhesus monkeys. *Primates* 14:249–254, 1973.

122. Altmann J: *Baboon Mothers and Infants*. Cambridge, MA, Harvard University Press, 1980.

123. Dittus WPJ: The social regulation of population density and age-sex distribution in the toque monkey. *Behaviour* 63:281–322, 1977.

124. Gartlan JS: Adaptive aspects of social structure in *Erythrocebus patas*, in Kondo S, Kawai M, Ehara A, Kawamura S (eds): *Proceedings from the Symposia of the Fifth Congress of the International Primatological Society*. Tokyo, Japan Science Press, 1975, pp 161–171.

125. Henzi SP, Lucas JW: Observations on the inter-troop movement of adult vervet monkeys (*Cercopithecus aethiops*). *Folia Primatol* 33:220–235, 1980.

126. Ohsawa H: Takeover of a harem and the subsequent promiscuity in patas monkeys, in Ehara A, Kimura T, Takenaka O, Iwamoto M (eds): *Primatology Today*. New York, Elsevier, 1991, pp 221–224.

127. Packer C: Inter-troop transfer and inbreeding avoidance in *Papio anubis*. *Anim Behav* 27:1–36, 1979.

128. Pusey AE, Packer C: Dispersal and philopatry, in Smuts BB, Cheney DL, Seyfarth RM, *et al* (eds): *Primate Societies*. Chicago, University of Chicago Press, 1987, pp 250–266.

129. van Noordwijk MA, van Schaik CP: Male migration and rank acquisition in wild long-tailed macaques (*Macaca fascicularis*). *Anim Behav* 33:849–861, 1985.

130. Brain C: Deaths in a desert baboon troop. *Int J Primatol* 13:593–599, 1992.

131. Dittus WP: The socioecological basis for the conservation of the toque monkey (*Macaca sinica*) of Sri Lanka (Ceylon), in Rainier III PoM, Bourne GH (eds): *Primate Conservation*. New York, Academic Press, 1977, pp 238–265.

132. Dittus WPJ: The social regulation of primate populations, in Lindburg D (ed): *The Macaques: Studies in Ecology, Behavior and Evolution*. New York, Van Nostrand Reinhold, 1980, pp 131–157.

133. Southwick CH, Siddiqi MF: Population dynamics of rhesus monkeys in Northern India, in Bourne GH, Rainier III PoM (eds): *Primate Conservation*. New York, Academic Press, 1977, pp 339–362.

134. Kaplan JR, Fontenot MB, Berard J, *et al*: Delayed dispersal and elevated monoamine activity in free-ranging rhesus monkeys. *Am J Primatol* 35:229–234, 1995.

135. Vessey SH, Meikle DB, Drickamer LC: Demographic and descriptive studies at La Parguera, Puerto Rico, *P R Health Sci J* 8:121–127, 1989.

136. Higley JD, Mehlman PT, Taub DT, *et al*: Excessive mortality in young male nonhuman primates with low CSF 5-HIAA concentrations. *Arch Gen Psychiatry* 53:537–543, 1996.

137. Jacobs BL, Azmitia EC: Structure and function of the brain serotonin system. *Physiol Rev* 72:165–229, 1992.

138. Arnsten AF, Goldman-Rakic PS: Selective prefrontal cortical projections to the region of the locus coeruleus and raphe nuclei in the rhesus monkey. *Brain Res* 306:9–18, 1984.

139. Stanley M, Traskman-Bendz L, Dorovini-Zis K: Correlations between aminergic metabolites simultaneously obtained from human CSF and brain. *Life Sci* 37:1279–1286, 1985.

140. Knott P, Haroutunian V, Bierer L, *et al:* Correlations post-mortem between ventricular CSF and cortical tissue concentrations of MHPG, 5-HIAA, and HVA in Alzheimer's disease. *Biol Psychiatry* 25:112A, 1989.

141. Wester P, Bergstrom U, Eriksson A, *et al:* Ventricular cerebrospinal fluid monoamine transmitter and metabolite concentrations reflect human brain neurochemistry in autopsy cases. *J Neurochem* 54:1148–1156, 1990.

142. Doudet D, Hommer D, Higley JD, *et al:* Cerebral glucose metabolism, CSF 5-HIAA, and aggressive behavior in rhesus monkeys. *Am J Psychiatry* 152:1782–1787, 1995.

143. Coccaro EF: Impulsive aggression and central serotonergic system function in humans: An example of a dimensional brain–behavior relationship. *Int Clin Psychopharmacol* 7:3–12, 1992.

144. Molcho A, Stanley B, Stanley M: Biological studies and markers in suicide and attempted suicide. *Int Clin Psychopharmacol* 6:77–92, 1991.

145. Jarvie HF: Frontal lobe wounds causing disinhibition: A study of six cases. *J Neurol Neurosurg Psychiatry* 17:14–32, 1954.

146. Miller LA: Impulsivity, risk-taking, and the ability to synthesize fragmented information after frontal lobectomy. *Neuropsychologia* 30:69–79, 1992.

147. Heinrichs RW: Frontal cerebral lesions and violent incidents in chronic neuropsychiatric patients. *Biol Psychiatry* 25:174–178, 1989.

148. van Woerkom TC, Teelken AW, Minderhous JM: Difference in neurotransmitter metabolism in frontotemporal-lobe contusion and diffuse cerebral contusion. *Lancet* vol. 1, 812–813, 1977.

149. Goldman-Rakic PS: Motor control function of the prefrontal cortex. *Ciba Found Symp* 132:187–200, 1987.

150. Miller SE: Serotonin, carbohydrates, and atypical depression. *Pharmacol Toxicol* 1:61–71, 1992.

151. Oxenstierna G, Edman G, Iselius L, Oreland L, Ross SB, Sedvall G: Concentrations of monoamine metabolites in the cerebrospinal fluid of twins and unrelated individuals—A genetic study. *J Psychiat Res* 20:19–29, 1986.

152. Clarke AS: Long-term effects of prenatal stress on HPA axis activity in juvenile rhesus monkeys. *Biol Psychiatry.* 1995.

153. Cloninger CR, Bohman M, Sigvardsson S, von Knorring AL: Psychopathology in adopted-out children of alcoholics. The Stockholm Adoption Study. *Recent Dev Alcohol* 3:37–51, 1985.

154. Bernstein IS, Ehardt CL: Modification of aggression through socialization and the special case of adult and adolescent male rhesus monkeys (*Macaca mulatta*). *Am J Primatol* 10:213–227, 1986.

155. Harlow HF, Harlow MK: The affectional systems, in Schrier AM, Harlow HF, Stollinitz F (eds): *Behavior of Nonhuman Primates.* New York, Academic Press, 1965, pp 287–334.

156. Higley JD, Suomi SJ: Parental behavior in non-human primates, in Sluckin W (ed): *Parental Behavior in Animals and Humans.* Oxford, UK, Blackwell Press, 1986, pp 152–207.

157. Coelho AM, Bramblett CA: Early rearing experiences and the performance of affinitive and approach behavior in infant and juvenile baboons. *Primates* 25:218–224, 1984.

158. Coelho AMJ, Bramblett CA: Effects of rearing on aggression and subordination in Papio monkeys. *Am J Primatol* 1:401–412, 1981.

159. Capitanio JP: Behavioral pathology, in Mitchell G, Erwin J (eds): *Comparative Primate Biology: Behavior, Conservation and Ecology.* New York, Alan R. Liss, 1986, pp 411–454.

160. Mitchell G: Abnormal behavior in primates, in Rosenblum RA (ed): *Primate Behavior: Developments in Field and Laboratory Research.* New York, Academic Press, 1970, pp 195–249.

161. Suomi SJ: Abnormal behavior and primate models of psychopathology, in Fobes JL, King JE (eds): *Primate Behavior.* New York, Academic Press, 1982, pp 171–215.

162. Suomi SJ: The development of social competence by rhesus monkeys. *Ann Ist Super Sanita* 18:193–202, 1982.
163. Dishion TJ, Loeber R: Adolescent marijuana and alcohol use: The role of parents and peers revisited. *Am J Drug Alcohol Abuse* 11:11–25, 1985.
164. Offord DR, Boyle MC, Racine YA: The epidemiology of antisocial behavior in childhood and adolescence, in Pepler DJ, Rubin KH (eds): *The Development and Treatment of Childhood Aggression.* Hillsdale, New Jersey, Lawrence Erlbaum Associates, Publishers; 1991, pp 31–54.
165. Forgatch MS: The clinical science vortex: A developing theory of antisocial behavior, in Pepler DJ, Rubin KH (eds): *The Development and Treatment of Childhood Aggression.* Hillsdale, NJ, Lawrence Erlbaum, 1991, pp 291–316.
166. Mulder RT, Joyce PR, Cloninger CR: Temperament and early environment influence comorbidity and personality disorders in major depression. *Compr Psychiatry* 35:225–233, 1994.
167. Patterson GR, Stouthamer-Loeber M: The correlation of family management practices and delinquency. *Child Dev* 55:1299–1307, 1984.
168. Patterson GR, DeBaryshe BD, Ramsey E: A developmental perspective on antisocial behavior. *Am Psychol* 44:329–335, 1989.
169. Patterson GR, Capaldi D, Bank L: An early starter model for predicting delinquency, in Pepler DJ, Rubin KH (eds): *The Development and Treatment of Childhood Aggression.* Hillsdale, NJ, Lawrence Erlbaum, 1991, pp 139–168.
170. Eron LD, Huesmann LR, Zelli A: The role of parental variables in the learning of aggression, in Pepler DJ, Rubin KH (eds): *The Development and Treatment of Childhood Aggression.* Hillsdale, NJ, Lawrence Erlbaum, 1991, pp 169–188.
171. Farrington DP: Offending from 10 to 25 years, in Von Desen KT, Mednick SA (eds): *Prospective studies of crime and delinquency.* Boston, Kluver-Nijhoff, 1983, pp 17–37.
172. Steinberg L, Lamborn SD, Darling N, Mounts NS, Dornbusch SM: Over-time changes in adjustment and competence among adolescents from authoritative, authoritarian, indulgent, and neglectful families. *Child Dev* 65:754–770, 1994.
173. Werner EE: Resilient offspring of alcoholics: A longitudinal study from birth to age 18. *J Stud Alcohol* 47:34–40, 1986.
174. Windle M: The difficult temperament in adolescence: Associations with substance use, family support, and problem behaviors. *J Clin Psychol* 47:310–315, 1991.
175. Suomi SJ, Ripp C: A history of mother-less mother monkey mothering at the University of Wisconsin Primate Laboratory, in Reite M, Caine N (eds): *Child Abuse: The Nonhuman Primate Data.* New York, Alan R. Liss, 1983, pp 50–78.
176. Lucas K, Krusinger J, Suomi SJ, Linnoila M: Serotonin functioning, early rearing, and severe aggression are correlated with acquisition of social dominance rank. *Am J Primatol* 36:140, 1995.
177. Cadoret RJ, Yates WR, Troughton E, Woodworth G, Stewart MA: Genetic-environmental interaction in the genesis of aggressivity and conduct disorders. *Arch Gen Psychiatry* 52:919–924, 1995.

III

Psychology

Alfonso Paredes, Section Editor

Overview

Alfonso Paredes

In spite of popular assumptions about the close association between alcohol use and human violence, support for a causal relationship is lacking. Epidemiological and correlational data usually offered to document the association does not validate causal explanations. It is therefore necessary to review research specifically designed to elucidate the mechanisms responsible for this relationship. The chapters included in this section present three research perspectives. In Chapter 10, Brad J. Bushman describes laboratory experiments conducted with humans, including the methods of alcohol administration and the measurements used to assess aggressive behavior. The chapter illustrates how various assumptions have been operationalized for testing. The merit of explanations of alcohol-related aggression is examined including the role attributed to physiological disinhibition and personal expectancies. In this regard, an effect has been attributed to the person's belief of having drunk alcohol, contrasting it with the physiological effects of the substance. Indirect cognitive, emotional, and physiological factors also have been suggested. The author applied meta-analytic procedures to draw conclusions from the literature. In his opinion, alcohol "causes" aggression, but such effect cannot be attributed solely to pharmacological mechanisms. Expectancy effects must be considered. Furthermore, alcohol indirectly produces changes within the person that increases the probability of expressing this behavior. Bushman concludes that experimental manipulations that facilitate aggression, such as provocations, frustrations, and aggressive cues, have a stronger effect on intoxicated subjects than on their sober counterparts.

In Chapter 11, Mark W. Lipsey and associates provide a broad review of the literature. The findings from animal models are briefly examined, remind-

Alfonso Paredes • Laboratory for the Study of Addictions and UCLA Drug Abuse Research Center, West Los Angeles Veterans Administration, Los Angeles, California 90073.

Recent Developments in Alcoholism, Volume 13: Alcoholism and Violence, edited by Marc Galanter. Plenum Press, New York, 1997

ing us at the same time of the necessity of using human subjects in the experiments. The authors contend that it may not be justified to draw homologies between "neural circuits" and the physiological activities that mediate aggressive behavior in animals and those responsible in humans. These studies, however, may help to identify the neurochemical systems in the brain that mediate the effects of alcohol. Lipsey *et al.* emphasize the need of applying experimental approaches to address the possibility that observed differences in the expression of violence are related to factors other than alcohol consumption. Violent behavior is a relatively rare event; after all, most individuals who drink do not become violent. We are therefore dealing with low probabilities difficult to detect and compare. Nevertheless, it is important to identify the causal mechanisms by which alcohol consumption might influence these probabilities. There are many processes operating that may account for the effects of alcohol on violence. These include cognitive impairment, disinhibition of violent impulses, or the expectancy effects mentioned earlier. Interactions leading to violence involve alcohol as well as personality and situational variables. Research with human subjects within laboratory conditions is necessary in spite of methodological challenges and the contrived nature of laboratory drinking situations. Within such context it is possible to manipulate alcohol consumption as well as other relevant variables. Consumption is difficult to manipulate under naturalistic conditions. Human studies should help to determine if aggressive behavior can be caused by manipulating consumption under defined circumstances. If research specifically designed to reveal causal relationships does not demonstrate their existence, the plausibility of a causal associations under natural conditions would be less likely.

Lipsey *et al.* devote considerable attention to the methodological problems common in studies of alcohol–violence interactions. There are sampling problems when groups that characteristically exhibit violent behavior are investigated, as is the case with criminal system populations. Under these circumstances, comparisons with subjects with similar characteristics and patterns of alcohol consumption, but who do not exhibit violent behavior, cannot be done. The authors note that many investigations do not control for confounding variables like sociodemographic characteristics, personality disorder, other drug use, and early exposure to violence. Greater attention to these variables therefore is encouraged.

A better conceptualization of the issues involved and operational definitions of the key variables are necessary. In spite of the methodological deficiencies of the studies in the literature, the authors note that the relevant research does not yield consistently or predominantly negative or null results. The alcohol–violence assumptions ventured are generally consistent with a causal role of the neurophysiological action of alcohol. Factors beyond the pharmacological effects of the substance, however, play a role.

Maria Elena Khalsa-Denison and associates, in Chapter 12, begin by drawing a parallel between the views from the literature regarding the association between alcohol and violence and those between cocaine and violence. This brief review is followed by a study that examines characteristics of the violent behavior exhibited by cocaine-dependent patients. The authors point out that a significant proportion of cocaine-dependent individuals are also users of alcohol. Intake of alcohol in a large proportion of these cases is severe enough to justify a diagnosis of alcohol dependence. Alcohol is consumed by these individuals concurrently or alternatively. It is therefore important to consider the consequences of the combined intake, contrasting it with the use of only one drug. Applying a natural history methodology the cocaine use career of cocaine-dependent individuals was parceled out in segments of time defined by the use of the drug in combination or not with alcohol. The social behavior exhibited during these periods, including violence, was also recorded. According to the findings of the study, violent behavior was more frequent during periods of alcohol and/or cocaine use. On the other hand, this behavior was less likely to be manifested during abstinent periods. Alcohol intake periods were more likely to be accompanied by violent behavior whether or not cocaine was used concurrently. Violent behavior was not normative for this group; the subset of patients who exhibited this type of behavior was also more likely to have manifested this behavior prior to the onset of their addiction. This would suggest that individual factors other than the pharmacological effects of the drug were at play. Given the limitations of a study such as this, the conclusions are tentative and highlight a need for further research on this issue.

A greater effort comparing the mechanisms underlying violent behavior in users of alcohol and other drugs is needed. Such investigations may reveal interesting contrasts. In the future it may be possible to construct a matrix with the various drugs along one dimension and a sequence of neurobiological and psychosocial factors along another dimension. Within this matrix, the relative contribution of these factors could be presented. In the case of some drugs, pharmacological factors would play a predominant role, while cognitive, disinhibition, and personality or social–environmental variables may be of greater salience in others. With certain drugs, social systemic effects, such as violence resulting from acts aimed to obtain a supply of the drug or control over the distribution, may be more prominent.[1]

The nature of the association between alcohol and violence and the mechanisms involved has not been settled empirically as yet. This is perhaps reflected in Lipsey's statement indicating that only for some persons and/or under some circumstances a causal relationship exists between alcohol use and violent behavior. Precision in the definition of the assumptions regarding the mechanisms that play a causal role in the genesis and expression of violent behavior and application of appropriate research designs remain a major challenge for investigators.

Reference

1. Goldstein J: Cocaine and crime in the United States. Presentation for the United Nations Interregional Criminological Research Institute International Symposium on Cocaine, March 1991, Rome, Italy.

10

Effects of Alcohol
on Human Aggression

Validity of Proposed Explanations

Brad J. Bushman

Abstract. In the present review, meta-analytic procedures were used to test the validity of three explanations of alcohol-related aggression: physiological disinhibition, expectancy, and indirect cause. According to the physiological disinhibition explanation, alcohol increases aggression directly by anesthetizing the center of the brain that normally inhibits aggressive responding. According to the expectancy explanation, alcohol increases aggression because people expect it to. According to the indirect cause explanation, alcohol increases aggression by causing changes within the person that increase the probability of aggression (e.g., by reducing intellectual functioning). The results from the review were inconsistent with the physiological disinhibition and expectancy explanations, but were consistent with the indirect cause explanation. Experimental manipulations that increased aggression (e.g., provocations, frustrations, aggressive cues) had a stronger effect on intoxicated participants than on sober participants.

1. Introduction

Violent crime is the issue of greatest concern to Americans today.[1-3] There is probably good reason for this concern, because the US violent crime rate has been increasing over the past several years (see Fig. 1). One violent crime occurs ever 16 seconds in the United States.[4] Although it is not the only factor that contributes to violent crime, alcohol intoxication does make a significant contribution. Numerous correlational studies have found a strong relation

Brad J. Bushman • Department of Psychology, Iowa State University, Ames, Iowa 50011-3180.

Recent Developments in Alcoholism, Volume 13: Alcoholism and Violence, edited by Marc Galanter. Plenum Press, New York, 1997

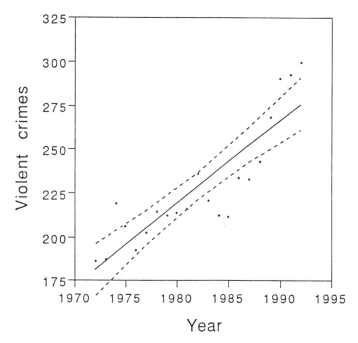

Figure 1. United States violent crime rate per 100,000 inhabitants, 1971–1992. NOTE: Data from US Department of Justice.[27] According to the FBI, violent crimes are offenses of murder, forcible rape, aggravated assault, and robbery. A regression line (solid line) and 95% confidence limits (dashed lines) were fit to these data. The least-squares regression line was $-9136.53 + 4.73(year)$, the coefficient of determination was $r^2 = .79$, and the coefficient of correlation was $r = .89$.

between alcohol intoxication and violent crime. These studies generally find that over 50% of the assailants were intoxicated at the time the violent crimes were committed.[5–11]

Unfortunately, it is difficult to draw causal inferences about the relation between alcohol and aggression from correlational data. Some of the complications surrounding correlational studies of alcohol-related aggression are these: The aggressor may misreport alcohol ingestion as an excuse or to avoid punishment; alcohol consumption may accompany participation in group events that could lead to violence; alcohol containers (e.g., bottles, beer glasses) may be used as weapons; alcoholism may force people into a social stratum where crime is more probable; some alcoholics involve themselves in crimes to support their habits; alcohol-related bungling of crimes may increase the probability of capture; and alcohol and violent crime may be responses to an underlying social malaise.[12] The experimental method avoids these and many other pitfalls because the researcher controls the occurrence of events and randomly assigns participants to conditions. Consequently, it is much easier to draw causal inferences about the effects of alcohol on aggression from experimental data than from correlational data. It also is much easier to test explanations of alcohol-related aggression with experimental studies than with correlational studies. The data base for the present review was therefore limited to experimental studies of alcohol-related human aggression.[13,14]

2. Prototypical Methods of Administering Alcohol and Measuring Aggression in Experimental Studies

Although each experimental study of alcohol-related aggression has unique components, many experimental studies have common features. The typical laboratory procedures for administering alcohol and measuring aggression are described in the following sections.

2.1. Administration of Alcohol

To evaluate the effects of alcohol on aggression in humans, most researchers use a placebo design, in which all participants are told that they will receive alcohol. Only half the participants, however, are actually given alcohol; the other half are given a placebo. To enhance the credibility of the placebo drink, experimenters have poured the beverage from "legitimate" bottles and have placed a small amount of alcohol on the surface of the drink. Sometimes an additional group is added to the placebo design, in which participants are told that they will not receive alcohol and they are not given alcohol. This group serves as a control because participants receive neither alcohol nor the expectancy of alcohol. The major problem with comparing participants in the alcohol group with participants in the placebo or control groups is that the psychological (e.g., expectancy) and pharmacological effects of alcohol are confounded in these studies.

The balanced placebo design overcomes this confounding problem.[15] In the balanced placebo design, half of the participants are told that they will receive alcohol and half are told that they will not receive alcohol. Within each of these groups, half of the participants are given alcohol and half are not (see Fig. 2). To enhance the credibility of the antiplacebo drink, experimenters have poured the beverage from "legitimate" bottles, diluted the alcohol, used false Breathalyzer readings, and required participants to complete tasks that distract them from focusing on the interoceptive signs of intoxication. The pure pharmacological effects of alcohol on aggression can be determined by comparing the antiplacebo group with the control group. The pure effects of alcohol-related expectancies on aggression can be determined by comparing the placebo group with the control group. Because the balanced placebo design crosses level of alcohol with level of expectancy, the interaction of these two factors also can be tested. It is difficult, however, to use the bal-

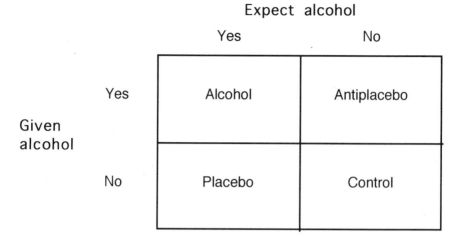

Figure 2. Balanced placebo design.

anced placebo design with large alcohol doses because participants become suspicious when they notice the physiological effects of alcohol.

2.2. Measurement of Aggression

Buss[16] defined aggression as "a response that delivers noxious stimuli to another organism" (p. 1). Green[17] clarified this definition by adding two elements: (1) the aggressor delivers the noxious stimuli with the intent to harm the victim, and (2) the aggressor expects that the noxious stimuli will have their intended effect. Buss further proposed that acts of human aggression can be classified using combinations of three dichotomous variables: physical versus verbal, direct versus indirect, and active versus passive. Although there are eight possible combinations of the three dichotomous variables proposed by Buss, none of the four "passive" types of aggression are common in experimental studies of alcohol-related aggression. This chapter therefore focuses on the four "active" types of human aggression. In physical aggression the noxious stimuli delivered to the victim are pain and injury, whereas in verbal aggression the noxious stimuli delivered to the victim are rejection and threat. In direct aggression the aggressor is easily identified by the victim, whereas in indirect aggression the aggressor is not easily identified by the victim. There are two ways in which an aggressive act can be indirect. First, the victim is not present and the noxious stimuli are delivered via the negative reactions of others. Second, the victim is not injured or threatened, but his or her belongings are stolen or damaged.

In the "real world," most extreme acts of aggression are violent crimes, which the FBI classifies as murder, forcible rape, aggravated assault, and robbery. According to Buss's framework, murder, forcible rape, and aggravated assault are examples of direct physical aggression, whereas robbery is

Table I. "Real World" and Laboratory Examples of the Direct and Indirect Types of Physical and Verbal Aggression

Type of aggression	"Real world" examples	Laboratory examples
Physical-Direct	Assaulting someone with body parts (e.g., limbs, teeth) or weapons (e.g., clubs, knives, guns).	Using intense shocks to punish a confederate whenever he or she makes an error on a task. Using shocks to evaluate a confederate's solution to a problem Delivering intense shocks to a confederate on a competitive reaction-time task.
Physical-Indirect	Stealing or damaging someone's property Setting a booby trap for someone Hiring an asassin to kill someone	Subtracting money from a confederate in an experiment
Verbal-Direct	Criticizing, derogating, or cursing someone Making obscene gestures to someone Threatening someone	Making negative verbal statements to a confederate
Verbal-Indirect	Spreading vicious rumors about someone	Negatively evaluating someone on a questionnaire.

an example of indirect physical aggression. Table I gives real world and laboratory examples of each of the four types of active aggression proposed by Buss (i.e., direct physical, indirect physical, direct verbal, indirect verbal). Prototypical procedures for measuring each type of active aggression are given below.

2.2.1. Direct Physical Aggression. The aggression machine paradigm has been the primary laboratory procedure used to measure direct physical aggression, although it is used less frequently now than it was in the past.[16] In this procedure, a participant and a confederate are generally told that the study is concerned with the effects of alcohol on teaching and learning abilities. Using a rigged lottery, the real participant is selected to be the teacher and the confederate is selected to be the learner. The participant presents stimulus materials to the confederate who attempts to master them. Before the learning task begins, the participant is sometimes angered by the confederate. When the confederate makes an incorrect response on a trial, the participant is told to punish him or her by means of electric shock. By using different buttons, the participant can control the intensity and duration of shock given to the confederate. The shocks, for example, may range in intensity from "just perceptible" (e.g., button 1) to "excruciatingly painful" (e.g., button 10). In some experiments, shock duration is controlled by holding down the shock button for the desired duration. The dependent variables are the intensity and the duration of shock given to the confederate. Some researchers have used noxious stimuli other than electric shocks, such as noise blasts.

The competitive reaction-time paradigm is another method commonly employed to study the effects of alcohol on direct physical aggression.[18] In this procedure, a participant and a confederate are generally told that the study is concerned with the effects of alcohol on perceptual motor skills. The participant competes with the confederate on a reaction-time task in which the slower-responding person receives electric shock. At the beginning of each trial, the participant sets the level of shock he or she wants the confederate to receive if the confederate's response is slower. At the end of each trial, the participant is informed of the level of shock the confederate set for him or her to receive on the trial. The slower-responding person then receives the indicated intensity of shock. In actuality, the experimenter determines who wins and loses and the feedback/shocks delivered. Sometimes provocation is manipulated by increasing the intensity of shock set by the "opponent" across trials on the reaction-time task. The dependent measure is the intensity of shock the participant sets for the opponent. Some researchers have used noise blasts rather than electric shocks as noxious stimuli.

2.2.2. Indirect Physical Aggression. The laboratory paradigms used to measure direct physical aggression also have been modified to measure indirect physical aggression. In one study, for example, male college students were given $2.00 and course credit for their participation.[19] Participants were told to subtract between zero cents (button 0) and nine cents (button 9) from a confederate whenever he made a mistake on a trial. This paradigm measures indirect physical aggression because the participant takes the confederate's belongings (i.e., his money).

The free-operant paradigm is another method commonly employed to study the effects of alcohol on indirect physical aggression.[20] In this procedure, the participant can press one of two buttons on an apparatus. Pressing button A results in the accumulation of points exchangeable for money. Pressing button B results in the subtraction of points from a fictitious second participant. Sometimes provocation is manipulated by subtracting points from the participant; the point loss is attributed to the fictitious second participant. The fixed ratios associated with each button also can be manipulated (e.g., a fixed-ratio of 100 responses might be required for button A, whereas a fixed-ratio of 10 responses might be required for button B).

2.2.3. Direct Verbal Aggression. In the laboratory, direct verbal aggression is measured by recording a participant's vocal comments to one or more confederates and counting the frequency of attacks or other negative verbal statements. In one study, for example, male participants were told that they would be participating in a study of alcohol's effect on creativity with five other participants whom they would not know.[21] Two of the group members were confederates. One confederate was a social facilitator who tried to develop cohesiveness among group members by initiating conversation and telling jokes. The other confederate tried to antagonize participants by complaining and insulting their intelligence (e.g., he said that this was the dumbest group of people he had ever encountered). The experimental sessions were videotaped and later coded for verbally aggressive statements made by the participants.

2.2.4. Indirect Verbal Aggression. Indirect measures of verbal aggression are more common in laboratory experiments than are direct measures of verbal aggression. Generally, a confederate or experimenter first provokes the participant. Rather than confronting the confederate or experimenter face-to-face, the participant uses a pencil-and-paper measure to evaluate him or her. The participant is led to believe that negative ratings will harm the confederate or experimenter in some way. In one study, for example, a male participant was told to trace a circle as slowly as possible.[22] After this task was completed, a male experimenter burst in the room, introduced himself as the supervisor who had been observing through a one-way mirror, and contemptuously stated, "Obviously, you don't follow instructions. You were supposed to trace the circle as slowly as possible without stopping but you clearly didn't do this. Now I don't know if we can use your data." The experimenter paused, then continued (interrupting the participant if he or she tried to respond), "Do it over again." After the experiment, the participant completed an evaluation form for each member of the lab staff, including the obnoxious experimenter. The form asked the participant to rate each staff member on 7-point scales as to whether he or she was effective in performing duties, was a capable employee, was likeable, made the participant feel comfortable, showed respect for the participant, and should be rehired. The evaluations were placed in a sealed envelope and were allegedly sent to the principal investigator to be used in future hiring decisions.

3. Explanations of Alcohol-Related Aggression

Although several explanations have been proposed to account for alcohol-related aggression, most can be placed into one of three categories depending on the role each assigns to alcohol: physiological disinhibition, expectancy, and indirect cause.

3.1. Physiological Disinhibition

Normally, people have strong inhibitions against behaving aggressively, because society strongly sanctions such behavior. According to the physiological disinhibition explanation, alcohol increases aggression directly by anesthetizing the center of the brain that normally inhibits aggressive responding. Disinhibition theorists argue that alcohol facilitates aggression "not by 'stepping on the gas' but rather by paralyzing the brakes" (p. 40).[23]

If alcohol directly causes aggression by reducing inhibitions, then participants in the antiplacebo group should behave more aggressively than participants in the control group. The antiplacebo versus control comparison provides the best test of the validity of the physiological disinhibition explanation of intoxicated aggression because it gives the pure pharmacological effects of alcohol on aggression (i.e., the effects of alcohol-related expectancies on aggression are removed).

3.2. Expectancy

According to the expectancy explanation, alcohol increases aggression because people expect it to. Those who behave aggressively while intoxicated can therefore "blame the bottle" for their actions. According to MacAndrew and Edgerton,[24] violence and other antisocial behaviors occur when alcohol is consumed because, in many societies, drinking occasions are culturally agreed-on "time-out" periods when people are not held accountable for their actions.

If alcohol-related expectancies cause aggression, then participants in the placebo group should behave more aggressively than participants in the control group. The placebo versus control comparison provides the best test of the validity of the expectancy explanation of intoxicated aggression because it gives the pure effects of alcohol-related expectancies on aggression (i.e., the pharmacological effects of alcohol on aggression are removed).

3.3. Indirect Cause

According to the indirect cause explanation, alcohol increases aggression by causing certain cognitive, emotional, and physiological changes that increase the probability of aggression. For example, some of the cognitive changes that accompany alcohol consumption are impaired intellectual functioning, inaccurate assessment of risks, and reduced self-awareness.

If alcohol indirectly causes aggression, then manipulations that increase aggression in laboratory experiments, such as provocations, frustrations, and aggressive cues, should have a greater effect on intoxicated participants than on sober participants. Support for the indirect cause explanation of intoxicated would be provided by a significant Alcohol × Manipulation interaction, followed up by contrasts that show that the experimental manipulation increased aggression more in participants who were given alcohol than in participants who were not given alcohol.

4. Present Review

The primary purpose of the present review was to test the validity of the physiological disinhibition, expectancy, and indirect cause explanations of intoxicated aggression. There are two general approaches to reviewing the literature: the narrative (or qualitative) approach and the meta-analytic (or quantitative) approach. In the traditional narrative review, the reviewer uses "mental algebra" to integrate the findings from a collection of studies and describes the results in a narrative manner. In the meta-analytic review, the reviewer uses statistical procedures to integrate the findings from a collection of studies and describes the results using numerical effect size estimates. Traditional narrative reviews are more likely than meta-analytic reviews to depend on the subjective judgments, preferences, and biases of the reviewer.[25] In the present review, meta-analytic procedures were used to test the validity of the proposed explanations of intoxicated aggression.

5. Method

5.1. Literature Search Procedures

All experimental studies retrieved in previous meta-analytic reviews of alcohol and aggression by Bushman and his colleagues were included.[13,14] To obtain more recent experimental studies, the PsycLIT computer data base was searched from January 1992 to March 1995. The terms used to describe aggression (aggression, agonistic, anger, attack, dominant, fight, hostility, violence) were the same descriptors used by the International Society for Research on Aggression in their journal, *Aggressive Behavior*. The aggression keywords were paired with three alcohol terms: alcohol, ethanol, and intoxicant. Various forms of the keywords also were used (e.g., aggress, aggression, aggressive, aggressor). The search was restricted to studies that used human participants. The literature review retrieved 60 research reports that included 66 independent samples of participants.*

5.2. Criteria for Relevance

Because the primary purpose of this review was to determine the validity of causal explanations of intoxicated aggression, two exclusion criteria were used. First, correlational studies were excluded from the review. Second, studies that used aggressive state measures were excluded unless they also used behavioral measures of aggression. An aggressive state is a combination of thoughts, feelings, behavioral tendencies, and physiological arousal levels that are elicited by stimuli capable of evoking aggression. Although an aggressive state should heighten the likelihood of aggression, it would not be classified by most psychologists as aggressive "behavior."

* Extreme outliers were removed from the data set. In the study by Zeichner and Pihl,[26] the noise intensity standardized mean estimates were 6.64 and 6.81 for the alcohol versus placebo comparisons, respectively. In the study by Zeichner and Pihl,[27] the noise intensity standardized mean estimates were 11.63 and 7.00 for the alcohol versus control and alcohol versus placebo comparisons, respectively.

5.3. Coding Frame

The information listed in the Appendix was extracted from the report of each study. These data were divided into three categories: participant characteristics, experiment characteristics, and primary study results. (For a detailed description of the source, participant, and experiment characteristics that moderate the relation between alcohol intoxication and aggression, see the meta-analysis by Bushman and Cooper.[13,14])

5.4. Meta-Analytic Procedures

The effect size estimate used in this review was the standardized mean difference, d (see Appendix). The standardized mean difference gives the number of standard deviation units between the sample means of two groups (e.g., placebo and control). According to Cohen,[28] a "small" d is 0.20, a "medium" d is 0.50, and a "large" d is 0.80. The average weighted sample standardized mean differences, where each standardized mean difference was weighted by the inverse of its variance, was used to estimate the common population standardized mean difference, δ. (Average standardized mean differences, 95% confidence intervals, and moderator tests were calculated using the procedures described in Hedges and Olkin.[29]) A 95% confidence interval also was calculated for δ.[29] If studies did not provide enough information to compute an effect size estimate, but did report the direction or statistical significance of results, vote-counting procedures were used to obtain an effect size estimate.[30] The procedure proposed by Bushman and Wang[31] was then used to combine the estimates based effect size and vote-counting procedures.

One problem that arises in estimating average effect size estimates is deciding what constitutes an independent hypothesis test. The present review used a shifting unit of analysis.[32] Each statistical test was coded as if it were an independent event. For example, if a single study contained two measures of aggression (e.g., intensity of shock given to a confederate and amount of money subtracted from a confederate), two effect size estimates would be coded. For the estimate of alcohol's overall effect on aggression, the two effect size estimates would be averaged so that the study would contribute only one effect size estimate. For an analysis in which the effects of alcohol are compared for different measures of aggression, the study would contribute two effect size estimates (e.g., direct physical aggression and indirect physical aggression). Thus, the shifting unit of analysis retains as much data as possible without violating two greatly the independence assumption that underlies the validity of meta-analytic procedures.

6. Results

6.1. Sex Differences in Intoxicated Aggression

The results showed that alcohol increased aggression more in men than in women, $\chi^2 (1, k = 65) = 4.64, p < 0.05$, where k is the number of independent samples of participants.[29] The average weighted effect size estimate for the 59 samples of male participants was 0.50 with 95% confidence interval [0.41, 0.58]. The average weighted effect size estimate for the six samples of female participants was 0.13 with 95% confidence interval [−0.20, 0.45]. Because alcohol increased aggression more in men than in women, subsequent analyses were based on the results from men only.

6.2. Measurement of Aggression

The type of aggression measure used (i.e., direct physical, indirect physical, direct verbal, indirect verbal) did not significantly influence the results reported in this review. Thus, the four types of aggression measures were pooled for subsequent analyses.

6.3. Validity of Proposed Explanations of Alcohol-Related Aggression

6.3.1. Physiological Disinhibition. If alcohol directly causes aggression by reducing inhibitions, then the level of aggression should be higher for participants in the antiplacebo group than for participants in the control group. The average weighted effect size estimate for the 13 antiplacebo versus control comparisons was −0.01, with 95% confidence interval [−0.21, 0.19]. Because the confidence interval contains the value zero, it appears that alcohol does not directly cause aggression.

6.3.2. Expectancy. If alcohol-related expectancies cause aggression, then the level of aggression should be higher for participants in the placebo group than for participants in the control group. The average weighted effect size estimate for the 20 placebo versus control comparison was 0.11, with 95% confidence interval [−0.06, 0.28]. Because the confidence interval contains the value zero, it appears that alcohol-related expectancies do not cause aggression.

As can be seen in Fig. 3, the effects of alcohol on aggression cannot be attributed solely to the pharmacological effects of alcohol nor to the effects of alcohol-related expectancies. Figure 3 also shows the results from studies in which the psychological and pharmacological effects of alcohol are confounded (i.e., alcohol versus placebo and alcohol versus control comparisons combined). In the real world, of course, the pharmacological and psychological effects of alcohol are confounded. For these confounded studies, the level of aggression was significantly higher for intoxicated participants than for sober participants. The average weighted effect size estimate based on 75 comparisons was 0.43 with 95% confidence interval [0.44, 0.62]. As can be seen in Fig. 3, the pharmacological and psychological effects of alcohol on aggression are not additive nor are they multiplicative. Thus, alcohol-related aggression cannot be explained by the independent or joint pharmacological and psychological effects of alcohol; another explanation is required.

6.3.3. Indirect Cause. If alcohol indirectly causes aggression by producing internal changes that increase the probability of aggression, then experimen-

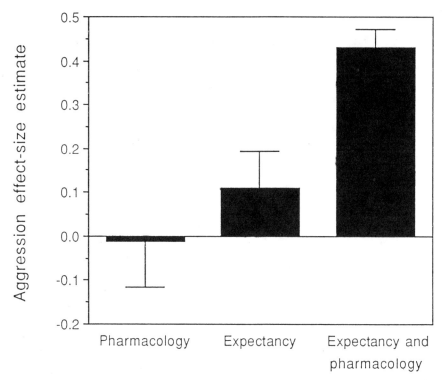

Figure 3. Psychological and pharmacological effects of alcohol on human aggression. NOTE: Capped vertical bars denote 1 standard error. Pharmacology, antiplacebo versus control comparison. Expectancy, placebo versus control comparison. Expectancy and pharmacology confounded, alcohol versus placebo and alcohol versus control comparisons combined.

tal manipulations that increase aggression should have a greater impact on intoxicated participants than on sober participants. Eighty-two percent of the studies included in this review used such manipulations. For this subset of studies, raters coded whether the Alcohol × Manipulation interaction was significant or nonsignificant. If the manipulation increased aggression, raters coded whether the effect was stronger for participants who received alcohol than for participants who did not receive alcohol.

The results from studies with nonsignificant and significant Alcohol × Manipulation interactions are shown in Fig. 4.* For nonsignificant interactions, 36 results were positive (i.e., in the predicted direction) and 14 results were negative (i.e., in the opposite direction). A sign test showed that the proportion of positive results was significantly greater than .5, $p < 0.05$. The corresponding effect size estimate was $g = .22$, a value close to Cohen's[28] conventional value for a "large" effect (i.e., $g = .25$). For significant interactions, 14 results were positive and 2 results were negative. A sign test showed

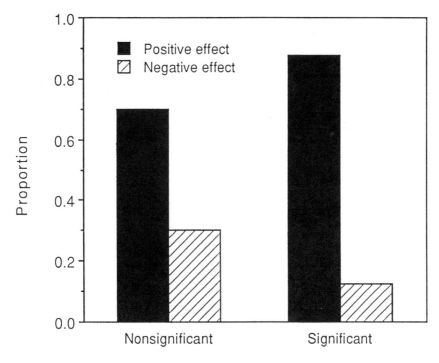

Figure 4. Effects of experimental aggression manipulations on intoxicated and sober participants. NOTE: Positive effect, aggression-eliciting manipulation was stronger for participants who received alcohol than for participants who did not receive alcohol. Negative effect, aggression-eliciting manipulation was stronger for participants who did not receive alcohol than for participants who received alcohol.

that the proportion of positive results was significantly greater than .5, $p <$ 0.05. The corresponding effect size estimate was $g = .38$, a value greater than Cohen's conventional value for a large effect. These results are entirely consistent with the indirect cause explanation of intoxicated aggression.

7. Conclusions

Does alcohol cause aggression? The results from this review suggest that it does. In experimental studies, intoxicated participants were more aggres-

---

* Four studies manipulated variables that decreased aggression (i.e., nonaggressive norms, non-aggressive cues, pain feedback). The Alcohol × Manipulation interaction was significant for one of the four studies. All four studies found that aggression reducing manipulations had a weaker effect on intoxicated participants than on sober participants.

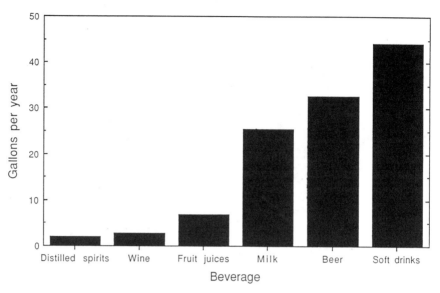

Figure 5. United States per capita consumption of selected beverages. NOTE: Data from US Department of Agriculture.[28] Milk includes plain and flavored. Fruit juices excludes vegetable juices. Alcoholic consumption rates are for the adult population.

sive, on average, than were sober participants. Larger effects might be obtained for higher alcohol doses on human aggression. The effects of alcohol on aggression are as large as the effects of other independent variables on aggression (e.g., media violence, anonymity, hot temperatures).[33] Alcohol also influences aggressive behavior as much as it influences other social (e.g., risk taking, moral judgment, sexual interest) and nonsocial (e.g., information processing, self-reported mood, physiological arousal) behaviors.[34]

Why does alcohol increase aggression? The results from this review suggest that intoxicated aggression cannot be solely attributed to the pharmacological or expectancy effects of alcohol. Another possibility, however, is that the null effects for the antiplacebo versus control and placebo versus control comparisons are due to methodological problems associated with the antiplacebo and placebo groups. These groups both involve deception. Participants in the antiplacebo group do not expect to receive alcohol and might become suspicious when they taste, smell, and notice the physiological effects of alcohol. Participants in the placebo group expect to receive alcohol and might become suspicious when they do not experience the physiological effects of alcohol. When participants in the antiplacebo and placebo groups realize that the experimenter has attempted to deceive them concerning the contents of their beverage, they also might become suspicious about other facets of the experiment and become more aware of their behavior. Because aggression is not a socially desirable response, participants in the antiplacebo and placebo groups might inhibit their behavior consciously.

The results from this review are consistent with the idea that alcohol indirectly causes aggression by producing changes within the person that increase the probability of aggression. Experimental manipulations that facilitate aggression, such as provocations, frustrations, and aggressive cues, were shown to have a stronger effect on intoxicated participants than on sober participants. This may explain why "barroom brawls" are so common. Bars often are crowded, noisy, smoky, and provocative environments.

The relation between alcohol and aggression would be of little concern if people rarely drank alcohol. But in the United States, alcohol is the beverage of choice for many people. As can be seen in Fig. 5, the average American adult drinks more beer than milk each year. What would happen to violent crime rates in the United States if people drank less alcohol? A study by Cook and Moore[35] reported that if alcohol consumption per capita decreased by just 10%, there would be a corresponding 1% decrease in murders, 6% decrease in forcible rapes, 6% decrease in aggravated assaults, and 9% decrease in robberies.* Thus, one way to obtain a kinder, gentler society would be to decrease alcohol consumption.

8. Appendix

8.1. Participant Characteristics

1. Sex of participants.
2. Number of participants.

8.2. Experiment Characteristics

1. Type of comparison (i.e., antiplacebo versus control, placebo versus control, alcohol versus placebo, alcohol versus control).
2. Type of aggression (i.e., direct physical, indirect physical, direct verbal, indirect verbal).
3. If the study contained an experimental manipulation that was expected to influence aggression, was the Alcohol × Experimental manipulation significant or nonsignificant at the $\alpha = 0.10$ level? (Due to low statistical power, the $\alpha = 0.10$ level was used rather than the $\alpha = 0.05$ level) What was the direction of the contrast analysis (i.e., *positive,* if the manipulation increased aggression, the effect was stronger for participants who received alcohol than for participants who did not receive alcohol; *negative,* if the manipulation

* Cook and Moore[35] calculated these estimates using regression analysis from US violent crime rates from 1979 to 1988.

increased aggression, the effect was stronger for participants who did not receive alcohol than for participants who received alcohol; *null*, the effect was the same for participants who did and did not receive alcohol)?

8.3. Primary Study Results

1. Direction of effect (i.e., positive, negative, null effect).
2. Significance of effect (i.e., significant, nonsignificant at the $\alpha = 0.05$ level).
3. Magnitude of effect (i.e., standardized mean differences estimate, *d*). The standardized mean difference estimate was defined as $d = (M_1 - M_2)/SD$, where M_1 and M_2 are the respective sample means for groups 1 and 2, and SD is the pooled standard deviation. When means and standard deviations were not reported, but *t* tests or *F* tests with 1 degree of freedom in the numerator were reported, *d* was calculated using Friedman's formula.[29] If *F* tests with multiple degrees of freedom in the numerator were reported, means and standard deviations were requested from authors.

References

1. Adler J: Kids growing up scared. *Newsweek* 43–50, 1994, January 10.
2. Lacayo R: Lock 'em up! *Time* 50–53, 1994, February 7.
3. Shannon E: Crime: Safer streets, yet greater fear. *Time* 63–65, 1995, January 30.
4. Shannon E: Crime: Safer streets, yet greater fear. *Time* 63–65, 1995, January 30.
5. Beck AJ: *Profile of Jail Inmates, 1989.* Washington, DC, Bureau of Justice Statistics, 1991.
6. Beck AJ, Kline SA, Greenfield LA: *Survey of Youth in Custody, 1987.* Washington, DC, Bureau of Justice Statistics, 1988.
7. Greenberg SW: Alcohol and crime: A methodological critique of the literature, in Collins JJ (ed): *Drinking and Crime: Perspectives on the Relationships between Alcohol Consumption and Criminal Behavior.* New York, Guilford, 1981.
8. Innes CA: *Drug Use and Crime.* Washington, DC, US Department of Justice, 1988.
9. MacDonald JM: *The Murderer and His Victim.* Springfield, IL, Charles C. Thomas, 1961.
10. Murdoch D, Pihl RO, Ross D: Alcohol and crimes of violence: Present issues. *Int J Addict* 25:1065–1081, 1990.
11. Pernanen K: *Alcohol in Human Violence.* New York, Guilford Press, 1991.
12. Brain PF: Multidisciplinary examinations of the "causes" of crime: The case of the link between alcohol and violence. *Alcohol Alcohol* 21:237–240, 1986.
13. Bushman BJ: Human aggression while under the influence of alcohol and other drugs: An integrative research review. *Curr Direct Psychol Sci* 2:148–152, 1993.
14. Bushman BJ, Cooper HM: Effects of alcohol on human aggression: An integrative research review. *Psychol Bull* 107:341–354, 1990.
15. Ross S, Krugman AD, Lyerly SB, Clyde DJ: Drugs and placebos: A model design. *Psychol Rep* 10:383–392, 1962.
16. Buss AH: *The Psychology of Aggression.* New York, Wiley, 1961.
17. Green RG: *Human Aggression.* Pacific Grove, CA, Brooks/Cole, 1990.
18. Taylor SP: Aggressive behavior and physiological arousal as a function of provocation and the tendency to inhibit aggression. *J Pers* 35:297–310, 1967.

19. Barnett RK: The effects of alcohol, expectancy, provocation, and permission to aggress upon aggressive behavior. *Dissertation Abstracts International* 40:4993B (University Microfilms No. ADG80-09229, 0000), 1979.
20. Cherek DR, Spiga R, Egli M: Effects of response requirement and alcohol on human aggressive responding. *J Exp Anal Behav* 58:577–587, 1992.
21. Murdoch D, Pihl RO: Alcohol and aggression in a group interaction. *Addict Behav* 10:97–101, 1985.
22. Rohsenow DJ, Bachorowski J: Effect of alcohol and expectancies on verbal aggression in men and women. *J Abnorm Psychol* 93:418–432, 1984.
23. Muehlberger CW: Medicolegal aspects of alcohol intoxication. *Mich State Bar J* 35:38–42, 1956.
24. MacAndrew C, Edgerton RB: *Drunken Comportment: A Social Explanation.* Chicago, Aldine, 1969.
25. Cooper H, Rosenthal R: Statistical versus traditional procedures for summarizing research findings. *Psychological Bulletin* 87:442–449, 1980.
26. Zeichner A, Pihl RO: Effects of alcohol and behavior contingencies on human aggression. *J Abnorm Psychol* 88:153–160, 1979.
27. Zeichner A, Pihl RO: Effects of alcohol and instigator intent on human aggression. *J Stud Alcohol* 41:265–276, 1980.
28. Cohen J: *Statistical Power Analysis for the Behavioral Sciences,* 2nd ed. Hillsdale, NJ, Lawrence Erlbaum, 1988.
29. Hedges LV, Olkin I: *Statistical Methods for Meta-analysis.* New York, Academic Press, 1985.
30. Bushman BJ: Vote-counting procedures in meta-analysis, in Cooper H, Hedges LV (eds): *The Handbook of Research Synthesis.* New York, Russell Sage Foundation, 1994, pp 193–213.
31. Bushman BJ, Wang MC: A procedure for combining sample standardized mean differences and vote counts to estimate the population standardized mean difference in fixed effects models. *Psychol Methods* 1:66–80.
32. Cooper HM: Integrating research: *A Guide for Literature Reviews,* 2nd ed. Hillsdale, NJ, Erlbaum, 1989.
33. Anderson CA, Bushman BJ: External validity of "trivial" experiments: The case of laboratory aggression. *General Psychology Review,* in press.
34. Steele CM, Southwick L: Alcohol and social behavior I: The psychology of drunken excess. *J Pers Soc Psychol* 48:18–34, 1985.
35. Cook PJ, Moore MJ: Violence reduction through restrictions on alcohol availability. *Alcohol Health Res World* 17:151–156, 1993.
36. Maguire K, Pastotre AL (eds): *Sourcebook of Criminal Justice Statistics, 1993.* US Department of Justice, Bureau of Justice Statistics. Washington, DC, US Government Printing Office, 1994.
37. US Bureau of the Census: *Statistical Abstract of the United States: 1994,* 114th ed. Washington, DC, US Government Printing Office, 1994.
38. Friedman H: Magnitude of an experimental effect and a table for its rapid estimation. *Psychol Bull* 70:194–197, 1968.

11

Is There a Causal Relationship between Alcohol Use and Violence?

A Synthesis of Evidence

Mark W. Lipsey, David B. Wilson, Mark A. Cohen, and James H. Derzon

Abstract. This chapter reviews the evidence bearing on the question of whether those individuals who consume alcohol have an increased probability of subsequent violent behavior. Four bodies of relevant research are examined: experimental studies with animals, experimental studies with humans, individual-level correlational studies, and macro-level correlational studies. All these research approaches provide some evidence of an association between alcohol consumption and violent behavior, but no firm conclusion can be drawn about whether alcohol plays a causal role in such behavior. Various limitations, deficiencies, and ambiguities of available research that contribute to this state of affairs are discussed.

1. Introduction

Ample evidence demonstrates that alcohol consumption frequently accompanies incidents of intentional violence.[1-3] Roizen,[4] for instance, summarized a large number of studies showing that offenders were variously estimated to have consumed alcohol prior to 28–86% of homicides, 24–37% of assaults, 7–

Mark W. Lipsey, David B. Wilson, and James H. Derzon • Vanderbilt Institute for Public Policy Studies, Vanderbilt University, Nashville, Tennessee 37212.   **Mark A. Cohen** • Owen Graduate School of Management, and Vanderbilt Institute for Public Policy Studies, Vanderbilt University, Nashville, Tennessee 37212.

Recent Developments in Alcoholism, Volume 13: Alcoholism and Violence, edited by Marc Galanter. Plenum Press, New York, 1997

72% of robberies, 13–60% of sex offenses, and 6–57% of incidents of marital violence. What makes the alcohol–violence relationship especially interesting, of course, is the possibility that alcohol consumption may have a distinct causal influence on subsequent violent behavior. For example, if a causal influence of alcohol abuse on violence can be demonstrated, we not only gain some important information about the adverse effects of alcohol and the etiology of violence, but also identify treatment for alcohol abuse as a potentially important component of any strategy for preventing or reducing violent behavior.

As Roizen[4] noted, "alcohol's presence [in violent incidents] is often considered presumptive of a causal relationship" (p. 6). In the research community, however, it is widely recognized that correlation does not establish causality, and considerable skepticism has been voiced about the state of current evidence on the causal link. As Roizen[4] further remarks, "more is written about the possible contributions alcohol might make to violent and criminal behavior than is written from research that attempts to establish whether there is an empirical relationship and what that relationship might be" (p. 6). Similar sentiments have been expressed by Fagan,[5] Greenberg,[6] Pernanen,[7] Walfish and Blount,[8] and others.

It is the purpose of this chapter to review the current state of empirical evidence bearing on the question of whether consumption of alcohol increases the likelihood that those individuals who consume it will subsequently engage in violent behavior toward others. Our focus is on the psychopharmacological effects of alcohol ingestion upon the behavior of drinkers, including both their directly aggressive behavior and other behavior that might be closely related to the likelihood of those persons engaging in violence, e.g., risk-taking. We do not include, however, effects on accidental violence (e.g., motor vehicle accidents), violence toward self (e.g., suicide), or violence incidentally associated with alcohol distribution (e.g., violence in attempts to obtain money to purchase alcohol). While these are interesting topics, we wish to limit our focus to the important public issue of interpersonal, especially criminal, violence and ask if alcohol consumption is one of its causes.

1.1. The Nature of the Causal Question

The concept of causality is an inherently complex one, especially in the behavioral sciences,[9] and no less so in application to the question of the causal effects of alcohol on violent behavior. To bring some structure to the issue for present purposes, we differentiate three aspects of the causal question:

1. Is there an overall causal relationship, i.e., a main effect? This is a question of whether alcohol consumption results in an increased likelihood generally that the drinkers will subsequently engage in violent behavior. Demonstration of a general causal effect requires evidence that, all other things equal, typical persons who consume alcohol have an incrementally higher probability of engaging in subsequent violent behavior than if they

had not consumed the alcohol. A variant is to demonstrate that persons who consume alcohol have a higher probability of engaging in violence than essentially similar other persons in essentially similar circumstances.

It is the phrases "all other things equal" and "essentially similar" in the above statements that provide the greatest difficulty in establishing credible evidence on the causal question. Any comparison that involves ambiguity about how well these conditions are met leaves open the possibility that any observed differences in violence stem from factors other than alcohol consumption. We will have more to say about this critical and refractory matter later. It is also pertinent to note that causality in this context has to do with the probability of behavior, that is, the relative frequency of occurrence in sets of persons, incidents, observations, and the like. Since violent behavior in most circumstances is a relatively rare event, it follows that we are necessarily dealing chiefly with low probabilities that will be correspondingly difficult to detect and compare.

2. Is there a causal relationship for some persons and/or some circumstances, that is, a moderator or interaction effect? This is a question of whether it can be demonstrated empirically that alcohol consumption results in an increased likelihood of violent behavior for persons identifiable by some distinctive characteristics or for persons in certain identifiable situations, or both.[10] Many researchers believe that causal effects come essentially in the form of an alcohol × person × situation interaction.[7,11–13] That is, alcohol consumption increases the probability of violent behavior only for some persons in some situations. The challenge here is twofold: to identify the characteristics of those persons and/or those situations that represent high risk and, for those cases, to demonstrate an increased likelihood of violence when alcohol is consumed (as in no. 1, above).

3. Is there an identifiable causal mechanism by which alcohol consumption might influence the probability of violent behavior? This is a contingent question that is meaningful only if a causal relationship of some sort can be demonstrated, but it is nevertheless very important to the causal question. An empirical demonstration of a causal link between alcohol and violence would make a limited, albeit fundamental, contribution to our understanding in the absence of any indication of how such an effect comes about. A considerable literature of research and theory identifies many possible causal processes that may account for an effect of alcohol on violence. These include a variety of physiological or psychological effects that alcohol ingestion might have on an individual, e.g., cognitive impairment, disinhibiting violent impulses or risk-taking, creating expectancies, serving as a cue for counternormative behavior, "deviance disavowal," and so forth.[7,11,14]

In this chapter, we focus primarily on the first two questions having to do with evidence that alcohol consumption increases the probability of subsequent violent behavior generally or that it increases it differentially for some persons in some situations. These questions are fundamental to the study of the alcohol–violence relationship[13] and answers continue to be elusive. As various researchers have observed, the evidence for a significant causal link between alcohol use and violent behavior is ambiguous, complex, and problematic.[11,15–17]

1.2. The Complexities of Empirically Demonstrating a Causal Link

If there were a simple and direct causal relationship between alcohol and violence, virtually everyone who drank (at least over some threshold) would become violent, a proposition refuted by everyday experience. For instance, in over 600 hr of observation in pubs and bars, Grayham et al.[18] observed no instances of fights or physical injury. We know, therefore, that at most there is a rather loose causal coupling between alcohol consumption and violence. It follows that the relationship of interest is difficult to observe empirically and is most assuredly complex, as the experience of many researchers attests.

The methodological challenges inherent in studying this complex relationship are formidable. First, we must distinguish two rather different versions of the causal hypothesis at issue with different implications for study design. The version that first comes to mind when one thinks of alcohol causing violence involves incidents as the unit of analysis. In this case, the focus is on persons who drink and the likelihood that they will engage in violent behavior shortly thereafter (an "incident"), within the time frame defined by the presence of alcohol in psychoactive form in their systems. Studies of this situation typically examine incidents of a selected sort, e.g., crime incidents, and attend to whether alcohol was consumed and whether violence occurred. This line of study is often referred to as investigation of the "acute" effects of alcohol on violence.[1,4,15] The other version focuses on persons as the unit of analysis with attention to their patterns of alcohol use and violent behavior over time. The linkage of interest here is whether persons who chronically use (or abuse) alcohol are more likely to engage in violent behavior, irrespective of alcohol consumption immediately prior to a particular instance of violence. This line of study investigates the "chronic" effects of alcohol on violence. Clearly, the nature of the causal connection posited, the mechanisms through which it might occur, and the methods by which it can be studied differ quite considerably for these two lines of inquiry.

Perhaps the most problematic aspect of studying the effects of alcohol on violence is the inherent trade-off between internal and external validity. Well-controlled experimental designs in which participants are randomly assigned to alcohol and no-alcohol conditions and observations are made of subsequent aggression unquestionably have the highest internal validity for testing the causal inference at issue. However, for compelling practical and ethical reasons, researchers cannot control the alcohol consumption of people in everyday life and then monitor their violence levels in natural situations. Instead, laboratory-drinking situations must be employed and, most especially, proxy or surrogate measures of violence must be contrived. Thus strong testing of the causal role of alcohol consumption on violent behavior occurs only in a form that is quite unrepresentative of the violence in society that is the major concern of policymakers, law enforcement, and many citizens.

Stronger external validity, or generalizability, to violence in natural situations comes from correlational or observational studies of such violence. For instance, survey studies have frequently been used to examine the association between reported alcohol use and violent behavior for various population groups. Assuming reasonable validity to those reports (which cannot always be assumed), such studies have the advantage of dealing with the types of drinking and violence that are of concern as social problems. What associations they find between alcohol use and violent behavior, however, are inherently ambiguous with regard to causality. An alcohol–violence correlation may result from alcohol causing violent behavior, from violent behavior or its intentions causing alcohol use (e.g., to build courage, to forget), or from other factors that influence both drinking and violence (e.g., risk-taking personality, disadvantaged economic circumstances). It is also possible for such correlations to be spurious, that is, to result from coincidence or artifact rather than from a meaningful causal process. Alcohol abusers, for instance, may be more inclined to embellish the extent of their violent behavior in research interviews than nonusers, creating a spurious association between reported alcohol use and violence. Determining which of these accounts applies is difficult and almost never conclusive. Study of the causal role of alcohol in violence thus presents a perverse quandary: Either strong testing of causal inference or generalizability to the circumstances of principal interest must be sacrificed in any empirical research design that attempts to address the issue.

A third area of difficulty in alcohol–violence research has to do with the definition and operationalization of the constructs selected to represent alcohol use and violent behavior, the independent and dependent variables, respectively, in such study. If the focus is on alcohol use in a single instance (the "acute" case), issues of dosage and timing apply. Alcohol has few discernable physiological effects in very small doses and in sufficiently large doses renders drinkers comatose and incapable of violence. There is a wide range in between, however, over which alcohol may have different effects on the likelihood of violence. Similar concerns apply to the timing between alcohol consumption and the point of observation for violence. Assuming some decay curve in alcohol's effects, any given dose of alcohol might have quite different effects at different intervals subsequent to consumption.

Where the long-term effects of alcohol use are at issue (the "chronic" case), there is also great variety in the possible drinking patterns that may be at issue, often distinguished with phrases such as "social drinking," "abuse," "alcoholism," "binge drinking," and the like. In neither the chronic nor the acute case does the research literature show any consistency in the definition and operationalization of alcohol use nor has there been much systematic exploration of the relative importance of dose, timing, or drinking pattern as dimensions of the alcohol use construct and its variants. As a result, the alcohol construct appears as something of a "fuzzy set" in research studies with corresponding ambiguity for the researcher attempting to properly operationalize the construct or the reviewer attempting to interpret the research results.

A further complication is that alcohol use is almost inevitably a highly bundled construct; that is, most observations or measurements incorporate several distinctly different aspects of drinking packaged together in a single index. At the narrowest level is the pharmacological aspect of alcohol consumption, e.g., as represented in blood alcohol content. This cannot generally be manipulated and measured in isolation, however. In most practical measurement circumstances, drinkers are aware of their alcohol consumption, introducing such psychological aspects as expectancy and cultural meanings into the picture, variables that may have their own effects independent of the pharmacological effects of alcohol. In addition, drinking is generally embedded in a social context involving a mix of circumstances, locations, companions, and the like that may also separately influence the likelihood of violence. It is quite difficult to isolate these different aspects of alcohol use in any operationalization of the construct or even to attain some consistency in the mix of aspects from one research study to another. Correspondingly, when relationships between alcohol use and violent behavior are found, it is generally difficult to know which of the quite different ingredients of the alcohol use construct package is responsible. While some attention has been given to this issue, especially in experimental studies of alcohol consumption, it continues to confound the study of alcohol and violence.

Turning to the dependent variable in the equation, we find similarly thorny problems associated with the definition and operationalization of the violence construct in this research area. The commonsense notion that violence, at least in its clearest and most extreme version, involves intentional behaviors that physically harm another person is at the core of most definitions, but for very good reasons operationalizations frequently include more and sometimes less than this core concept. One problem is with the notion of intent, which invokes aspects of the internal or cognitive states of individuals that cannot be easily measured. However, without this element in the definition, even if it cannot be explicitly verified, accidental harm to another person falls under the violence construct and it takes on a different meaning in relation to alcohol effects (given the well-documented motor impairment alcohol produces). If intent is viewed as a defining feature, on the other hand, then it may be of less relevance whether actual physical harm was done. Thus, many definitions and operationalizations include threats or attempts as well as completed violence. Another area of variation has to do with the target of the violence. Some operationalizations include violence against property or violence against self along with violence against another person. Further variation comes in around the notion of physical harm—some operationalizations include verbal abuse, arguments, and the like as violence, albeit perhaps psychological violence.

Moreover, violence is often measured using multi-item or composite measures designed to increase the reliability of measurement compared to single items or to better reflect the multifaceted nature of violent behavior. Frequently, such composite measures encompass a range of antisocial behaviors with physical violence generally viewed as an extreme form of such behavior. Depending on the mix of items or facets included, however, the portion of such measures related to the intentional physical harm of another person can be quite small. In sum, then, a broad range of relatively distinct and disparate behaviors, individually and in aggregates, are encompassed under one or another operationalization of the violence construct in alcohol–violence studies. The design, review, and interpretation of such studies, correspondingly, suffers from ambiguity about the construct at issue and what meaning to attribute to its diverse operationalizations.

With these issues in mind, we turn to a review of the four distinct bodies of empirical evidence bearing most directly on the question of the causal influence of alcohol consumption on the likelihood of violent behavior. Two of the relevant research paradigms chiefly use controlled experimental design—animal studies and laboratory simulations with humans. Two use observational or correlational methods—surveys of drinking and violent behaviors and community level analyses of the covariation between alcohol availability and violence.

2. Experimental Approaches

2.1. Animal Studies

Studies of the effects of alcohol on animals necessarily have uncertain generalizability to human behavior. However, they do offer an opportunity to explore the possibility that there is a very general pharmacological link between alcohol ingestion and aggressive behavior, at least in mammals whose neurophysiology may be similar in important respects to humans. In addition, of course, animal studies offer possibilities of laboratory control and experimentation with dosage, stimuli, and aggressive contexts that would be impossible with human subjects. Experimental studies of the effects of alcohol on the aggressive behavior of animals have been itemized and thoroughly reviewed by Miczek et al.[3] and Berry and Smoothy,[19] and no attempt will be made here to do more than summarize some of the conclusions that can be drawn from their efforts.

Perhaps the most important conclusion to be drawn from these reviews is that examination of the alcohol–violence link in animals does not yield any simple picture that might guide the understanding of this issue for human behavior. To begin with, there are many different forms of animal aggression—conflict in relation to status hierarchies, defense of territory, male rival fighting, female defense of young, predatory aggression, antipredator defense, and various forms of aggression under such stresses as isolated housing, crowding, restricted access to food, and noxious stimulation.[20] Moreover, there is evidence that many of these forms of aggression are related to specific brain mechanisms unlikely to respond the same way to alcohol.[3,21] Nor do such brain mechanisms bear any necessary resemblance to those in humans. As Miczek *et al.*[3] put it, "There is no direct evidence . . . that demonstrates homology between the neural circuitry and physiologic activity that mediate aggressive behavior in animals and those responsible for human violence" (p. 381).

Another complication in the animal studies is evidence of significant individual differences in the aggressive response to alcohol among members of the same species in similar circumstances. Miczek, Weerts, and DeBold[22] reviewed a variety of studies in which subpopulations of rodents and primates showed reliable increases in aggressive behavior when given alcohol, while other individuals exhibited no such effect or even a suppression of aggression. Among primates, these differences in response seem to be related to social status (see also ref. 20). Some evidence also links these individual differences in aggressive response to differences in specific neurotransmitter systems.[22,23] Thus, the animal studies reveal important moderator and interaction effects involving alcohol, even though the specific variables involved in those interactions have not yet been fully identified.

As a result of the variation in types of aggression and neurological mechanisms, individual differences in aggressive response to alcohol, and other possible sources of variation (e.g., methodological differences[20]), animal studies of alcohol and aggression have not produced consistent results. The studies itemized by Berry and Smoothy[19] and Miczek *et al.*[3] include a notable portion that show no effects of alcohol on aggression and some show reduced aggression with the same alcohol doses that are associated with increases in other studies. Miczek, DeBold, and VanErp[23] described the experimental research with animals on the effects of alcohol on aggression as "largely inconclusive" (p. 407), and Brain, Miras, and Berry[20] characterized it as "somewhat disappointing" (p. 140).

Nonetheless, there are some instructive results from the animal studies. Despite the varied animal subjects, forms of aggression, and research paradigms, a substantial proportion of these studies do show increased aggressive behavior relative to control animals with administration of alcohol. Moreover, where alcohol effects appear, they are at lower and moderate doses; higher doses generally sedate the animals and depress aggression, as in humans. Thus, there are causal pathways from alcohol ingestion to increased aggressive behavior, at least in some animals, at some doses, in some circumstances, and for some forms of aggression. Further, animal studies have produced evidence that the effects of alcohol are mediated by certain neurochemical systems in the brain.[24] Some of these neurochemical systems, in turn, have been linked to aggressive behavior, though no specific role for these mechanisms has yet been established in mediating alcohol's effects on such behavior.

Also, some studies in mice, rats, and primates have shown effects of chronic alcohol consumption on aggressive behavior under stress conditions.[3,24] Rats administered three daily doses of alcohol, for instance, attacked intruders more severely than control animals.[25] Relatively few animal studies have investigated chronic alcohol consumption, however, so evidence on this matter is limited.

Thus, there are experimentally demonstrable effects of both acute and chronic alcohol ingestion on aggression among some animal subjects. Such effects, however, do not appear consistently or universally. Individual differences among the test subjects and variations in the conditions, methods, doses, forms of aggression, and the like appear to interact with alcohol in a complex way that sometimes elevates aggression and sometimes does not.

2.2. Human Studies

A considerable number of experimental studies of the effects of acute alcohol ingestion on human subjects has been conducted with attention to a range of outcome variables. For purposes of reviewing the results of the subset of those studies that examined effects on aggression, we rely on a meta-analysis we[26] have recently completed in order to update similar efforts by others.[27–30] For this meta-analysis, we made a thorough search for published and unpublished study reports, retrieved those identified as potentially eligible for inclusion, systematically coded the characteristics of each eligible study and its statistical findings, and analyzed the resulting database. Since the studies at issue all employed experimental designs, the metric we used to record their findings was the standardized mean difference on an aggression measure between the experimental group receiving alcohol and the control or placebo group not receiving alcohol. This metric, known as an effect size or Cohen's d, is conventional in meta-analysis and indexes the difference between groups in standard deviation units.[31] Thus, in this application, an effect size of .50 indicates that the group that was administered alcohol yielded a mean aggression score that was half a standard deviation higher than the mean for the control group with which it was compared. For purposes of computing mean effect sizes and other such statistics, each individual effect size was weighted by its inverse variance to give larger weight to those based on larger samples.[32]

We coded 52 independent studies from 50 reports that met criteria requiring: (1) human subjects, (2) experimental design in which alcohol consumption was the independent variable and some measure described as aggression or a proxy for aggression was the dependent variable, and (3) the study was reported in English and contained sufficient information to permit calculation of appropriate effect sizes for its key results. (A bibliography of the coded studies is available from the authors.) The aggression measure in eight of these studies, however, did not involve any physical stimulus or actual implied potential of physical harm (e.g., monetary penalties, harsh evaluation ratings). In order to keep a focus on physical aggression, we eliminated these from the pool and retained the 44 studies using some physical stimulus as an aggressive response. Of these, one used noxious noise and all the others used electric shock.

With one exception, all of these studies used one of two laboratory paradigms: the competitive reaction time paradigm (31 studies) or the teacher–learner paradigm (12 studies). In the competitive reaction time paradigm, the subject is led to believe that he or she is competing with another subject in a series of tasks set up to examine the influence of alcohol on reaction time. When the subject wins a reaction time trial, he or she delivers a shock to the opponent at an intensity level selected by the subject immediately prior to the trial. The intensity of these shocks serves as the dependent measure for the study. In actuality, the opponent does not exist and the wins and losses are controlled by the experimenter. The degree of threat or provocation is manipulated in some of these studies by varying the frequency and/or intensity of the shocks received by the subjects on the trials they lose. Depending on the researcher's hypothesis, of course, other features of the paradigm may be varied as well.

In the teacher–learner paradigm, the subject is informed that the experiment is studying the effects of alcohol on teaching and learning abilities. A rigged drawing determines that the subject will serve as the teacher in a visual discrimination or paired association memory task. The learner is actually a confederate of the experimenter (or a computer) who follows a predetermined pattern of right and wrong answers. Each time the learner makes an error, the subject (teacher) can choose to correct the learner via an "aggressive" response (a shock in 11 studies, a noxious noise in 1) or a "neutral" response (a red feedback light). In this paradigm the learner cannot retaliate toward the subject (ref. 33 is the one exception). The frequency, intensity, or duration of these shocks (or noise) serves as the primary dependent measure for these studies.

The one study that departed from these two paradigms[34] examined the influence of alcohol, arousal, and aggressive cues on aggressive behavior by asking subjects in various conditions to assist the experimenter in "stimulating" a bogus subject. The subject could choose to stimulate the bogus subject with either a tone or an electric shock. The duration of the shocks served as the measure of aggression.

2.2.1. External Validity. The major strength of these studies, of course, is their ability to manipulate alcohol consumption in a randomized trial under relatively controlled conditions and, hence, directly investigate the causal influence of the alcohol manipulation on the response variables. Their greatest weakness is uncertainty regarding the extent to which the results can be generalized from the laboratory conditions in which they were obtained to real instances of alcohol consumption and violence in natural situations. From the standpoint of ecological validity, we would prefer that there be some straightforward mapping that could be made between the circumstances of these experimental paradigms and the natural situations to which we would like to generalize. Clearly, however, there are a number of notable differences between these laboratory paradigms and the typical circumstances of naturally occurring drinking and violence that make such a mapping problematic. Intentionally administered electric shock, for instance, is a relatively rare violent response in natural situations. While some limited evidence suggests that it may be an acceptable proxy,[35] this issue has not been explored carefully and the results to date are not especially convincing. Also, while interpersonal violence is generally face-to-face and intimately personal, the "violence" in the laboratory paradigms is largely depersonalized: shock is administered to an unseen subject in another room by pushing a button. Additionally, these paradigms depend on some artificial constraints on respondents' options. In the competitive reaction time paradigm, the respondents are required by the experimental protocol to administer shock, i.e., to be aggressive. The only choice allowed is with regard to how aggressive they will be. The teacher–learner paradigm does generally permit a "neutral" or nonaggressive option, but the demand characteristics of the experimental situation work against its exclusive use by a subject who does not desire to be aggressive.

Another constraint on the generalizability of the results of these studies arises from the subject selections typically made by the experimenters and the alcohol doses administered to those subjects. Of the 44 eligible studies in our meta-analysis, 34 used college student subjects exclusively and 4 others used a mix in which college students were a large proportion. In addition, 41 of these studies used exclusively male subjects. The latter selection may not be especially damaging with regard to generalization issues since most naturally occurring violence is committed by males. It is not the case, however, that college students commit a large proportion of such violence.

Alcohol doses in these studies were typically reported in terms of milliliters per kilogram of body weight, but more than half also reported blood alcohol concentrations (BAC). By using the high correlation between milliliters per kilogram and BAC ($r = .82$), we were able to estimate mean BAC levels for the subjects in most of the studies. Some subjects attained BAC levels that would only be considered in the mild impairment range (13 studies with an estimated BAC from 0.03 to 0.08). Most of the studies (31), however, used dose levels around the per se drunk level established in many states (0.08–0.10), though none exceeded 0.10. Thus, the subjects given alcohol ranged from moderately intoxicated to legally drunk, but none were in the range of severe intoxication often found in cases of criminal violence.[13]

2.2.2. Alcohol–Violence Relationship. Despite uncertainty about the ecological validity and subject representativeness of these studies in relation to naturally occurring drinking and violence, they do provide an opportunity to determine if ostensibly aggressive behavior can be caused by manipulating alcohol consumption under at least some circumstances. If some form of an alcohol–violence causal relationship cannot be shown in laboratory situations specifically designed to reveal it, the plausibility of such a link under more complex and varied natural conditions is undermined. If such a link can be shown under laboratory conditions, then more focused inquiry can be made into the nature of that linkage and the other circumstances in which it might occur.

The mean effect size found in our meta-analysis for the major comparisons between the aggression levels shown by subjects to whom alcohol was administered and the control subjects who received no alcohol was 0.54. This overall mean indicates that subjects to whom the alcohol conditions were applied in this body of studies scored, on average, about half a standard deviation higher on the aggression measure than the control subjects who participated in the same task but did not consume any alcohol. If we use the 10-point shock intensity scale from the competitive reaction time paradigm as a frame of reference, a half standard deviation effect size indicates that subjects in the alcohol conditions, on average, administered shocks that were about one scale step higher than subjects in the nonalcohol conditions. Our effect size result is in agreement with earlier meta-analytic work by Bushman,[27] Bushman and Cooper,[28] Hull and Bond,[29] and Steele and Southwick,[30] all of whom reported positive effects of the alcohol conditions on measures of aggression.

On the face of it, this overall mean effect size can be interpreted as relatively strong evidence for the causal effect of alcohol consumption on at least one form of aggressive behavior. Researchers in this area have recognized, however, that the situation is more subtle than that. The manipulations used in these experiments have various aspects, as do the reactions of subjects to those manipulations. Before drawing a firm conclusion about the causal role of alcohol, it is necessary to seek some assurance that it was the alcohol part of these manipulations that was primarily responsible for the effect on aggression and not some other aspect that was bundled with alcohol in these manipulations. We therefore used the information coded in our meta-analysis to examine differences among studies that might shed some light on the potential for misleading confounds or artifacts in their results.

2.2.3. Potential Artifacts. We first compared the mean effect sizes resulting from the two different research paradigms that dominate these studies. As Table I shows, the competitive reaction time paradigm produced significantly larger effect sizes than the teacher–learner paradigm (statistically significant between-groups Q). The use of shock-based aggression measures and the alcohol doses administered were similar for the studies in the two major paradigms, suggesting that some other difference between them may be responsible for the difference in results. We therefore further differentiated the procedures in each paradigm to explore any association between them and the effect sizes found. We did this on an exploratory basis, recognizing that the Q statistics already showed homogeneous results within each paradigm

Table I. Effect Size Statistics for Alcohol versus Nonalcohol Conditions by Experimental Paradigm[a]

Experimental paradigm	Weighted mean ES	95% CI[b]	$Q_w{}^c$	n
Competitive reaction time	0.61	0.49, 0.74	30.2	29
Teacher–learner	0.41	0.20, 0.62	13.0	12
Other	0.04	−0.47, 0.55	NA	1
Total	0.54	0.43, 0.64	49.8	42

[a]Two studies (Zeichner and Pihl[57,58]) were removed from the analysis due to their having extreme outliers (effect sizes greater than 6.0).
[b]CI, Confidence interval (see Hedges and Olkin[32]).
[c]Q_w, Homogeneity within groups (*$p < 0.05$, reject homogeneity). The between-groups Q indicates that there is heterogeneity between groups ($Q_B(2) = 6.7$, $p < 0.05$).

(Table I). For such small numbers of studies, however, Q has relatively little statistical power to reject the hypothesis of homogeneity.

A major variation in the competitive reaction time paradigm had to do with the shocks the subject received. Twenty-two studies used some version of the standard format in which all subjects received shocks back from the "opponent." In three studies, the subjects received no shocks. In the remaining four studies, half the subjects received the standard format, while the other half received no shocks. As Table II shows, the effects of the alcohol condition on aggression were much lower when the subjects were not shocked. Note that the small number of studies requires that this comparison be interpreted cautiously but, as Gustafson[36] suggested, it may be that alcohol–violence effects only appear under provocation when nonaggressive options are unavailable.

The major variations among the smaller number of studies using the teacher–learner paradigm were as follows: one used a noxious noise for the aggressive stimulus instead of shock, three involved a provocation (e.g., an insulting comment or negative evaluation from the learner or a threat of a retaliatory shock), and three studies did not offer the nonaggressive response

Table II. Effect Size Statistics for the Competitive Reaction Time Studies by Whether the "Opponent" Shocked the Subjects

Provocation condition[a]	Weighted mean ES	95% CI[b]	$Q_w{}^c$	n
Subjects shocked	0.72	0.58, 0.86	21.9	26
Subjects not shocked	0.22	−0.03, 0.48	3.2	7

[a]Four studies contributed an effect size to both provocation conditions.
[b]CI, Confidence interval (see Hedges & Olkin[32]).
[c]Q_w, Homogeneity within groups (*$p < 0.05$, reject homogeneity). The between-groups, Q indicates that there is heterogeneity between groups ($Q_B(1) = 11.3$, $p < 0.05$).

option (red feedback light). As Table III shows, these variations appear to produce rather different mean effect sizes, though, with the small numbers of studies involved, none of these differences attained statistical significance. There appear to be especially modest effects for conditions involving a provocation and for conditions involving no nonaggressive response option. Note that in this regard the results from the teacher–learner paradigm show an apparent reversal of the results from the competitive reaction time paradigm. Provocation in the competitive reaction time studies (exclusively shock) was associated with larger effects; provocation (shock threat and verbal) in the teacher–learner studies was associated with smaller effects. Similarly the competitive reaction time studies obtained relatively large effects while inherently allowing no nonaggressive response option, while the teacher–learner studies found their largest effects when a nonaggressive response option was allowed.

Unfortunately, not enough studies have been conducted for most of the paradigm variations to give stable results regarding their different effects. It does appear, however, that the alcohol effect is rather dependent on the particular procedures used in the research paradigm. Moreover, the paradigms seem to yield inconsistent results with regard to the effects associated with provocation and nonaggressive response options. It also appears that the alcohol effect is rather modest in many of the variations.

One other procedural aspect of these research paradigms was examined.

Table III. Effect Size Statistics for the Teacher–Learner Studies by Major Procedural Variation[a]

Procedural variation	Weighted mean ES	95% CI[b]	Q_w[c]	n
Dependent variable				
Shock intensity	0.40	0.13, 0.67	8.1	7
Number of shocks	0.63	0.28, 0.99	5.5	4
Shock duration	0.67	0.33, 1.02	1.6	4
Shock composite	0.51	0.12, 0.90	3.7	4
Noise composite	0.13	−0.44, 0.69	NA	1
Threat/provocation				
No provocation	0.45	0.22, 0.69	14.9	12
Verbal provocation	0.05	−0.52, 0.62	0.003	2
Shock provocation	−0.24	−1.12, 0.64	NA	1
Nonaggressive response options				
Yes	0.50	0.27, 0.74	9.3	9
No	0.08	−0.36, 0.52	1.0	3

[a]Four studies had an effect size for shock intensity, number, and duration.
[b]CI, Confidence interval (see Hedges and Olkin[32]).
[c]Q_w, Homogeneity within groups (*$p < 0.05$, reject homogeneity). The between-groups Q statistic for the dependent variable was not computed, because the inclusion of the same subjects in multiple distributions violates the assumptions of this statistic. The between-groups Q for provocation indicates that there is homogeneity between groups ($Q_B(2) = 3.6$, $p > 0.05$). The between-groups Q for nonaggressive response options indicates that there is homogeneity between groups ($Q_B(1) = 2.7$, $p > 0.05$).

Table IV. Effect Size Statistics for Each Paradigm by Whether Experimenter Blinding Was Used

Breakout by paradigm	Mean ES	Weighted 95% CI[a]	$Q_w{}^b$	n
Competitive reaction time				
Blinding	−0.30	−1.10, 0.51	NA	1
No blinding	0.64	0.51, 0.76	25.1	28
Teacher–learner				
Blinding	0.11	−0.39, 0.60	1.0	2
No blinding	0.47	0.24, 0.70	10.2	10

[a]CI, Confidence interval (see Hedges and Olkin[32]).
[b]Q_w, Homogeneity within groups (*$p < 0.05$, reject homogeneity). The between-groups Q statistic for the competitive reaction time breakout indicates that there is heterogeneity between groups ($Q_B(1) = 5.1$, $p < 0.05$). The between-groups Q statistic for the teacher–learner breakout indicates that there is homogeneity between groups ($Q_B(1) = 1.8$, $p > 0.05$).

For this, we determined whether the researcher administering the instructions and collecting the data from the subjects was kept unaware ("blind") of the experimental condition in which the subject had been placed. In these studies experimenter blinding is important to control for subtle clues the experimenter may give the subject on how the researcher expects the subject to behave, e.g., unintentionally cuing subjects in the alcohol condition to behave aggressively.[37] Only three of the studies reported that they employed this methodological control (Table IV). In each research paradigm, the few studies using experimenter blinding found notably smaller effects than those studies that did not employ that control. Unfortunately, too few studies applied experimenter blinding to reach a firm conclusion here, but these results leave open the possibility that the apparent alcohol effect is little more than subjects' response to experimenter demand.

Last, we looked at an issue that has received a fair amount of attention in this research literature: alcohol expectancy effects. If the subjects in a placebo control condition believe they have consumed alcohol, then the difference between the alcohol and placebo condition should reflect the pharmacological effects of alcohol, rather than subjects' expectations about the effects of alcohol. The balanced placebo design was developed to explore directly the influence of expectations on aggressive responding. This design is a 2 × 2 factorial with four conditions: (1) alcohol (expect alcohol, receive alcohol); (2) placebo (expect alcohol, receive tonic); (3) control (expect tonic, receive tonic); and (4) antiplacebo (expect tonic, receive alcohol). This design yields a main effect for alcohol, a main effect for expectancy, and an interaction between alcohol and expectancy. Of the six studies that used the balanced placebo design, five were teacher–learner studies and one was a competitive reaction time study. Table V shows the mean effect sizes for the various effects separately for each paradigm.

Table V. Effect Size Statistics for the Balanced Placebo Design
by Experimental Paradigm

Factor	Mean ES	Weighted 95% CI[a]	Q_w^{b}	n
Alcohol factor				
Competitive reaction time	0.24	−0.33, 0.81	NA	1
Teacher–learner	0.11	−0.12, 0.33	14.0*	5
Expectancy factor				
Competitive reaction time	0.61	0.03, 1.18	NA	1
Teacher–learner	0.19	−0.03, 0.42	12.7*	5
Interaction				
Competitive reaction time	−0.54	−1.12, 0.03	NA	1
Teacher–learner	0.06	−0.17, 0.28	6.4	5

[a]CI, Confidence interval (see Hedges and Olkin[32]).
[b]Q_w, Homogeneity within groups (*$p < 0.05$, reject homogeneity). A positive interaction effect size indicates that high expectancy increases the effect of alcohol.

As Table V reveals, the careful attempt of the balanced placebo designs to separate out the effect of actually consuming alcohol from the effect of thinking you have consumed alcohol produces some rather surprising results. First, the main effect of alcohol is notably small in both the research paradigms. Also, the main effect for alcohol is smaller than the main effect for expectancy for all the studies. In other words, the largest part of the subjects' increased aggressiveness in these studies appears to come from their belief that they have drunk alcohol, not from the actual effects of the alcohol itself.

2.2.4. Individual Differences. A particularly noteworthy feature of the results of these experimental studies is the great variability reported for subjects in their aggressive responses.[10,12] Individual difference variables have been relatively neglected in this area of research, however, so little can be said about the characteristics of those who respond more or less aggressively under the influence of alcohol. Some modest evidence suggests that predisposition for aggressiveness and related constructs such as unfriendliness, quickness to anger, and trait hostility may differentiate those who respond more aggressively to alcohol,[10] but other plausible factors have not yet been investigated.

2.2.5. Conclusions about Experimental Studies of Humans. The research paradigms used in experimental studies of the effects of alcohol consumption on aggression in human subjects are not good simulations of socially important forms of drinking and violence. Moreover, the subjects used in those studies (mostly male college students) and, to a lesser extent, the alcohol doses administered do not well represent the populations and doses of greatest practical interest. Nonetheless, this body of research does demonstrate that there are some laboratory manipulations of alcohol consumption that exert causal influence on the aggressiveness of responses that subjects believe are directed at another person. Unfortunately, the role of alcohol per se in those manipulations remains uncertain. The measured effects of alcohol on aggressive responses in these studies appear to vary inconsistently according to the research paradigm and its particular conditions, diminish when controls for experimenter demand are employed, and largely reflect the belief that alcohol has been consumed rather than actual consumption. It will remain difficult to interpret the results of this body of research until further studies are done to better disentangle the actual effects of alcohol from the variety of other aspects of subjects' perceptions and expectations, experimenter demand characteristics, and procedural particulars with which alcohol consumption is packaged in these studies.

3. Correlational Approaches

The research that most directly investigates the association between alcohol use and socially significant forms of violence is necessarily observational or correlational. Such studies yield information about the covariation of real-world alcohol use and violent behavior and generally represent one of two different levels of analysis. Most frequent are studies with individual persons as the unit of analysis which investigate the relationship between the varying degrees of alcohol use by those individuals and the extent of their violent behavior, e.g., a survey of convicted felons about whether they drank prior to committing their offenses. A second and less common type of study investigates the alcohol–violence relationship at a more macro-level. These macro or community studies examine aggregate statistics for regions or political jurisdictions to investigate covariation between alcohol availability and violence over time or across different communities. Such a study might, for instance, examine whether communities with higher levels of alcohol consumption experienced more criminal violence than communities with lower levels.

Correlation, of course, is not necessarily causality, and the major challenge faced by correlational studies investigating the causal role of alcohol in violence is to rule out alternate explanations of any alcohol–violence correlation. Since experimental control of the factors related to such alternate explanations is not possible in these studies, statistical controls must be employed instead. The essence of statistical control is to introduce one or more control variables into the analysis of the relationship between the alcohol independent variable and the violence dependent variable. The results are then examined for indications that the control variable is sufficient to explain all or part of the zero-order alcohol–violence relationship.

The difficulty with statistical controls, other than technical issues associated with using them correctly, is that they can only be employed with specific, measured variables. Thus, a researcher must be able to identify in advance every variable that might account for an alcohol–violence correlation in his or her sample and research circumstances, measure it, and use it in subsequent data analysis. The practical impossibility of such a complete specification means that, even in the most favorable circumstances, there is some uncertainty about whether all of the relevant control variables have been included. And with that comes uncertainty about whether any remaining alcohol–violence correlation represents a causal relationship or merely the confounding influence of some unmeasured control variable.

We turn now to an examination of the major bodies of correlational research and consider how they have handled the difficult problem of assessing the causal influence of alcohol on violence.

3.1. Individual-Level Studies

The typical individual-level correlational study is a survey of a sample of persons who are questioned with regard to their alcohol consumption (acute or chronic) and their involvement in violent behavior. The data relevant to the alcohol–violence relationship yielded by these studies come in the form of one or more alcohol variables on which alcohol use varies across the individuals in the sample and one or more violence variables whose values similarly vary across the sample. The key correlation in these studies reflects whether those individuals with higher alcohol use also exhibit higher levels of violent behavior and, conversely, whether those with lower alcohol use exhibit lower levels of violence.

The reason we spell out the nature of the correlation at issue in these studies so specifically is that there is widespread reporting of simple, but potentially misleading, co-occurrence statistics. Various studies show, for instance, that alcohol was consumed by large proportions of violent offenders prior to their offense.[4] Statistics about the co-occurrence of alcohol use and violent behavior, however, do not constitute a correlation between alcohol and violence, since there is no variation on the violence variable—everyone in the sample is violent. Put another way, there is no base rate information in these statistics about the level of alcohol use among those comparable persons who were not violent. Thus, if alcohol is involved in 50% of violent offenses, we do not know if it is involved in 10, 50, or 90% of nonviolent offenses by otherwise comparable persons. Without the "other half" of the data required for a correlation, no strength of association information can be garnered from co-occurrence statistics.

To summarize the relatively large body of individual-level correlational studies on alcohol and violence, we draw once again on our own meta-analytic work (details in ref. 26). Studies were deemed eligible for this meta-analysis if (1) the report contained quantitative information on the relationship between a measure of alcohol use and a measure of violent or aggressive behavior by individual persons; (2) the quantitative information was sufficient to compute a product-moment correlation between alcohol use and violence, or multivariate results were presented with statistics describing the alcohol–violence relationship; and (3) the report was in English. A combination of bibliographic search strategies was applied to locate and retrieve as many eligible published and unpublished reports as possible. Using these strategies, 870 documents were located and screened, yielding 129 studies that met the eligibility criteria for the meta-analysis (a bibliography of these studies is available from the authors).

Over 100 items of information were coded for each eligible study. This included effect size information for all alcohol–violence relationships reported in a study (coded as correlation coefficients), all control variable information, and various particulars of the study methods, measurements, samples, settings, and so forth. The coded studies were divided into those that dealt with acute alcohol use (consumption associated with a single incident) or chronic alcohol use (a pattern of consumption over some time period). A second distinction was made between studies involving criminal violence and those involving domestic violence. For our purposes, domestic violence was any type of interpersonal violence against family members within the home, such as spouse or child abuse. Criminal violence was any other type of interpersonal violence potentially chargeable as a crime, whether defined in a legal context (e.g., murder, assault, rape) or not (e.g., fighting).

Table VI describes the general characteristics of this body of studies, categorized according to the type of alcohol–violence relationship. The vast majority were conducted in the United States, most since 1980. Criminal and general population samples characterized the criminal-chronic studies, while most of the criminal-acute studies sampled criminal populations and most of the domestic-chronic studies involved clinical populations (e.g., marital or family therapy clients, alcohol or drug treatment clients). The type of sampling varied considerably and relatively few studies were based on true probability samples. Face-to-face interviews were the most common method of obtaining data; few studies used physical measures, e.g., blood alcohol concentration. Note that only two studies reported on the relationship between acute alcohol use and domestic violence.

Effect sizes were coded as correlation coefficients for all the alcohol–violence relationships reported in each study; some studies contributed only a single effect size, while others contributed several. We randomly selected one of the relevant correlations within each study for each category of relationship using the most general and differentiated measures of alcohol consumption and violence and the largest aggregate sample in each study. The characteristics of each respective alcohol and violence measure represented in these summary effect sizes are reported in Table VII. Alcohol measures chiefly represented level of alcohol use or distinctions regarding problem drinking (e.g., alcoholism). This information was most often collected using questionnaires or standardized instruments for self-report by respondents. Most of the violence measures reflected physical violence. Like the alcohol measures,

Table VI. Study Descriptors for Correlational Studies by Type of Relationship[a,b]

	Criminal		Domestic	
	Chronic	Acute	Chronic	Acute
Variable	n (%)	n (%)	n (%)	n (%)
Country/region				
United States	53 (77)	18 (58)	33 (89)	2 (100)
Scandinavia	1 (1)	2 (7)	1 (3)	
United Kingdom	8 (12)	5 (16)		
Canada	5 (7)	4 (13)		
Other/cannot tell	2 (3)	2 (7)	3 (8)	
Publication year				
1950–69	3 (4)	2 (7)		
1970–74	6 (9)			1 (50)
1975–79	7 (10)	5 (16)	1 (3)	
1980–84	19 (28)	7 (23)	8 (22)	1 (50)
1985–89	20 (29)	10 (32)	15 (41)	
1990–94	14 (20)	7 (23)	13 (35)	
Population sampled				
Criminal	29 (42)	24 (77)	2 (5)	2 (100)
Criminal/psychiatric	8 (12)	4 (13)	1 (3)	
Clinical/treatment	8 (12)	2 (7)	25 (68)	
General population	24 (35)	1 (3)	9 (24)	
Sample size				
25–49	3 (4)		5 (14)	
50–99	10 (15)	2 (7)	9 (24)	
100–199	7 (10)	6 (19)	11 (30)	
200–499	17 (25)	7 (23)	7 (19)	1 (50)
500–999	14 (20)	6 (19)	2 (5)	
1,000–9,999	15 (22)	5 (16)	3 (8)	1 (50)
10,000+	3 (4)	4 (13)		
Cannot tell		1 (3)		
Type of sampling				
Convenience	17 (25)	5 (16)	24 (65)	1 (50)
Probability	22 (32)	9 (29)	5 (14)	
Quasi-probability	5 (7)	2 (7)		
Census	3 (4)	3 (10)	1 (3)	
Time-sampling	18 (26)	12 (39)	5 (14)	1 (50)
Cannot tell	4 (6)		2 (5)	
Survey method				
Face-to-face	35 (51)	14 (45)	21 (57)	1 (50)
Self-report	23 (33)	6 (19)	14 (38)	
Physical measure	1 (1)	1 (3)		
Archival	8 (12)	9 (29)	2 (5)	1 (50)
Cannot tell	2 (3)	1 (3)		
Total	69	31	37	2

[a]Percentages may not sum to 100 due to rounding error.
[b]Nine studies provided both criminal-chronic and criminal-acute relationships and one study provided both a domestic-chronic and criminal-chronic relationship. There were 129 studies and 139 relationships.

these were most often questionnaires or standardized instruments for self-report, but a large proportion came from archives or official records (e.g., arrest data).

We turn now to an overview of the results of this meta-analysis bearing on the nature and magnitude of the relationship between alcohol use and violence. The first line of evidence is the summary correlations between alcohol and violence reported in these studies. We averaged these across studies, using a sample-size weighting procedure,[31,38] to yield the figures in Table VIII. The largest overall mean correlation was in the domestic-chronic category with a weighted mean of 0.22; the criminal-chronic category had a weighted mean of 0.15, while the criminal-acute category had a mean of 0.10. (There were too few studies to calculate a mean for the domestic-acute category.) The confidence intervals indicated that all of these mean correlations were statistically significant. Taken together, these findings show that greater alcohol use among individuals is clearly associated with higher levels of violent behavior.

It is useful to appraise the magnitude of the alcohol–violence correlations in Table VIII using terms more intuitively meaningful than the product-moment correlation. Assuming a normal distribution on the violence measure, a transformation analogous to that called U3 by Cohen[39] provides one useful approach. To apply this transformation, we imagine dividing the aggregate sample represented in each mean effect size into two groups: those with no or low alcohol use and those with moderate to high use. If we imagine further that 10% of the low-use group demonstrates violent behavior, we can then ask what proportion of the high-use group must show violent behavior to yield a relationship of the same magnitude as the mean correlations in Table VIII.

For the largest weighted mean correlation in Table VIII, $r = .22$ for the relationship between chronic alcohol use and domestic violence, the corresponding proportion is .20. That is, if 10% of the low-alcohol-use group engaged in domestic violence, then 20% of the high-alcohol-use group would also. Thus, the correlation of .22 can be understood as representing a 10-percentage-point increase in the proportion of the sample engaged in violence, or a doubling of the likelihood of violence. Similarly, the criminal-chronic mean correlation of .15 is equivalent to a contrast between a low-alcohol-use group that is 10% violent and a high-use group that is 17% violent. The mean correlation of .10 for the criminal-acute relationship, in turn, corresponds to a contrast between 10% and 14% violent.

We see, therefore, that even though the correlations in Table VIII are numerically modest, the relationships they index are not trivial. What we do not know is how much of the difference in violence between high- and low-alcohol users is really due to the causal influence of alcohol and how much is due to other factors confounded with alcohol use. We must, therefore, find ways to probe more deeply into the nature of the correlations in Table VIII before drawing any conclusions about the causal influence of alcohol consumption on violence. Of particular importance in this regard is the evidence

Table VII. Alcohol and Violence Measure Descriptors for Correlational Studies by Type of Relationship[a]

	Criminal		Domestic	
	Chronic	Acute	Chronic	Acute
Measure descriptor	n (%)	n (%)	n (%)	n (%)
Alcohol Measure				
Construct (Chronic)				
Binge use	2 (3)		1 (3)	
Problem use	8 (12)		7 (19)	
Alcoholism	25 (36)		18 (49)	
Level of use	25 (36)		9 (24)	
Role impairment	2 (3)			
Other	4 (6)		2 (5)	
Construct (acute)				
Presence/absence	3 (4)	21 (68)		2 (100)
Level of consumption		8 (26)		
Impairment		1 (3)		
BAC		1 (3)		
Type of alcohol measure				
Psychometric	11 (16)		20 (54)	
Published questionnaire	8 (12)	1 (3)	3 (8)	
Researcher questionnaire	36 (52)	18 (58)	9 (24)	
Judgment rating	4 (6)	1 (3)	3 (8)	1 (50)
Archival	8 (12)	10 (32)	2 (5)	1 (50)
Other/cannot tell	2 (3)	1 (3)		
Source for measure				
Self-report	55 (80)	17 (55)	24 (65)	
Archive	11 (16)	11 (36)	4 (11)	1 (50)
Observation		1 (3)	7 (19)	1 (50)
Instrument/BAC	1 (1)	1 (3)		
Other	2 (3)	1 (3)	2 (5)	
Violence measure				
Type of violence				
Physical	36 (52)	9 (29)	32 (87)	2 (100)
Sexual	4 (6)	5 (16)		
Physical and sexual	26 (38)	16 (52)	4 (11)	
Other/cannot tell	3 (4)	1 (3)	1 (3)	
Type of violence measure				
Psychometric	5 (7)	1 (3)	11 (30)	
Published questionnaire	6 (9)		5 (14)	
Researcher questionnaire	28 (41)	2 (7)	9 (24)	
Judgment rating	1 (1)		4 (11)	1 (50)
Archival	27 (39)	27 (87)	6 (16)	1 (50)
Other/cannot tell	2 (3)	1 (3)	2 (5)	
Source for measure				
Self-report	39 (57)	2 (7)	18 (49)	
Archive	28 (41)	28 (90)	7 (19)	1 (50)
Observation		1 (3)	9 (24)	1 (50)
Other	2 (3)		3 (8)	
Totals	69	31	37	2

[a]Percentages may not sum to 100 due to rounding error.

in Table VIII from the standard deviation and homogeneity test. These results show that there was substantial variability across the effect size estimates aggregated into these mean values. This indicates that different studies are yielding effect size estimates that differ from one another much more than would be expected on the basis of sampling error alone. We turn, then, to consideration of some of the differences among studies that may be associated with the variability in results.

As noted earlier, the main problem in interpreting the mean correlations between alcohol use and violent behavior is the uncertainty about the confounding influence of other variables. In observational studies, groups differing in level of alcohol use (or level of violence) are likely to also differ on any of a number of other relevant variables. The research literature in this area provides limited discussion of the types of variables that are most likely to be confounded in the alcohol–violence correlation. While there are many variables that might be candidates, we chose to focus on three rather fundamental categories of variables that are known to be empirically associated with either alcohol use or violent behavior, which represent conditions temporally prior to the violent behavior of interest and which plausibly play a rather direct role in any differences among persons who drink more or less or who are more or less violent. These three categories of variables are (1) stable sociodemographic characteristics that differentiate persons likely to be more or less involved in alcohol and violence, (2) major risk factors for violence that precede and may also influence alcohol use, and (c) use of other drugs along with alcohol that could independently affect the probability of subsequent violent behavior.

The types of statistical control procedures that may be employed for such confounding variables include simple ones like sample restrictions (e.g., restricting the study sample only to males), matching (e.g., matching persons who had or had not committed violent crimes on age and gender), cross-tabulations (e.g., a cross-tabulation between violence and alcohol use by gen-

Table VIII. Individual Level Cross-Sectional Correlations (r) by Type of Relationship[a]

Type of relationship	Weighted mean r	95% CI[b]	Unweighted SD	$Q_w{}^c$	n
Criminal-chronic	0.15	0.14, 0.16	0.15	470.7*	67
Criminal-acute	0.10	0.08, 0.12	0.16	231.5*	29
Domestic-chronic	0.22	0.20, 0.24	0.16	132.7*	34

[a]Only one correlation (r) per study was used for each type of relationship. When multiple correlations were available, one was randomly selected. Each correlation was weighted by its sample size less three (see Hedges and Olkin[32]), with samples sizes greater than 1000 recoded to 1000. An alcohol–violence correlation could not be obtained for two criminal-chronic and criminal-acute studies, three domestic-chronic studies, and one domestic-acute study. These studies had multivariate analyses of the alcohol–violence relationship and were analyzed separately.
[b]CI, Confidence interval (see Hedges and Olkin[32]).
[c]Q_w = Homogeneity within groups (*$p < 0.05$, reject homogeneity).

der), and more sophisticated multivariate techniques (e.g., multiple regression with alcohol use and one or more control variables entered to predict violent behavior). If confounding variables play a role in the alcohol–violence correlation, we would expect different results from studies attempting more control of such variables than those with less control.

The frequency with which the simple control procedures of sample restriction, matching, and cross-tabulations were applied in the studies represented in our meta-analysis can be seen in Table IX. The most common types of controls were restrictions of the study sample by gender (typically restricted to males), age, criminal status (i.e., restriction to convicted offenders, delinquent youth, etc.), or socioeconomic status (usually restricted to low ranges). Matching and cross-tabulation were seldom used. Beyond sample restrictions on the few variables indicated, there was little use of simple control techniques in this literature.

If there is little application of simple control procedures in the research reporting on the empirical correlation between alcohol use and violence, we might hope to find a correspondingly greater use of sophisticated multivariate analysis to produce more highly controlled estimates. Our search strategy, however, turned up only 14 criminal and 13 domestic violence studies that conducted a multivariate analysis with alcohol use and one or more other

Table IX. Frequency of Simple Control Procedures for Confounding Variables across All Relationship Types ($n = 139$)

Variable category	Sample restriction n (%)	Matching between groups n (%)	Cross-tabulation n (%)
Demographics			
Gender	81 (58)	2 (1)	7 (5)
Age	38 (27)	5 (4)	5 (4)
Ethnicity	9 (7)	2 (1)	1 (1)
SES	31 (22)	2 (1)	0 (0)
Income level	1 (1)	0 (0)	0 (0)
Education level	12 (9)	1 (1)	0 (0)
Employment status	2 (1)	0 (0)	1 (1)
Marital status	17 (12)	0 (0)	0 (0)
Risk factors for violence			
Prior violence measure	7 (5)	0 (0)	0 (0)
Criminal status	64 (46)	0 (0)	0 (0)
Long-term recidivism	0 (0)	0 (0)	0 (0)
Observed violence in home	0 (0)	0 (0)	0 (0)
Abused as child	0 (0)	0 (0)	0 (0)
Childhood aggression	0 (0)	0 (0)	0 (0)
Alcohol and drug use			
Prior alcohol use	8 (6)	0 (0)	0 (0)
Prior drug use	5 (4)	0 (0)	0 (0)

Table X. Variables Used in the Criminal Violence Studies That Reported Multivariate Analyses of the Alcohol–Violence Relationship

Study	Violence measure	Alcohol measure	Sociodemographics	Risk for violence	Drug use	Other
Abram[59]	Number of arrests for violence	Alcoholism	2[a]	1[a]	1[a]	0
Collins and Schlenger[60]	Violent versus nonviolent offense	Drinking at time of offense[b]	4[a]	2	0	0
Dermen and George[61]	Frequency of physical aggression	Drinking habits[b]	1[a]	2[a]	0	2[a]
Fagan et al[62]	Self-reported violent delinquency	Drinking problems	0	2[a]	1[a]	8[a]
Fagan et al[63]	Domestic versus domestic and extradomestic violence	Drinking while abusive[c]	4[c]	6[c]	1[c]	0
Harrison and Gfroerer[64]	Violence in past year; Booked for violence in past year	Intoxicated monthly in past year[b]	8	0	2[a]	0
Kandel et al[65]	Fighting	Months used alcohol	0	2[a]	1	9[a]
Lawton[66]	Current violence score	Current alcohol score; Past alcohol score	2[a]	1	0	0
Mann et al[67]	Total self-reported violence	Alcohol use	2[a]	4[a]	1	6[a]
Mason[68]	Number of commitments and convictions for violent offenses	Alcohol influence during most recent crime[b]	0	3[a]	1[a]	1[a]
Miller and Welte[69]	Person versus property offending	Alcohol prior to crime[b]	6[a]	0	0	0
Rathus et al[70]	Fist fighting; Carrying a weapon; Fighting w/weapon; Using force to steal	MacAndrew Alcoholism Scale[b]	1[a]	0	0	0
Simonds and Kashani[71]	Person versus property offending	Alcohol use[b]	0	0	12[a]	0
Watts and Wright[72]	Violent delinquency	Alcohol use[b]	0	0	3[c]	0

[a] At least one variable was a significant predictor of the violence measure.
[b] Significant independent predictor of violence measure.
[c] Significance levels not reported.

variables as predictors and a measure of violence as the dependent (or predicted) variable. Table X summarizes the studies reporting a multivariate analysis in a criminal violence study, while Table XI summarizes the studies reporting a multivariate analysis in a domestic violence study. The categories and numbers of control variables that were reported in the multivariate analyses are noted, along with an indication of whether or not any were found to be statistically significant.

Two general findings can be observed in the collection of criminal violence studies summarized in Table X. First, virtually all the studies found control variables that accounted for a significant portion of the variance in violence independent of the effect of alcohol. Thus, while persons with higher levels of alcohol consumption tended to display more violence than those with lower levels, there were other differences between the groups that were also capable of accounting for the differences in violence, e.g., differences in drug use or prior history of violence. Second, in 6 of these 14 studies, no statistically significant relationship between alcohol and violence remained after the influence of the control variables was removed. In contrast to the criminal studies, the domestic violence studies showed a different pattern of findings (Table XI). While many control variables did exercise a significant influence, 11 of the 13 studies that reported significance levels indicated that a significant alcohol–violence relationship remained after controlling for other variables.

Perhaps the most important finding shown in Tables X and XI, other than how few studies there are that make sophisticated attempts to produce a controlled estimate of the alcohol–violence relationship, is the limited selection of control variables in those studies. Only 5 of the 27 studies included control variables from all three of the categories shown (sociodemographics, risk for violence, and drug use). These findings, therefore, confirm the observations made by recent reviewers regarding the shortage of sophisticated information about the nature of the statistical association between alcohol use and violent behavior (e.g., refs. 4, 7, 40).

In order to integrate the limited information on the results of application of the simple control techniques shown in Table IX and the few sophisticated multivariate control studies shown in Tables X and XI, we created a crude index of the amount of control of potentially confounding factors in each study. In brief, we assigned points to each study for various degrees and types of control and added those into a scale ranging from −2 to +7, with higher values representing more control. We then correlated this "statistical control index" with the study level effect sizes. The weighted correlation of this index with effect size across all the studies was −0.20. This shows a tendency for more controlled studies to yield smaller alcohol–violence correlations. Since the application of well-chosen statistical controls is so infrequent in this literature, however, and such a limited range of control variables is used, this result gives only a weak indication of what effects adequate control might have. Nonetheless, it gives additional empirical confirmation to

Table XI. Variables Used in the Domestic Violence Studies That Reported Multivariate Analyses of the Alcohol–Violence Relationship

Study	Violence measure	Alcohol measure	Sociodemographics	Risk for violence	Drug use	Other
Berk et al[73]	Severity of female's injuries	Male drinking; Male's number of alcohol priors[b]	5[a]	4	0	5
Chapa et al[74]	Mexican-American child abusers versus nonabusers; Anglo-American child abusers versus nonabusers	Use of alcohol[b]	4[a]	0	2[a]	8[a]
Coleman et al[75]	Conjugal violence versus no conjugal violence	Husband's alcohol use[b]	1[a]	2[a]	1[a]	0
Diacatou et al[76]	Father's aggressiveness toward family members	Alcohol consumption[b]	2[a]	0	0	0
Fagan et al[63]	Most serious past injury to domestic partner	Drinking while abusive[c]	4[c]	8[c]	1[c]	0
Famularo et al[77]	Physical child maltreatment; Sexual child maltreatment	Alcohol abuse[b]	0	0	3[a]	0
Hofeller[78]	Severity of abuse; Violent versus nonviolent marriages	Man's use of alcohol[b]	2[a]	3[a]	0	2
Julian and McKenry[79]	Physically abusive vs. nonabusive male partner	Alcohol usage[b]	1[a]	0	0	3[a]
Kantor and Straus[80]	Minor spouse abuse; Severe spouse abuse	Husband drunk[b]	3[a]	0	2[a]	1[a]
Leonard and Blane[81]	Marital aggression	Alcohol Dependence Scale score[b]	0	1	0	1
Leonard and Senchak[82]	Premarital aggression	Husband heavy drinking[b]	4[a]	1[a]	0	3[a]
Miller et al[83]	Parolee-to-spouse violence	Alcohol problems	3	0	2	2
Wahl[84]	Physically abusive vs. nonabusive husbands	Alcohol abuse (SMAST)[b]	0	2[a]	0	2[a]

[a] At least one variable was a significant predictor of the violence measure.
[b] Significant independent predictor of violence measure.
[c] Significance levels not reported.

the view that confounding variables inflate the alcohol–violence correlation in this literature and contribute to the heterogeneity of results reported.

3.1.1. Individual Differences.

One consequence of the limited application of control variables to analysis of correlational alcohol–violence data is a shortage of information on possible moderating variables that might differentiate persons or circumstances in which alcohol and violence were more closely linked. Much current theorizing emphasizes the idea that alcohol may have a causal influence on violence only for certain persons and/or situations.[5,7,41] The correlational research reviewed above, however, pays scant attention to exploring individual differences or situational variables that may moderate the alcohol–violence relationship. A full accounting of the variables that might differentiate the persons or situations in which alcohol has significant causal effects would have to include various neurobiological,[12,24,42] psychological,[10] psychiatric,[1,11,12,43,44] and environmental[5,7] factors, among others.

Combing through our meta-analysis data revealed little investigation of such variables, and hence little that could be gleaned on the issue of moderating variables. Juvenile samples (under age 21) produced larger alcohol–violence correlations than older samples. We also found a slight tendency for criminal–psychiatric samples (e.g., psychiatric wards of criminal institutions) to show larger alcohol–violence correlations than general criminal samples (e.g., incarcerated felons) or clinical treatment samples (e.g., alcoholism patients). Alcohol dose is so poorly described in these studies that no statements about dose relationships can be made. Relatively few studies even examined the difference between alcohol consumption and alcohol abuse in characterizing the alcohol–violence relationship. Other variables may well differentiate cases of closer alcohol–violence association but are not sufficiently well represented in this body of studies to be examined.

3.1.2. Conclusions about Individual-Level Correlational Studies.

The most general finding of this research synthesis of individual-level correlational studies is that the overall statistical association between alcohol use and violent behavior is positive and of nontrivial magnitude for the relationships of chronic alcohol use to criminal behavior, acute alcohol use to criminal behavior, and chronic alcohol use to domestic violence, with the latter showing the largest correlation. Insufficient studies are available to appraise the correlation for acute alcohol use and domestic violence.

A number of potentially important confounding variables, of course, could easily inflate the zero-order alcohol–violence correlation. Our attempts to explore the role of such variables was disappointing. The available research base simply does not include sufficient control variables to permit analysis. Even the relatively small number of studies that used multivariate techniques often represented a very limited selection of control variables. Nonetheless, their results tended to show a reduction in the alcohol–violence relationship when other variables were controlled. Our own index of the overall amount of control in each study showed a similar trend. In the few studies that did apply sophisticated multivariate techniques to statistically control selected confounding variables, the alcohol–violence correlation was generally reduced, and, in some cases, went to zero. In particular, it appears that well-selected controls may reduce the residual correlation between alcohol and criminal violence, although less reduction is apparent in the domestic violence relationship.

There is thus good reason to believe that the positive correlation between alcohol and violent behavior represents a relationship that is confounded by other variables (e.g., sociodemographics, other drug use, early exposure to violence, and other variables such as personality disorders). There is also reason to believe that this correlation varies by situational context and by level of alcohol consumption. Unfortunately, the body of literature reporting alcohol–violence correlations does not adequately examine these potentially confounding and moderating variables in a systematic fashion. Despite the large volume of studies, there is little in this body of research that bears convincingly on the issue of causality in the alcohol–violence relationship.

3.2. Macro-Level Studies

Macro-level or aggregate level studies examine the covariation between alcohol consumption or availability and violence at the level of some social grouping (community, city, state, etc.). Such studies make no attempt to link the violent behavior they examine specifically to the individuals whose consumption of alcohol is implicit in their aggregate measures of alcohol availability. Thus, they do not directly address the question of whether individuals who consume alcohol are more likely to behave violently. It is reasonable to assume, however, that if alcohol has such effects on drinkers, the results will show up in the aggregate statistics used in macro-level studies. In addition, of course, such studies will reflect any other pathways by which alcohol might lead to violence, e.g., by making potential victims more vulnerable, by attracting potential offenders or victims to high risk environments, and the like.

As with individual-level correlational studies, the challenge to this form of research is to rule out the possibility that any alcohol–violence covariation is spurious or is the result of some other factor that independently affects both alcohol consumption and violence levels in a given region (e.g., poverty rates).

While a number of studies of the macro-level relationship between alcohol availability and traffic fatalities, health indicators, and the like have been conducted,[45,46] relatively few studies have examined violent behavior as a dependent variable. These generally use one of three approaches: investigating covariation between alcohol availability and rates of violence (1) across groups, (2) across time (time series), or (3) some combination of group and time comparisons.

3.2.1. Across-Group Studies. Study of covariation across social groupings is illustrated by one of the two studies reported in Parker and Rebhun.[47] Parker analyzed data from 256 US cities on alcohol availability (number of liquor stores per 1000 people), homicide rates from the Uniform Crime Reports (UCR), and a set of control variables selected on theoretical grounds and including median age, median family income, racial composition, population density, region, migration, a social bonds composite, female labor force participation, percent of children with one parent, and volume of retail eating and drinking establishments. Separate models were fit for data from 1960, 1970, and 1980, with the 1970 and 1980 models including homicide rates from the 10-year prior data, so that the dependent variable reflected change in homicide rates over that period.

Parker found a significant relationship between alcohol availability and homicide in the 1970 model, representing a period of rapid increase in alcohol consumption, but not in the 1960 or 1980 model. He also showed that many other factors in his models were related to levels and changes in homicide rates, particularly racial composition and female labor force participation (a proxy for amount of work and leisure time spent out of home).

In another illustrative study examining covariation across groups, Dull and Giacopassi[48] analyzed 37 cities in Tennessee with local alcohol control ordinances of varying strength. They found positive correlations between the permissiveness of the ordinances and the rates for each of the UCR index crimes, but these reached statistical significance only in the cases of rape and robbery (notably, not murder and assault). Moreover, when control variables were introduced for poverty, age, racial composition, and the like, no significant relationships remained between the alcohol variable and any of the UCR index crimes. Similar results appeared for a second alcohol variable: number of alcohol outlets per 100,000 population.

Similarly mixed results have emerged in studies analyzing covariation at the state level for US data. Parker[49] found that statewide alcohol consumption was related to indices of two of five types of homicide and interacted with other important predictors. Lester[50] found that suicide rates were higher in states with weaker alcohol restrictions, but that homicide rates were higher in states with the strongest alcohol restrictions. Lester,[51] using measures of alcohol availability, use, and abuse, however, found these to have no relationship to statewide homicide rates.

3.2.2. Across-Time Studies. Lenke[52] reported that time-series analyses of alcohol and violence have been around since at least 1896, when Ferri is said to have found increased violence following good wine harvests in France. In his own analyses, Lenke discovered significant covariation between annual per capita alcohol sales and rates of assault and homicide in Sweden (approx.

1921–1984), rates of assault in Finland (1950–1980) and Norway (1931–1977), and between alcohol production and assaults in France (1831–1869, 1873–1913, 1919–1958). However, significant relationships were not found between alcohol production and homicides in France (1865–1913, 1946–1982) or between per capita alcohol sales and assaults in Denmark (1950–1978). Similarly, Lester[53] reported significant covariation between annual per capita alcohol consumption and both male and female homicide rates in Australia from 1966 to 1985. When control variables for divorce rates and unemployment were included in the model, however, only the relationship for males continued to be significant.

Ensor and Godfrey[54] attempted to fit a particularly sophisticated model to the rates of six crime categories in England and Wales over the years 1960–1988. They controlled for the probability of being caught and prosecuted and for prosperity using variables chosen to reflect opportunities for crime and the opportunity cost of crime in a model designed to represent interactions between alcohol, crime levels, and the criminal justice system response to crime. Per capita alcohol consumption was found to be a significant predictor of rates of violent crime as well as rates of several types of property crimes. Alcohol consumption was also found to be a predictor of the probability of being caught for violent crimes, suggesting one way in which alcohol involvement might be overrepresented among apprehended offenders.

3.2.3. Across-Time and -Group Studies. Some macro-level studies provide a combined analysis of covariation across both social groups and time. Cook and Moore,[55,56] for instance, examined the relationship between state-level beer taxes and alcohol consumption (based on sales data) and rates of homicide, rape, robbery, and assault (from the UCR). They analyzed annual data for each of the contiguous 48 states for the years 1979–1988 using dummy variables for each state to control for unobserved, persistent state-specific determinants of crime rates. They found that variations in the beer tax were associated with alcohol consumption, which was lower when taxes were higher. Most important for present purposes, they found significant covariation between alcohol consumption and crime rates for rape, assault, and robbery, but not for murder.

Parker[41] criticized the Cook and Moore study for omitting variables such as poverty, routine activity levels, racial composition, and the like that are linked to violence rates and were themselves changing over the time period at issue. Parker and Rebhun,[47] in one of their two studies, examined the relationship of changes in state minimum age of purchase laws for alcohol with homicide rates over the period 1976–1983. Prior to this period, 29 states lowered the minimum age below 21 years and others already had lower minimum ages. By 1988, all of these states had raised the minimum age to 21 years. Parker used a pooled cross-section time series analysis on data for each of the 50 states plus the District of Columbia for each year from 1976 through 1983, using a dummy code to identify the year in which the drinking age was raised. Other variables in the model included alcohol consumption (beer sales in barrels per capita), infant mortality (as a poverty index), an index of inequality, racial composition, region, and total state population.

Parker and Rebhun[47] applied this model to six different homicide rates: "primary" when victim and offender knew each other, "nonprimary" when there was no known relationship between them, with each of these further divided according to offender age (15–18, 19–20, and 21–24). The results showed that beer consumption was positively and significantly related to all categories of homicide except primary, age 21–24 (though the coefficient for the latter was in the same direction). In addition, change in the minimum age of purchase law was significantly related to reductions in homicide for the primary, age 21–24 category, but not to the others (though these coefficients were in the same direction). Other significant variables across the models were infant mortality (poverty index), racial composition, region (South vs. other), and total state population.

3.2.4. Natural Experiments. Studies like Cook and Moore[55,56] and Parker and Rebhun,[47] in which relatively sudden events restrict the availability of alcohol, constitute a kind of natural experiment. Whereas there are many cooccurring trends in typical time series that could plausibly account for the covariation in alcohol consumption and violence (e.g., unemployment), few of these trends are likely to show sudden changes that coincide with the timing of such "external" events as new legislation or other social incidents that restrict access to alcohol. Such episodes, therefore, provide an especially good opportunity to examine the macro-level relationship between alcohol and violence.

Lenke[52] summarized an interesting group of natural experiments set in Sweden: (1) the rationing of alcohol during World War I, (2) the repeal of the general alcohol restriction system in 1955, (3) the strike at the Alcohol State Monopoly in 1963, (4) the legalization of sales of medium beer in grocery stores in 1965, (5) the legalization of sales of strong beer in grocery stores in some provinces in 1967, and (6) the discontinuation of Saturday open hours at the Alcohol Monopoly Stores in 1981. While the results were not totally consistent, Lenke summarized as follows:

> The general conclusion from the cases described . . . is that changes and variation in the availability and consumption of alcohol tend to affect crimes of violence. When availability of alcohol has been reduced or increased, the rates of violent crimes have tended to follow the same direction. (p. 103)

Similar results were found in several, but not all, analogous natural experiments in Finland and Norway (summarized in refs. 52, 55, 56).

3.2.5. Conclusions about Macro-Level Correlational Studies. The authors of many of these macro-level studies argue plausibly that their various results have important policy implications. Demonstration of covariation between alcohol availability and rates of violence and, especially, evidence that policy actions such as alcohol taxes and drinking age laws may affect violence rates are indeed provocative. For purposes of assessing the causal role of alcohol consumption in violent behavior, however, the macro-level studies available are less than conclusive. First, not all of these investigations have revealed a significant covariation between alcohol availability and rates of violence. In addition, there is uncertainty regarding the appropriate control variables to include in the models to account for other factors that may co-occur with greater or lesser levels of alcohol availability, and relatively few of the range of possibilities have been examined. Also, these studies do not distinguish between alcohol consumption per se and other co-occurring factors (such as male gatherings) that might be responsible for any effects found. Nonetheless, given the level of aggregation represented in these studies, it is notable that the alcohol–violence relationship appears with sufficient strength that it cannot be readily dismissed.

It is unfortunate that few of the macro-level studies have attempted any probing of their data to better pinpoint the particular persons or circumstances most responsible for the overall alcohol–violence relationships discovered. One exception is Lenke,[52] who included a liver cirrhosis mortality variable to distinguish rates of heavy, long-term drinking. This variable was found to be significantly related to homicide rates, but not assaults, in his Swedish time series. Lenke also cited evidence from several of the natural experiments he reviewed that indicated that heavy drinkers may have played a disproportionate role in the changes in the rates of violent crime that were recorded.

4. Overall Conclusions

Aside from the many specific conclusions drawn above regarding the research in each of the broad categories reviewed, we believe three general conclusions are warranted:

1. The research base relevant to the question of the causal role of alcohol consumption in violent behavior, despite its overall volume, is very unsatisfactory. It is permeated by problems of inadequate experimental and statistical control, questionable generalizability to socially important forms of violence, limited attention to individual differences and moderator variables, weak conceptualizations of the issue, and capricious operationalizations of the key variables. As a result, the causal issue is still cloudy and uncertain. Some of the difficulties are inherent in the nature of the issue under study, but much is remediable. The alcohol–violence relationship is not merely an academic issue, it is one with important social implications that deserves more systematic, careful, and probing attention from researchers.

2. While granting the inadequacies of available research, it is nonetheless important to recognize that none of the relevant bodies of research yield a

consistently or even predominately negative or null result on the causal question. Each provides substantial evidence of an alcohol–violence *association* that is consistent with a causal interpretation and none yet provides evidence sufficient to rule out such an interpretation. One is tempted to say that where there is this much smoke, there must be some fire. Such a conclusion would clearly be premature given the deficiencies of the empirical evidence, but the possibility highlights the importance of continued research on this issue.

3. While a causal influence of alcohol consumption on violence cannot be ruled out with present evidence, it seems apparent that there is no broad, reliable, "main effect" of alcohol on violence, analogous to the easily demonstrated and almost ubiquitous effects on motor and cognitive functioning that occur at sufficient doses. If alcohol has any causal effects on violence, they almost certainly occur only for some persons and/or some circumstances. The most important research question regarding the alcohol–violence relationship, therefore, is not one of global causal influence. Rather, it is the more focused question of what individual differences, moderator, and situational variables characterize circumstances in which alcohol might potentiate violent behavior. The greatest failure of the research reviewed in this chapter is the inadequate attention to this question and, as a consequence, the inability to address the most pressing social issues involving alcohol and violence.

ACKNOWLEDGMENT. Support for the preparation of this chapter has been provided in part by the Washington Technical Information Group, Inc. and the Dean's Fund of the Owen Graduate School of Management, Vanderbilt University. The views stated in this chapter are those of the authors and do not necessarily represent the positions of Washington Technical Information Group, Inc.

References

1. Collins JJ: Drinking and violence: An individual offender focus, in Martin SE (ed): *Alcohol and Interpersonal Violence: Fostering Multidisciplinary Perspectives* (Research Monograph No. 24). Washington, DC, National Institute on Alcohol Abuse and Alcoholism, 1993, pp 221–235.
2. Reiss AJ, Roth JA: Alcohol, other psychoactive drugs, and violence, in Reiss AJ, Roth JA (eds): *Understanding and Preventing Violence.* Washington, DC, National Academy Press, 1993, pp 182–220.
3. Miczek KA, DeBold JF, Haney M, *et al*: Alcohol, drugs of abuse, aggression, and violence, in Reiss AJ, Roth JA (eds): *Understanding and Preventing Violence:* vol 3, *Social Influences.* Washington, DC, National Academy Press, 1994, pp 377–570.
4. Roizen J: Issues in the epidemiology of alcohol and violence, in Martin SE (ed): *Alcohol and Interpersonal Violence: Fostering Multidisciplinary Perspectives* (Research Monograph No. 24). Washington, DC, National Institute on Alcohol Abuse and Alcoholism, 1993, pp 3–36.
5. Fagan J: Set and setting revisited: Influences of alcohol and illicit drugs on the social context of violent events, in Martin SE (ed): *Alcohol and Interpersonal Violence: Fostering Multidisciplinary Perspectives* (Research Monograph No. 24). Washington, DC, National Institute on Alcohol Abuse and Alcoholism, 1993, pp 161–192.
6. Greenberg SW: Alcohol and crime: A methodological critique of the literature, in Collins JJ (ed): *Drinking and Crime.* New York, Guilford Press, 1981, pp 70–109.

7. Pernanen K: Alcohol-related violence: Conceptual models and methodological issues, in Martin SE (ed): *Alcohol and Interpersonal Violence: Fostering Multidisciplinary Perspectives* (Research Monograph No. 24). Washington, DC, National Institute on Alcohol Abuse and Alcoholism, 1993, pp 37–70.

8. Walfish S, Blount WR: Alcohol and crime: Issues and directions for future research. Special Issue: Alcohol and the criminal justice system. *Criminal Justice Behav* 16:370–386, 1989.

9. Mackie JL: Causes and conditions. *Am Philosoph Q* 2:245–264, 1965.

10. Lang AR: Alcohol-related violence: Psychological perspectives, in Martin SE (ed): *Alcohol and Interpersonal Violence: Fostering Multidisciplinary Perspectives* (Research Monograph No. 24). Washington, DC, National Institute on Alcohol Abuse and Alcoholism, 1993, pp 121–147.

11. Fagan J: Intoxication and aggression, in Tonry M, Wilson JJ (eds): *Drugs and Crime*. Chicago, University of Chicago Press, 1990, pp 241–320.

12. Lang AR, Sibrel PA: Psychological perspectives on alcohol consumption and interpersonal aggression: The potential role of individual differences in alcohol-related criminal violence. *Criminal Justice Behav* 16:299–324, 1989.

13. Pernanen K: Research approaches in the study of alcohol-related violence. *Alcohol Health Res World* 17:101–107, 1993.

14. Collins JJ: Suggested explanatory frameworks to clarify the alcohol use/violence relationship. *Contemp Drug Problems* 15:107–121, 1988.

15. Collins JJ: Alcohol and interpersonal violence: Less than meets the eye, in Weiner NA, Wolfgang, ME (eds): *Pathways to Criminal Violence*. Newbury Park, CA, Sage, 1989, pp 49–57.

16. Evans CM: Alcohol and violence: Problems relating to methodology, statistics, and causation, in Brain PF (ed): *Alcohol and Aggression*. Dover, NH, Croom Helm, 1986, pp 138–160.

17. McCord J: Considerations of causes in alcohol-related violence, in Martin SE (ed): *Alcohol and Interpersonal Violence: Fostering Multidisciplinary Perspectives* (Research Monograph No. 24). Washington, DC, National Institute on Alcohol Abuse and Alcoholism, 1993, pp 71–79.

18. Grayham K, La Rocque L, Yetman R, et al: Aggression and bar-room environments. *J Stud Alcohol* 41:277–292, 1980.

19. Berry MS, Smoothy R: A critical evaluation of claimed relationships between alcohol intake and aggression in infra-human animals, in Brain PF (ed): *Alcohol and Aggression*. Dover, NH, Croom Helm, 1986, pp 84–137.

20. Brain PF, Miras RL, Berry MS: Diversity of animal models of aggression: Their impact on the putative alcohol/aggression link. *J Stud Alcohol Suppl* 11:140–145, 1993.

21. Berry MS, Brain PF: Neurophysiological and endocrinological consequences of alcohol, in Brain PF (ed): *Alcohol and Aggression*. Dover, NH, Croom Helm, 1986, pp 19–54.

22. Miczek KA, Weerts EM, DeBold JF: Alcohol, benzodiazepine–GABA$_A$ receptor coomplex and aggression: Ethological analysis of individual differences in rodents and primates. *J Stud Alcohol Suppl* 11:170–179, 1993.

23. Miczek KA, DeBold JF, VanErp AM: Neuropharmacological characteristics of individual differences in alcohol effects on aggression in rodents and primates. *Behav Pharmacol* 5:407–421, 1994.

24. Miczek KA, Weerts EM, DeBold JF: Alcohol, aggression, and violence, in Martin SE (ed): *Alcohol and Interpersonal Violence: Fostering Multidisciplinary Perspectives* (Research Monograph No. 24). Washington, DC, National Institute on Alcohol Abuse and Alcoholism, 1993, pp 83–119.

25. Peterson JT, Pohorecky LA: Effect of chronic ethanol administration on intermale aggression in rats. *Aggress Behav* 15:201–215, 1989.

26. Cohen MA, Lipsey MW, Wilson DB, Derzon JH: *The Role of Alcohol Consumption in Violent Behavior: Final Report*. Research Report, VIPPS, Vanderbilt University, 1994.

27. Bushman BJ: Human aggression while under the influence of alcohol and other drugs: An integrative research review. *Curr Direct Psychol Sci* 2:148–152, 1993.

28. Bushman BJ, Cooper HM: Effects of alcohol on human aggression: An integrative research review. *Psychol Bull* 107:341–354, 1990.

29. Hull JG, Bond CF: Social and behavioral consequences of alcohol consumption and expectancy: A meta-analysis. *Psychol Bull* 99:347–360, 1986.
30. Steele CM, Southwick L: Alcohol and social behavior I: The psychology of drunken excess. *J Pers Soc Psychol* 48:18–34, 1985.
31. Cooper H, Hedges LV (eds): *The Handbook of Research Synthesis.* New York, Russell Sage Foundation, 1994.
32. Hedges LV, Olkin I: *Statistical Methods for Meta-Analysis.* New York, Academic Press, 1985.
33. Gustafson R: Threat as a determinant of alcohol-related aggression. *Psychol Rep* 58:287–297, 1986.
34. Heermans HW: The effect of alcohol, arousal and aggressive cues on human physical aggression in males (doctoral dissertation, Rutgers University, 1980). *Dissertation Abstracts International* 41:3630B (University Microfilms No. 81-05011), 1981.
35. Taylor SP: Experimental investigation of alcohol-induced aggression in humans. *Alcohol Health Res World* 17:108–112, 1993.
36. Gustafson R: Alcohol and aggression. *J Offender Rehab* 21:41–80, 1994.
37. Rosenthal R, Rosnow RL (eds): *Artifact in Behavioral Research.* New York, Academic Press, 1969.
38. Hunter JE, Schmidt FL: *Methods of Meta-Analysis: Correcting Error and Bias in Research Findings.* Newbury Park, CA, Sage, 1990.
39. Cohen J: *Statistical Power Analysis for the Behavioral Sciences,* 2nd ed. Hillsdale, NJ, Lawrence Erlbaum, 1988.
40. Fagan J: Interactions among drugs, alcohol, and violence. *Health Aff* 12:65–79, 1993.
41. Parker RN: Rational choice and pooled cross-section time series: Theoretical and methodological pathways to new understanding of the alcohol/violence relationship, in Martin SE (ed): *Alcohol and Interpersonal Violence: Fostering Multidisciplinary Perspectives* (Research Monograph No. 24). Washington, DC, National Institute on Alcohol Abuse and Alcoholism, 1993, pp 213–220.
42. Roth JA: *Psychoactive Substances and Violence.* Washington, DC, National Institute of Justice (NCJ Document Reproduction Service No. 145534), 1994.
43. Murdoch D, Pihl RO, Ross D: Alcohol and crimes of violence: Present issues. *Int J Addict* 25:1065–1081, 1990.
44. Swanson JW: Mental disorder, substance abuse, and community violence: An epidemiological approach, in Monahan J, Steadman HJ (eds): *Violence and Mental Disorder: Developments in Risk Assessment.* Chicago, University of Chicago Press, 1994, pp 101–136.
45. Grossman M, Chaloupka FJ, Saffer H, Laixuthai A: Effects of alcohol price policy on youth: A summary of economic research. *J Res Adolesc* 4:347–364, 1994.
46. Gruenewald PJ, Millar MS, Treno AJ: Alcohol availability and the ecology of drinking behavior. *Alcohol Health Res World* 17:39–45, 1993.
47. Parker RN, Rebhun L: *Alcohol and Homicide: A Deadly Combination of Two American Traditions.* Albany, NY, State University of New York Press, 1995.
48. Dull RT, Giacopassi DJ: The impact of local alcohol ordinances on official crime rates: The case of Tennessee. *Justice Q* 4:311–323, 1987.
49. Parker RN: Bringing "booze" back in: The relationship between alcohol and homicide. *J Res Crime Delinq* 32:3–38, 1995.
50. Lester D: Restricting the availability of alcohol and rates of personal violence (suicide and homicide). *Drug Alcohol Depend* 31:215–217, 1993.
51. Lester D: Alcohol availability, alcoholism, and suicide and homicide. *Am J Drug Alcohol Abuse* 21:147–150, 1995.
52. Lenke L: *Alcohol and Criminal Violence: Time Series Analysis in a Comparative Perspective.* Stockholm, Almqvist & Wiksell, 1990.
53. Lester D: Alcohol consumption and rates of personal violence in Australia. *Drug Alcohol Depend* 31:15–17, 1992.
54. Ensor T, Godfrey C: Modelling the interactions between alcohol, crime and the criminal justice system. *Addiction* 88:477–487, 1993.

55. Cook PJ, Moore MJ: Economic perspectives on reducing alcohol-related violence, in Martin SE (ed): *Alcohol and Interpersonal Violence: Fostering Multidisciplinary Perspectives* (Research Monograph No. 24). Washington, DC, National Institute on Alcohol Abuse and Alcoholism, 1993, pp 193–212.

56. Cook PJ, Moore MJ: Violence reduction through restrictions on alcohol availability. *Alcohol Health Res World* 17:151–156, 1993.

57. Zeichner A, Pihl RO: Effects of alcohol and behavior contingencies on human aggression. *Journal of Abnormal Psychology* 88:153–160, 1979.

58. Zeichner A, Pihl RO: The effects of alcohol and instigator intent on human aggression. *J Stud Alcohol* 41:265–276, 1980.

59. Abram KM: Effect of co-occurring disorders on criminal careers: Interaction of antisocial personality, alcoholism, and drug disorders. *International Journal of Law & Psychiatry* 12:133–148, 1989.

60. Collins JJ, Schlenger WE: Acute and chronic effects of alcohol use on violence. *Journal of Studies on Alcohol* 49:516–521, 1988.

61. Dermen KH, George WH: Alcohol expectancy and the relationship between drinking and physical aggression. *Journal of Psychology* 123:153–161, 1989.

62. Fagan J, Piper ES, Moore M: Violent delinquents and urban youth. *Criminology* 23:439–466, 1986.

63. Fagan J, Hansen KV, Stewart DK: Violent men or violent husbands? Background factors and situational correlates of violence toward intimates and strangers. In Finkelhor D, Gelles RJ, Hotaling GT, Straus MA (eds): *The dark side of families: Current family violence research.* Beverly Hills, CA, Sage, 1983, p 49–68.

64. Harrison L, Gfroerer J: The interaction of drug use and criminal behavior: Results from the National Household Survey on Drug Abuse. *Crime and Delinquency* 38:422–433, 1986.

65. Kandel D, Simcha-Fagan R, Davies M: Risk factors for delinquency and illicit drug use from adolescence to young adulthood. *Journal of Drug Issues* 16:67–90, 1986.

66. Lawton EG: Persons who injure others: A study of criminally assaultive behavior in Philadelphia (Doctoral dissertation, Temple University). *Dissertation Abstracts International* 40:3549A, 1979.

67. Mann F, Friedman CJ, Friedman AS: Characteristics of self-reported violent offenders versus court identified violent offenders. *International Journal of Criminology and Penology* 4:69–87, 1976.

68. Mason FH: Demographic and psychological test variables associated with prior offender violence (Doctoral dissertation, University of South Carolina). *Dissertation Abstracts International* 47:1790B, 1986.

69. Miller BA, Welte JW: Comparison of incarcerated offenders according to use of alcohol and/or drugs prior to offense. *Criminal Justice and Behavior* 13:366–392, 1986.

70. Rathus SA, Fox JA, Ortins JB: The MacAndrew Scale as a measure of substance abuse and delinquency among adolescents. *Journal of Clinical Psychology* 36:579–583, 1980.

71. Simonds JF, Kashani J: Specific drug use and violence among delinquent boys. *American Journal of Drug & Alcohol Abuse* 7:305–322, 1979.

72. Watts WD, Wright LS: The drug use-violent delinquency link among adolescent Mexican-Americans. In De La Rosa M, Lambert EY, Gropper B (eds): *Drugs and violence: Causes, correlates, and consequences* (Research Monograph Series No. 103). Washington, DC, National Institute on Drug Abuse, 1990, pp 136–159.

73. Berk RA, Berk SF, Loseke DR, Rauma D: Mutual combat and other family violence myths. In Finkelhor D, Gelles RJ, Hotaling GT, Straus MA (Eds): *The dark side of families: Current family violence research.* Beverly Hills, CA, Sage, 1983, pp 197–212.

74. Chapa D, Smith PL, Rendon FV, Valdez R, Yost M, Cripps T: The relationship between child abuse and neglect and substance abuse in a predominantly Mexican-American population. In Lauderdale ML, Anderson RN, Cramer SE (eds): *Child abuse and neglect: Issues on innovation and implementation* (Proceedings of the Second Annual National Conference on Child Abuse

and Neglect, vol. 1). Washington, DC, National Center on Child Abuse and Neglect, 1978, pp 116–125.

75. Coleman KH, Weinman ML, Hsi BP: Factors affecting conjugal violence. *Journal of Psychology* 105:197–202, 1980.

76. Diacatou A, Mamalakis G, Kafatos A, Vlahonikolis J, Bolonaki I: Alcohol, tobacco, and father's aggressive behavior in relation to socioeconomic variables in Cretan low versus medium income families. *International Journal of the Addictions* 28:293–304, 1993.

77. Famularo R, Kinscherff R, Fenton T: Parental substance abuse and the nature of child maltreatment. *Child Abuse & Neglect* 16:475–483, 1992.

78. Hofeller KH: *Social, psychological, and situational factors in wife abuse.* Palo Alto, CA, R&E Research Associates, 1982.

79. Julian TW, McKenry PC: Mediators of male violence toward female intimates. *Journal of Family Violence* 8:39–56, 1993.

80. Kantor GK, Straus MA: Substance abuse as a precipitant of wife abuse victimizations. *American Journal of Drug & Alcohol Abuse* 15:173–189, 1989.

81. Leonard KE, Blane HT: Alcohol and marital aggression in a national sample of young men. *Journal of Interpersonal Violence* 7:19–30, 1992.

82. Leonard KE, Senchak M: Alcohol and premarital aggression among newlywed couples. *Journal of Studies on Alcohol* 54(Suppl. No. 11):96–108, 1993.

83. Miller BA, Nochajski TH, Leonard KE, Blane HT, Gondoli DM, Bowers PM: Spousal violence and alcohol/drug problems among parolees and their spouses. *Women and Criminal Justice* 1:55–72, 1990.

84. Wahl JA: Self-esteem, attitudes toward women, alcohol abuse and history of family violence in spouse battering males (Doctoral dissertation, Oklahoma State University, 1987). *Dissertation Abstracts International* 19:1961B, 1988.

12

Alcohol and Cocaine Interactions and Aggressive Behaviors

M. Elena Denison, Alfonso Paredes, and Jenia Bober Booth

Abstract. This chapter presents (1) a review of several studies on the relationship between violent/aggressive behavior and the use of cocaine and/or the use of alcohol; and (2) findings from our study of cocaine-dependent men, illustrating deviant and violent behavior before and during cocaine addiction careers. As had been found in previous research, use of alcohol and cocaine seemed to increase the likelihood of the cocaine users in our sample engaging in deviant or violent behaviors. The extent of deviant or violent behavior, in our sample, during periods of cocaine use, periods of cocaine–alcohol use, periods of alcohol use only, and periods of abstinence for both alcohol and cocaine are discussed. Changes in the nature of the deviant or violent behaviors prior to and after the onset of cocaine addiction are also described.

1. Introduction

Deviant behaviors including crime occur at high rates among cocaine users, and violence has long been associated with alcohol use; a better understanding of the behavioral correlates of combined and individual use of alcohol and cocaine is needed. In this chapter, we outline findings from several studies that examined the relationships between violent/aggressive behavior and the use of alcohol and other drugs. This brief overview is followed by a presentation of results derived from our study of cocaine-dependent men to illustrate

M. Elena Denison, Alfonso Paredes, and Jenia Bober Booth • Laboratory for the Study of Addictions and UCLA Drug Abuse Research Center, West Los Angeles Veterans Administration, Los Angeles, California 90073.

Recent Developments in Alcoholism, Volume 13: Alcoholism and Violence, edited by Marc Galanter. Plenum Press, New York, 1997.

some of the relationships between violence and use of cocaine and alcohol that manifest in cocaine-dependent individuals.

2. Alcohol and Violence

Epidemiological investigations have found a close association between human violence and alcohol use. Drinking of alcohol has been implicated in domestic violence, homicide, sexual assaults, suicide, and traffic accidents. Aggressive behavior also seems to be concomitant with the use of drugs such as cocaine.[1] The mechanisms responsible for these putative interactions are complex. Alcohol and other drugs may act through pharmacological mechanisms that inhibit neurobehavioral systems, which under normal circumstances control aggression. For instance, impulsive alcoholic violent offenders appear to have a deficit of brain serotonin metabolism and low concentration of 5-hydroxyindoleacetic acid in the cerebrospinal fluid.[2] At a behavioral level, alcohol may facilitate aggressive behavior by reducing awareness and by impairing intellectual functioning and risk assessments.[3]

Individuals with certain personality features are more likely to exhibit heightened destructiveness when under the influence of alcohol. For example, adolescents with conduct disorder, in general [as defined in the Diagnostic and Statistical Manual of Mental Disorders, 4th edition (DSM-IV)], consume more alcohol and show increased violence; even those without conduct disorder demonstrate heightened aggression if they are alcohol users.[4]

The mechanisms involved in the alcohol–violence relationship have been investigated experimentally.[5,6] These investigators suggest that alcohol effects are selective and do not disrupt higher cognitive functions "across the board." When exposed to low levels of personal threat, inebriated individuals allocated equal attention to all situational cues, in which case alcohol did not impair the salience of relevant information; subjects did not respond aggressively. Under high levels of personal threat, however, alcohol-intoxicated individuals give greater attention to negative or personally threatening cues and display more intense aggression. Under placebo conditions, subjects do not respond differentially to positive and negative personal information and, in general, showed low levels of aggression.[5] However, Zeichner et al.[6] also found that the consumption of alcohol had a dampening effect on the physiological effects of situational stress (decrease in heart rate and systolic blood pressure). Thus, aggressive reactions of hostile men under the influence of alcohol may be due more to the psychological effects than the physiological effects of alcohol.

3. Cocaine and Violence

Violence may be strongly influenced by social circumstances. In the case of cocaine, individuals moved by their compulsion to use the drug may engage in violence to obtain resources for drugs. In addition, violence is often an outcome of territorial struggles of groups or individuals who try to control procurement and distribution of illicit drugs.[7] In some urban centers where cocaine use prevalence is high, firearm aggression, including homicide, increased as much as 123% within a 5-year period.[1] The association of cocaine and violent crime as an economically motivated event was suggested by the authors, but this relationship was apparently found to be weak. Notably, violence observed among cocaine users was not a function of compulsive drug seeking, while concomitant use of alcohol was related to more than 70% of the severe violent events observed in these individuals.

The nature of the interactions between alcohol and violence and between cocaine and violence differs in important ways. It has been suggested that the alcohol relationship to violence appears to be primarily pharmacological, while the cocaine relationship to violence is primarily "social–systemic."[8] In another study,[9] daily use of crack cocaine and the frequency of illicit criminal activities aimed to obtain a supply of the drug appeared to be interrelated, but dose–response effects were difficult to demonstrate. The level of violence is only partially related to the method of cocaine administration. Violence of greater intensity tended to be associated with freebase crack cocaine smoking or intravenous administration in contrast with intranasal use, but this relationship was not strong. Violent actions requiring sustained activity such as rape, burglary, and armed robbery are not found to be related to the route of administration of the drug used by the perpetrator.[10]

Drug-related activities such as trafficking are accompanied by increased mortality and account for one third to one half of homicide-related deaths among cocaine users.[11] The authors found that drug dealing was associated with other high-risk behaviors, including nonfatal violence and the probability of being incarcerated. The authors stated that, in spite of commonly held beliefs, drug involvement and weapon carrying are not normative among youth. Young men involved in drug dealing or weapon carrying are a subset of individuals more likely to participate in a wide variety of delinquent (or high-risk) behaviors. The subjects in Stanton and Galbraith's[11] study show poor school performance and greater likelihood of receiving disciplinary dismissals. These men usually reported poor relationships with their parents. The perception of drug dealing as the only viable income-generating option has also been found to predict drug trafficking and violence.[12] In contrast, among inner-city male adolescents in New York City, type of crime including violent crime was not related to drug dealing but to the use of alcohol and drugs (such as marijuana and intranasal heroin). Again, though, these youths reported multiple arrests, truancy, and psychological distress, gave history of sexual molestation as children, substance-abusing parents, and cocaine/crack-using friends.[13]

There is no progressive linear relationship between level of drug use and gun possession, number of guns owned, and routinely carrying guns as indicator of proneness to violence. On the other hand, individuals who sold drugs were more likely to own guns.[14] In Los Angeles, gang-related homicides have increased from 18 to 43% within the past 15 years, but drug trafficking has not been a major factor in this increase.[15-17] The authors suggest that in crack cocaine abusers, crack distribution and drug selling may not create violent or actively criminal individuals, but rather individuals who have a tendency toward violence may be attracted to this activity. However, in the Belenko et al.[18] study, crack addicts had significant increases in the seriousness of the crimes committed, as well as increases in the rate of criminal activity after initiation of crack use. In addition to this sample of crack addicts being more likely to be violent overall, the increase for violent arrests was more than three times larger than the increase among powder cocaine defendants. Belenko et al.[18] found a general acceleration in arrests following initiation into crack cocaine use, suggesting that the diversity and frequency of involvement in nondrug crime implies a more generalized pattern of deviance underlying their behavior.

Several investigators have identified two major subpopulations of cocaine-dependent individuals. One group uses mainly cocaine, while the other group (of approximately equal size in some samples) uses cocaine and alcohol severely enough to meet the diagnosis of abuse for both substances.[19,20]

Users of alcohol and cocaine and users of cocaine only differ along important dimensions. In a nationally representative sample of young adults, combined alcohol–cocaine abusers demonstrated higher levels of drug use in the prior 30 days and lifetime drug use, higher levels of delinquent activity, and higher rates of unemployment and marital instability. A decreasing order of problem severity was observed: cocaine and alcohol abusers had the most severe problems, followed by cocaine-only users and by alcohol-only abusers. Interestingly, however, the study noted that joint alcohol–cocaine abusers reported the lowest high school dropout rate and scored the highest on measures of verbal intelligence.[21]

4. Drug Use Status and Deviant Behaviors: Results of the Study

Our research offered an opportunity to conduct a preliminary exploration of some of these interactions. We had available a large database from subjects who participated in our investigations of the progression of cocaine dependence and factors that influence clinical and treatment outcomes. With these data, we initiated a preliminary examination of the behaviors of our subjects during periods of different states of drugs use: cocaine only, alcohol only, cocaine and alcohol in combination, and abstinence from both alcohol and cocaine. Retrospective data covering the period lasting an average of approximately 10 years from the first use of cocaine to admission to treatment for cocaine dependence were used in this investigation.

4.1. Characteristics of the Study Sample

The subjects selected for this study were veterans of military service who requested treatment for cocaine dependence at the Veterans Affairs Medical

Center in West Los Angeles. The population served by this hospital includes very few women; thus, the 320 subjects selected for this study were all men. Participants met DSM-III-R criteria for cocaine dependence and signed a consent form approved by the Human Subjects Subcommittee from the medical center. An additional 63 men from this population who were asked to participate in the research projects refused. The main reasons given were lack of interest, skepticism about assurance of confidentiality, unwillingness or apprehension about disclosing previous drug or criminal history, and lack of time to devote to research interview.

In regard to the sociodemographic characteristics of this group, at admission, 30% of the men were married, 25% divorced, 17% separated, 1% were widowed, and 27% had never married. Eighty-six percent completed at least twelfth grade. Twenty-eight percent did not work during the 4 weeks preceding entry into treatment, 58% worked full time, and the remaining 14% worked less than full time. Eighty-two percent had been incarcerated at some time in their lives and 13% were on probation at the time of the intake

Table I. Demographic Characteristics
of the Sample ($n = 320$)

Characteristic	Percent
Age at interview, years[a]	
21–30	21.8
31–40	56.7
>41	21.5
Ethnicity	
African American	67.5
Caucasian	24.7
Hispanic	6.9
Other	0.9
Education, years	
<12	13.8
12	42.8
>12	43.4
Main occupation at admission	
Skilled	15.0
Semiskilled	33.7
Unskilled	9.1
Unemployed	42.2
Ever incarcerated (self-report)	81.8
Age at first arrest, years[b]	
<18	12.3
18–24	39.4
>24	48.3
Ever married	72.2
Homeless at admission	10.9

[a]Mean age at interview = 35.5 years old (SD = 6.4).
[b]Mean age at first incarceration = 25.1 years old (SD = 7.2).

interview. Additional information on the sociodemographic profile of the sample is given in Table I.

4.2. Data Collection Methodology

Specially designed schedules were used at project intake to collect sociodemographic data, developmental history, and information on social functioning and history of treatment. Another instrument, the Natural History Interview, was the main source of detailed longitudinal information concerning the patterns of cocaine and other drug use. This instrument is an adaptation of a schedule developed by Nurco and his colleagues[22] and is described in detail elsewhere.[19] Briefly, a schematic time chart is prepared during a face-to-face interview showing important events in the subject's life, such as initiation of drug use, treatment episodes, dates of marriage, childbirths, geographic moves, arrests, and periods of incarceration and legal supervision. These events are used as time-anchoring points in order to facilitate the review of significant aspects of the subject's drug and social history as autobiographical sequences and have been shown to provide one method that subjects can use to organize and anchor their memories of personal events.[23]

With the assistance of the subject, a trained interviewer establishes the date of first cocaine use, records in on a time chart, and proceeds chronologically from 12 months before first use to the time of the interview. Data are collected on the use of cocaine, alcohol and other drugs, health status, drug treatment experience, employment, family adjustment, criminal behavior, and other social adjustment variables for the initial time period. Subsequent time periods are demarcated by changes in levels of cocaine use and significant life events such as any social adjustment variable, subject's drug treatment, or legal status. The interviewer proceeds to review each successive time segment, repeating the systematic process of collecting retrospective longitudinal data covering long periods of the addicts history.[24] From these raw data, monthly rates of various categories of behaviors become available within each segment. These rates are invariant or constant within each time period with respect to items such as type of drug use, methods of administration, work tenure, interpersonal relationships, drug dealing, and property crimes.

4.3. Cocaine Use Patterns

The mean age of the subjects at the time of first cocaine use was 24 years old (SD = 7 years). The main reasons given for initiating use were to satisfy curiosity (65%), to get a "good high" (8%), peer acceptance (7%), friends were using (7%), to enhance sexual pleasure or to procure sex partners (3%), and to relieve depression (3%). Subjects often gave more than one reason for initiating cocaine use.

In most cases a friend or acquaintance was instrumental in introducing the person to cocaine use (76%); in 12% of the cases a parent, sibling, or other relative played a role in the initiation; for 8%, either a dealer, a prostitute, or other person; and for 4%, a girlfriend or wife influenced first cocaine use. The first supply of cocaine was obtained free by 84% of the respondents and 16% reported purchasing the drug. Forty-two percent of the subjects reported that they were not high on any other drug when they first used cocaine, though 26% of them reported they were high on alcohol the first time they used cocaine, 22% were high on marijuana, and 10% were high on other drugs.

The favored route of administration at first cocaine use (FCU) was intranasal (75%). Less-preferred routes were smoking crack (11%), smoking cocaine as primo (marijuana cigarettes spiked with cocaine) or rails (tobacco cigarettes with cocaine) (both totaling 5%), intravenous (5%), and freebasing (4%).

The average time span from FCU to treatment entry (TE) for the group was 10 years (standard deviation = 6 years). The proportion of users using cocaine intranasally decreased from 75% at initiation of the cocaine use career to 7% at the time of TE and admission to the research program. On the other hand, crack use increased from 11% at initiation to 64% at the time of TE.

4.4. Other Drug Use

Table II shows the average drug histories for this group for cocaine, heroin, marijuana, downers, amphetamines, and other drugs. All subjects

Table II. Drug History: Cocaine, Heroin, Other Opiates, Marijuana, Downers, and Amphetamines (n = 319)

Drug group	Percent ever used	Age first used	Percent used regularly	Age first used regularly
Cocaine	100%	24 ± 7	99%	29 ± 7
Cocaine (intravenous)	25%	27 ± 7	18%	29 ± 7
Heroin (intravenous)	23%	23 ± 7	11%	23 ± 7
Speedball (cocaine and heroin, intravenous)	12%	28 ± 6	6%	28 ± 7
Other opiates (morphine, opium, codeine, Demerol, Percodan, etc.)	42%	22 ± 6	17%	24 ± 6
Marijuana or hashish	98%	16 ± 4	81%	18 ± 4
Downers (reds, rainbows, Quaaludes, etc)	56%	20 ± 5	21%	19 ± 5
Amphetamines (tablets or pills)/uppers (whites, Dexedrine, Ritalin, Preludin)	67%	20 ± 5	31%	21 ± 5
Hallucinogens (LSD, mescaline, peyote)	65%	20 ± 5	21%	19 ± 4
Tranquilizers (Valium, Librium, Miltown, etc.)	35%	24 ± 7	8%	26 ± 8
PCP (angel dust)	63%	23 ± 7	16%	23 ± 6
Synthetic drugs/designer drugs (Fentanyl or synthetic H)	6%	28 ± 7	1%	38 ± 1
Glue, spray cans, gasoline, etc.	25%	14 ± 3	7%	13 ± 3

had used cocaine and the majority were using crack at TE, but only 25% of them had ever used cocaine intravenously and only 18% had ever done so regularly.

While 25% of the subjects had used cocaine intravenously and 23% had used heroin intravenously, only 12% had ever "speedballed" (injected cocaine and heroin) and only 6% used this combination intravenously on a regular basis.

The majority of the subjects had tried marijuana (98%). Of the 81% who used marijuana regularly, the average age they started regular use was 18 years old (SD = 4). Sixty-seven percent of the subjects had used amphetamines and uppers, 31% had used them regularly. On average, these subjects started using amphetamines regularly (average age = 21 years old, SD = 5) before they started regular cocaine use. Fifty-six percent of the subjects had used downers and 21% had used them regularly. On average, these subjects also started regular use of downers (average age = 19, SD = 5) before they started regular cocaine use. Over more than 60% of the subjects had tried hallucinogens and PCP, but less than one fourth had ever used these drugs regularly. Less than 20% of all the subjects ever used other drugs regularly.

4.5. Use of Alcohol

Alcohol was consumed by a large proportion of the subjects. Ninety percent of the subjects reported drinking during their cocaine use careers (FCU to TE). The average age of first reported alcohol use was 14 years old (SD = 4). The majority of the subjects (76%) reported first getting drunk between the ages of 12 and 21. While 38% of the subjects reported that they used no other drug at the same time as they used cocaine, when subjects reported that they used at least one other drug at the same time that they used cocaine, 34% reported that this drug was alcohol. Thirty-seven percent of the subjects reported that they used alcohol after their cocaine use. Fourteen percent reported they used alcohol as a substitute for cocaine. However, when asked whether their alcohol use was related to their cocaine, 61% of these subjects reported that, during periods of cocaine use, there was no relation.

Thirty-six percent of sample reported that they had experienced at least one blackout from drinking, 17% had experienced "the shakes," and 3% had had delirium tremens. Thirty-six percent of these subjects reported having developed a tolerance for alcohol and 37% reported that they had drunk alcohol to relieve or avoid withdrawal symptoms. Sixty-four percent had tried, at least once, to cut down or control their alcohol use; only 36% were successful.

Alcohol also affected these subjects' lives in other manners. Thirty-two percent of the sample reported they had lost friends, missed social activities, or given up hobbies or sports because of alcohol. Thirty-eight percent reported that they continued to use alcohol despite having medical, family, financial, psychological, or other alcohol-related problems. The majority of the subjects (74%) reported they drove while drunk and 32% had been arrested for driving under the influence of alcohol.

4.6. Socially Disruptive or Deviant Behavior during Adolescence

Table III shows the number of subjects who engaged in socially disruptive or deviant behavior before the age of 18, their average ages when they first and last engaged in these activities, the frequency in which these subjects engaged in these behaviors, and the time frame of their participating in these activities in reference to their primary (cocaine) addiction. Note that many of these variables have large standard deviations (sometimes larger than the mean), illustrating the higher variability within the sample (see Table III).

These subjects engaged, in at least once before they were 18 years old, in the following activities: getting suspended and/or expelled from school (56%); going to school drunk and/or high (50%); and running away from home (33%). Deviant behaviors include: threatening an adult before age 18 (25%) and actually hitting an adult before the age of 18 (18%). Thirteen of these subjects had stolen from school and 11% had damaged school property.

Ninety-seven percent of all the subjects who had been suspended/expelled from school at least once had done so prior to their cocaine addiction. Only 2% had had this happen to them after their cocaine addiction had started and only 1% reported having this happen both before and after their cocaine addiction.

Before the age of 18, as many as 86% of the subjects who had gone to school drunk and/or high had done so prior to their cocaine addiction. Six percent had gone to school drunk/high only after their cocaine addiction had started, while 8% of these subjects had gone to school this way both before and after the commencement of their cocaine addiction. The first time these subjects ever went to school drunk/high they were, on average, 16 years old (SD = 3). Their average age the last time they went to school this way was 18 (SD = 4). Forty-five of the subjects who had gone to school drunk/high reported that they had done so too many times to remember how often, while five of the subjects estimated they had gone to school this way at least 1000 times. The other subjects who got drunk and/or high at school reported having done so an average of 52 times. Even so, the variability of the number of times these subjects went to school drunk/high was quite large (SD = 108), with the minimum number of reported times being one time but the maximum being an estimate of 500 times.

Most of the subjects who had threatened (95%) or had hit an adult (95%) had done so prior to the beginning of their cocaine addiction. The first time these subjects ever threatened an adult they were, on average, 15 years old (SD = 2). They were also, on average, 15 years old (SD = 2) the first time they ever hit an adult. The last time they threatened to hit an adult they were, on average, 16 years old (SD = 4), which was also the last time they reported they had hit an adult when they were under 18 years old. Four subjects reported

Table III. Criminal Activity in Cocaine Addicts before the Age of 18

Criminal activity prior to the age of 18: whether arrested or not	Percentage who ever engaged in this activity	Of the subjects who had engaged in this criminal activity — Average age when first engaged in this activity	SD	Of the subjects who had engaged in this criminal activity — Average age last time engaged in this activity	SD	Of the subjects who had engaged in this criminal activity — Number of subjects who reported they had engaged in the activity so many times they couldn't remember how often	Number of subjects who reported they had engaged in the activity 1,000 times or more	Of all the other subjects who knew or approximated how often they engaged in this criminal activity — Number of times ever done	SD	Percentage of the subjects who had engaged in this criminal activity — Before cocaine addiction (%)	After cocaine addiction (%)	Both before and after cocaine addiction (%)
Expelled/suspended from school	56%	14	3	15	3	2	0	2	3	97	2	1
Drunk/high in school	50%	16	3	18	4	45	5	52	108	86	6	8
Ran away	33%	12	3	13	3	1	0	2	3	97	0	0[a]
Threatened an adult (before the age of 18)	25%	15	2	16	4	4	0	5	9	95	1	4
Hit an adult (before the age of 18)	18%	15	2	16	4	1	0	4	8	95	2	2[a]
Stolen from school	13%	14	3	17	5	1	1	6	17	91	2	7
Damage school property	11%	13	3	14	3	1	0	2	2	97	0	3

[a]Subject(s) did not know if engaged in activity before or after cocaine addiction, or both.

they had threatened an adult so many times they could not remember how often. Yet, on average, the other subjects who had threatened an adult had done so five times (SD = 9). One subject reported that he had hit an adult so many times he could not remember how many. Still, most of the subjects who had hit an adult while they were under the age of 18 reported that, on average, they had done so four times, though the variability of their answers was a high (SD = 8), with a minimum number of times being one and the maximum being 50 times.

The majority of subjects who had stolen from (91%) school or damaged school property (97%) had done so prior to their cocaine addiction. The average age when subjects first stole from school was 14 years old (SD = 3). Their average age when they first damaged school property was even younger, 13 years old (SD = 3). While they did stop damaging school property at an earlier age, 14 years old (SD = 3), the last time these subjects ever stole from school they were, on average, 17 years old (SD = 5).

4.7. Social Deviance and Violence during Adulthood

A considerable amount of socially deviant behavior was reported by these subjects in adulthood. Table IV shows the percentage of subjects who reported engaging in criminal or unlawful activities, their average age when they first and last committed these acts, the number of times they engaged in these behaviors, and the percentage of subjects who reported having engaged in the behaviors either prior to, during, or before and during their cocaine addiction (see Table IV).

The most frequently reported unlawful activity these subjects engaged in was driving while under the influence of alcohol and/or drugs (85%). Seventy-two percent of the subjects who reported having driven under the influence had done so both prior to and during their cocaine addiction; 15% reported having only driven under the influence before their cocaine addiction; and 13% had only engaged in this behavior after they had become addicted to cocaine.

Subjects reported that their average age when they first drove under the influence was 19 years old (SD = 5). Their average age the last time they drove drunk and/or high was 32 years old (SD = 7). One hundred thirty-seven of these subjects reported that they had engaged in this behavior so many times that they could not remember how many; 23 reported they drove under the influence over 1000 times. Of the other subjects who had driven under the influence, the average number of times they engaged in this behavior was 69 times, though the variance in responses was still extremely high (SD = 132), indicating that some of these addicts engaged in this behavior a substantial number of times.

The pattern of nonviolent deviance was pronounced in this group. Sixty-five of the subjects reported stealing from stores. However, the majority of these subjects who reported stealing (74%) had done so before the onset of

Table IV. Criminal Activity in Cocaine Addicts

Criminal activity: whether arrested or not	Percentage who ever engaged in this activity	Of the subjects who had engaged in this criminal activity				Of the subjects who had engaged in this criminal activity		Of all the other subjects who knew or approximated how often they engaged in this criminal activity		Percentage of the subjects who had engaged in this criminal activity		
		Average age when first engaged in this activity	SD	Average age last time engaged in this activity	SD	Number who engaged in the activity so many times they couldn't remember how often	Number who had engaged in the activity 1,000 times or more	Number of times ever done	SD	Before cocaine addiction (%)	After cocaine addiction (%)	Both before and after cocaine addiction (%)
Driving when drunk high	85%	19	5	32	7	137	23	69	132	15	13	72
Stolen from store[a]	65%	12	5	19	10	30	4	18	55	74	6	21
Sold drugs	64%	23	8	31	7	93	20	78	141	16	36	47[b]
Gambling	61%	18	6	32	7	94	14	69	135	20	14	66
Carried a weapon	50%	20	7	30	8	78	14	57	104	28	23	49
Carried drugs for other	47%	24	8	31	8	33	4	34	76	21	38	39[b]

Damaged other's property[a]	28%	16	6	22	9	5	0	6	10	59	11	27[b]
Beat someone severely	28%	20	7	27	7	3	0	6	10	43	12	32[b]
Threatened with a weapon	27%	23	8	28	9	9	1	7	15	34	38	27[b]
Broken into a building[a]	23%	17	6	22	9	2	0	8	21	68	14	17[b]
Broken into a car	19%	18	6	21	7	5	0	6	9	74	18	8
Stolen a car	18%	19	6	20	6	1	0	8	34	63	23	13[b]
Prostitution/pimping[a]	13%	24	6	29	7	11	4	98	176	40	33	28
Used force for profit	12%	23	8	27	8	7	0	32	93	32	39	26[b]
Shot someone[a]	11%	23	6	26	7	0	0	2	3	49	31	20
Threatened for profit	8%	22	6	27	6	3	0	39	106	22	44	30[b]
Used weapon for profit[a]	6%	23	8	29	7	2	0	18	26	15	50	20[b]
Committed forcible rape	2%	23	7	24	7	0	0	1	0.4	33	67	0

[a]Subject(s) (1 to 3 subjects only) refused to answer whether engaged in activity at all.
[b]Subject(s) did not know if engaged in activity before or after cocaine addiction, or both.

cocaine use. Sixty-one percent of the subjects also reported engaging in gambling activities. This behavior was reported most frequently to have occurred both prior to and during their cocaine addiction (66% of these subjects).

Episodes of violent behavior and acknowledgment of carrying weapons were common, being reported by about 50% of the sample. Fifty percent of subjects reported carrying guns, knives, and blunt objects. Twenty-seven percent reported threatening others with a weapon and 8% reported threatening others for profit. Serious acts of violence were frequently mentioned: for example, beating another person severely was reported by 28% of the sample, shooting someone by 11%, and forcible rape by 2%.

A significant proportion of subjects reported participation in the illicit drug supply system. Sixty-four percent reported selling drugs and 47% carried drugs for others. Sixteen percent of the subjects who had sold drugs and 21% who had carried drugs for others did so before initiation of cocaine use. These activities increased after the use of cocaine became habitual; 36% of subjects sold drugs and 38% carried drugs for others only after the onset of their cocaine addiction.

4.8. Interactions of Cocaine and Alcohol Use

Subjects reported their alcohol and cocaine use in a total of 3608 (aggregate for the sample) monthly segments of their cocaine use history (FCU to TE). In 52% of these monthly periods, subjects used both alcohol and cocaine; in 27% of the segments, they used alcohol only; in 12%, they used cocaine only; and in 9% of the monthly periods, they used neither alcohol nor cocaine.

Table V shows the number of monthly episodes for each type use and percentage of monthly periods the subjects were engaged in drug dealing or other criminal activity. There was a statistically significant relationship between whether subjects were using cocaine, alcohol, both, or neither and whether they were engaged in criminal activity ($\chi^2 = 25.196$, $df = 3$, $P < 0.001$). When subjects used cocaine and alcohol in combination or just cocaine, they were more likely to engage in criminal activity (10% of those

Table V. Alcohol and Cocaine Use by Crime and Drug Dealing

Monthly segments where patients were using:	Frequency	Percent	Percent of monthly segments engaged in criminal activity[a]	Percent of monthly segments engaged in drug dealing[a]
Both alcohol and cocaine	1880	52	10	24
Cocaine only	439	12	10	21
Alcohol only	979	27	6	15
Neither alcohol nor cocaine	310	9	3	9
Total monthly segments	3608	100	9	20

[a]Statistically significant relationship at $P < 0.001$; χ^2 test.

monthly episodes) than when they were using neither cocaine or alcohol (3%) or when they were using alcohol only (6%). Also, when subjects were using both cocaine and alcohol (24%), or when they were using cocaine but not alcohol (21%), they were more likely to engage in drug dealing than when they were abstinent from both cocaine and alcohol (9%) or just using alcohol (15%), ($\chi^2 = 63.695$, $df = 3$, $P < 0.001$). Please note that amount used was not taken into consideration for this analyses in this section.

4.9. Violence in Cocaine Addicts according to Amount of Alcohol Used

Amount of alcohol used was calculated from the number and types of alcoholic beverages subjects reported they used per week in each monthly period. The number and types of alcoholic beverages were converted into number of ounces of alcohol absolute ethanol (100% pure alcohol) for each monthly period. Thus, the amount of alcohol variable reports the average ounces of alcohol consumed per month by subjects from first cocaine use to their treatment entry. These variables were obtained for 314 subjects. Consuming 120 ounces of alcohol per month or more (or an average of 4 ounces or more per day) was considered excessive alcohol use or excessive drinking.[25] Only 20% of the subjects were classified as excessive drinkers using this method, with the highest reported average amount of alcohol consumed over their cocaine use career being 207 ounces per week. Twenty-five subjects reported they did not consume any alcohol from their first cocaine use to their treatment entry.

Table VI shows criminal activities these subjects engaged in according to their alcohol use and the percentage of those who engaged in the behavior prior to, during, or both prior to and during their cocaine addiction. There was a statistically significant relationship between alcohol use and whether subjects had ever beaten someone severely ($\chi^2 = 5.370$, $df = 1$, $P = 0.020$). Forty percent of all subjects, who reported on average having consumed more than 28 ounces of alcohol per week, reported having beaten someone severely, while only 26% of subjects, who were not classified as engaging in excessive alcohol use over their cocaine use careers, reported having beaten someone severely. However, there was no statistically significant relationship between when, in the subjects' cocaine-using careers (only before, or after, or both before and after the onset of their cocaine addiction), they primarily engaged in this behavior ($\chi^2 = 0.015$, $df = 2$, $P = 0.992$).

There was also a statistically significant relationship between alcohol use and whether subjects ever threatened someone with a weapon ($\chi^2 = 5.898$, $df = 1$, $P = 0.015$). Thirty-nine percent of subjects, who reported on average having consumed more than 28 ounces of alcohol per week, reported having threatened someone with a weapon, while only 24% of subjects, who were not classified as engaging in excessive alcohol use over their cocaine use careers, reported having done so. Again, there was no statistically significant association between alcohol use and when in the subjects' cocaine using

Table VI. Violence in Cocaine Addicts by Alcohol Use ($n = 313$)

Criminal activity: whether arrested or not	Excessive alcohol use (≥28 ounces per week)[a]	Percentage who reported ever having engaged in this activity by excessive alcohol use	Percentage of those who engaged in excessive alcohol use or not and had engaged in this activity		
			Before cocaine addiction	After cocaine addiction	Both before and after cocaine addiction
Carried a weapon	Yes	56	23	26	51
	No	48	29	23	48
Beat someone severely[b]	Yes	40	44	24	32
	No	26	43	24	33
Threatened with a weapon[b]	Yes	39	25	42	33
	No	24	38	38	24
Damaged other's property	Yes	37	45	18	36
	No	27	65	9	26
Used force for profit	Yes	15	11	78	11
	No	12	39	29	32
Shot someone	Yes	13	38	25	38
	No	11	50	35	15
Threatened for profit	Yes	6	25	50	25
	No	9	23	45	32
Used weapon for profit	Yes	6	25	75	0
	No	6	15	54	31
Committed forcible rape	Yes	2	0	100	0
	No	2	40	60	0

[a]Average ounces of alcohol consumed per week over cocaine use history (FCU to TE)
[b]Statistically significant relationship between alcohol use and whether engaged in this violent behavior at $P <$ 0.05, χ^2 test.

careers they primarily engaged in this behavior ($\chi^2 = 1.427$, $df = 2$, $P = 0.490$). Under this classification of alcohol use, 50% (3 subjects) of the subjects who had committed forcible rape had engaged in excessive alcohol use; yet, all of these subjects who had committed rape had done so after the onset of their cocaine addiction.

Small sample sizes for each of the violent behaviors resulted in unreliable statistical comparisons in terms of alcohol use and when in the subjects' cocaine-using careers (only before, or after, or both before and after cocaine onset) they primarily engaged in each violent behavior; neither were any other statistically significant relationships found between each of the reported violent behaviors individually and the subjects' alcohol use.

5. Summary and Discussion

This chapter presents (1) a review of work done on the issue of cocaine–alcohol use and violence and (2) a longitudinal view of deviant and violent behaviors that occurred before and during the cocaine use careers of a group of cocaine-dependent veterans who sought treatment for their dependence.

Alcohol, by itself, has been found to have a calming effect physically but a disruptive effect psychologically. Inebriation, under high levels of personal threat, appears to focus attention on negative cues and lead to more intense aggression.[5,6] Cocaine, particularly crack cocaine, has also been associated with both an increase in the seriousness and rate of criminal activity,[18] with significant increases occurring after the onset of cocaine abuse. Few researchers have looked at the subpopulation of cocaine addicts who also abuse alcohol[19,20] and have found that cocaine–alcohol abusers are more likely to have higher rates of criminal behavior than both cocaine-only abusers and alcohol-only abusers.[21]

The study reported here looked further into the population of cocaine addicts to examine possible differences in levels and types of criminal, particularly violent, behaviors between cocaine addicts who abuse and those who did not abuse alcohol. It also looked at the differences in criminal activity for cocaine addicts when they were using both cocaine and alcohol, when they were using cocaine only or alcohol only, or when they were abstinent from both cocaine and alcohol. In addition, comparisons were made in order to try to distinguish between behavior these addicts engaged in prior to their cocaine addiction and during their cocaine use careers.

The sample in this study consisted of adult male cocaine addicts, average 36 years old, which is slightly older than the age of clinical populations of cocaine addicts examined by other studies. This age difference is most likely due to the study's prerequisite that subjects be veterans of the military service. African Americans were overrepresented in this study, which is consistent with other urban studies of cocaine users. While this could represent a sampling bias, there has been no evidence of ethnicity being a major influence on the variables studied.

These subjects also had an average level of education higher than that of the general population or the population of veterans, which is consistent with the findings of other investigators who have reported above-average levels of education in cocaine-using populations.[26–30] The average age at first cocaine use was 24 years old, which is also consistent with epidemiologic investigations that have reported that the period of high risk for cocaine experimentation is between the ages of 18 and 24.[31] Still, the variance in age of FCU was considerably high, with the age at first use ranging between 12 and 58 years old.

The average length of these subjects' cocaine careers from FCU to TE spanned 10 years. Most subjects reported that during the majority of this time they were also drinking alcohol, and 20% of these subjects were classified as excessive alcohol users when their alcohol use was averaged over the period of their cocaine careers. When subjects reported using another drug with cocaine, before or after their cocaine use, or as a substitute for cocaine, the most frequently reported drug was alcohol. These subjects' alcohol use started an average of 10 years prior to their FCU.

In addition to sociodemographic and drug use data, we examined patterns of behavior occurring during the cocaine-use career. Retrospective information covered a time span from FCU to the point at which the addiction became sufficiently severe to lead to help-seeking behavior and treatment for cocaine dependence. Most subjects began using cocaine intranasally, all of them progressed to smoking crack at some point in their cocaine career, but at the time of TE, 64% were smoking crack as their preferred route of administration. Most also had used alcohol and had been exposed to other drugs of abuse, particularly marijuana.

A subset of the sample exhibited socially deviant behavior, including violence. Deviant behaviors were present during early youth and adulthood, both before the onset of cocaine use as well as during the cocaine-use career. While the proportion of individuals who engaged in particular behaviors was relatively small, the frequency of the behaviors was large.

The extent of deviant or violent behavior during periods of cocaine use, periods of combined cocaine–alcohol use, periods of alcohol use, and periods of sobriety were described. These observations on cocaine-dependent individuals illustrate the complexity of the relationships between cocaine use, combined alcohol and cocaine use, and violent behavior. It should be noted that only a small segment of this cocaine-dependent sample engaged in violent behavior. Cocaine use did not appear to bring out tendencies that were not already existent, based on the fact that in most instances subjects who engaged in criminal behaviors were doing so prior to their cocaine use onset. Use of alcohol with cocaine seemed to increase the risk of a cocaine user engaging in violent behavior. The conclusions drawn from our results are preliminary; thus, further systematic inquiry of these issues is necessary.

Of all the delinquent behaviors these addicts participated in as juveniles, their variance in the frequency of participation remained high. While the majority of the subjects who had acted aggressively or violently as teenagers had done so prior to the onset of their cocaine addiction, the ages when they threatened an adult or hit an adult fall within the same time period as the initiation of their alcohol use. Further investigation within this population would need to be conducted in order to ascertain whether alcohol use during this time is correlated with these behaviors.

The nature of criminal activities in adulthood also changed as these subjects progressed in their cocaine addiction. The majority of the subjects who had ever broken into a building or car, stolen from a store, stolen a car, or damaged others' property had done so prior to the onset of their cocaine addiction. Those who had either beaten someone severely or shot someone had more often done so either prior to their cocaine addiction or both before and after the onset of their addiction. Driving while under the influence, gambling, carrying a weapon, and selling or carrying drugs for others were most often done both prior to and after the onset of their cocaine addiction. More violent crimes (such as threatening with a weapon or threatening for profit, using a weapon or force for profit, and committing rape), though reported by fewer subjects, were more frequently reported to have been committed after the onset of cocaine addiction.

As was expected, subjects reported having engaged in more criminal activities during periods of their cocaine career when they were also drinking alcohol. Subjects reported engaging in fewer criminal activities when they were drinking alcohol and abstinent from cocaine. When these addicts were abstinent from both alcohol and cocaine, they were least likely to engage in criminal activities.

In addition, those who had used alcohol to excess (an average of at least 4 ounces of pure alcohol per day) during their cocaine career were more likely to have engaged in serious violent behavior (beating someone severely and threatening with a weapon) than whose who had not used alcohol to excess. As would be expected, there was no difference in aggressive behaviors engaged in for profit by those who had used alcohol to excess and those who had not. There were also no significant differences between the number of cocaine addicts who drank alcohol to excess and those who did not in terms of shooting someone or committing rape; yet, all the subjects who drank alcohol excessively during their cocaine careers who had committed rape had done so only after the onset of their cocaine addiction, in comparison to 40% of those who did not drink excessively and had committed rape prior to the onset of their cocaine addiction.

6. Comments and Research Implications

These observations on deviant behavior among cocaine-dependent individuals, most of whom also drank alcohol during some point of their cocaine-using careers, illustrate the complexity of the relationships between cocaine use, alcohol use, and violent behaviors. Our findings indicate that only a small proportion of our cocaine-dependent sample engaged in violent behavior; cocaine use did not appear to induce behaviors that had not been engaged in previously. On the other hand, use of alcohol seemed to increase the likelihood of the cocaine user engaging in violent behavior. These conclusions drawn from our findings are preliminary; thus, further systematic inquiry of these issues is necessary and several research topics require much more explicit attention.

Further analyses need to be conducted with our data. For example, to distinguish between different levels of alcohol use during different periods in the cocaine career may provide better information on the dynamic links between both addictions and crime.

Further analyses are planned distinguishing between specific criminal activities subjects engaged in at different phases of the cocaine career (during the year prior to first cocaine use, between first cocaine use and first severe cocaine use, and between first severe cocaine use and treatment entry) in relation to the subjects' alcohol use during these time periods. These and other analyses will hopefully provide a better understanding of the interactions among drug-related behaviors and violence.

References

1. McGonigal MD, Cole J, Schwab CW, et al: Urban firearm deaths: A five year perspective. *J Trauma* 35:532–536, 1993.
2. Linnoila M, Virkkunen M, Scheinin M, et al: Low cerebrospinal 5-hydroxyindoleacetic acid concentration differentiates impulsive from impulsive violent behavior. *Life Sci* 33:2609–2614, 1983.
3. Bushman BJ, Cooper HM: Effect of alcohol on human aggression: An integrative research review. *Psychol Bull* 107:341–354, 1990.
4. Moss HB, Krisci L: Aggressively in adolescent alcohol abusers: Relationship with conduct disorder. *Alcohol Clin Exp Res* 19:642–646, 1995.
5. Zeichner A, Allen JB, Gianola PR, Lating JM: Alcohol and aggression: Effects of personal threat on human aggression and affective arousal. *Alcohol Clin Exp Res* 18:657–663, 1994.
6. Zeichner A, Giancola PR, Allen JD: Effects of hostility on alcohol stress-response dampening. *Alcohol Clin Exp Res* 19:977–983, 1995.
7. Goldstein PJ: The drug/violence nexus; A tripartite conceptual framework. *J Drug Issues* 15(4):493–506, 1985.
8. Goldstein J: Cocaine and crime in the United States. Presentation for the United Nations Interregional Criminological Research Institute International Symposium on Cocaine March 1991, Rome, Italy.
9. Miller NS, Gold MN: Criminal activity and crack addiction. *Int J Addict* 29:1069–1978, 1994.
10. Giannini AJ, Miller NS, Loiselle RH, Turner CE: Cocaine-associated violence and relationship to rout of administration. *J Subst Abuse Treat* 10:67–69, 1993.
11. Stanton B, Galbraith J: Drug trafficking among African American early adolescents: Prevalence, consequences, and associate behaviors and beliefs. *Pediatrics* 93:1039–1043, 1994.
12. Black MM, Richardo IB: Drug use-drug trafficking and weapon carrying among low-income African-American adolescent boys. *Pediatrics* 93:1065–1072, 1994.
13. Kang SY, Magura S, Shapiro JL: Correlates of cocaine/crack use among inner city-incarcerated adolescents. *Am J Drug Alcohol Abuse* 20:413–429, 1994.
14. Sheley JF: Drug and guns among inner-city high school students. *J Drug Educ* 24:301–321, 1994.
15. Hutson HR, Anglin D, Kyraicou D, et al: The epidemic of gang related homicides in Los Angeles county from 1979 through 1994. *J Am Med Assoc* 274(13):1031–1036, 1995.
16. Klein MH, Maxson CL, Cunningham LC: "Crack" street gangs and violence. *Criminology* 29:701–727, 1991.
17. Meehan PJ, O'Carrol PW: Gangs drugs and homicide in Los Angeles. *Am J Dis Child* 146:683–687, 1992.
18. Belenko S, Chin K, Fagan J: Typologies of criminal career among crack arrestees. Paper presented at the Annual Meeting of the American Society of Criminology, Reno, NV, 1989.
19. Khalsa ME, Paredes A, Anglin MD: Cocaine dependence behavioral dimensions and patterns of progression. *Am J Addict* 2:330–345, 1993.
20. Higgins S, Budney AJ, Bickel WK, et al: Alcohol dependence and simultaneous cocaine and alcohol use in cocaine-dependent subjects. *J Addict Dis* 13:177–189, 1994.
21. Windle M, Miller-Tutzauer C: Antecedents and correlates of alcohol, cocaine, and alcohol–cocaine abuse in early adulthood. *J Drug Educ* 21:133–148, 1991.
22. Nurco DN, Bonito AJ, Lerner M, Baller M: Studying addicts over time: Methodology and preliminary findings. *Am J Alcohol Abuse* 2:107–121, 1975.
23. Bradburn NM, Rips LJ, Shevell SK: Answering autobiographical questions: Impacts of memory and inference on surveys. *Science* 236(4798):157–161, 1987.

24. Khalsa ME, Anglin MD, Paredes A: Pre-treatment natural history of cocaine addiction. *NIDA Res Monogr* 105:494–500, 1991.
25. Barbor TF, Kvanzaler HR, Lauerman RJ: Social drinking as a health and psychosocial risk factor: Anstie's limit revisited, in Galanter M (ed): *Recent Developments on Alcoholism* New York, Plenum Press, 1987, pp 373–397.
26. Gawin FH: Cocaine addiction: Psychology and neurophysiology. *Science* 251(5001):1580–1586, 1991.
27. Gawin FH, Kleber HD: Cocaine use in a treatment population: Patterns and diagnostic distinctions. *NIDA Res Monogr* 61:182–192, 1985.
28. Gawin FH, Kleber HD: Abstinence symptomatology and psychiatric diagnosis in cocaine abusers. *Arch Gen Psychiatry* 43:107–113, 1986.
29. Schnoll SH, Carrigan S, Kitchen S, *et al:* Characteristics of cocaine abusers presenting for treatment, in Kozel NJ, Adams EH (eds): *Cocaine Use in America: Epidemiology and Clinical Perspectives.* NIDA Research Monograph 61. Rockville, MD, US Department of Health and Human Resources, 1988, pp 171–181.
30. Washton AM, Gold MS, Pottash AC, *et al:* Treatment outcome in cocaine abusers, in Harris LS (ed): *Problems of Drug Dependence.* NIDA Research Monograph 67. Rockville, MD, US Department of Health and Human Services, 1986, pp 381–384.
31. Anthony JC, Ritter CJ, Von Kerfett MR, *et al:* Descriptive epidemiology of adult cocaine use in four US communities, in Harris LS (ed): *Problems of Drug Dependence.* NIDA Research Monograph 67. Rockville, MD, US Department of Health and Human Services, 1985, pp 283–289.

IV

Family Issues

Edward Gottheil and Ellen F. Gottheil, Section Editors

Overview

Edward Gottheil and Ellen F. Gottheil

According to a recent bulletin of the Bureau of Justice Statistics, the number of prisoners in the custody of state correctional authorities for a variety of serious offenses increased from 1980 to 1993 by a factor of 2.8.[1] Of these, the largest increases, by a wide margin, were drug offenses (increasing by a factor of 9.79) and sexual assaults other than rape (by a factor of 6.68). In today's world, drug abuse and partner abuse have become increasingly significant public health issues.

Widely cited books by Pizzey,[2] Gelles,[3] and Steinmetz and Straus,[4] published only 22 years ago in 1974, markedly increased our attention on and concern about spouse abuse and helped promote an interest in research into the causes of marital violence. For the most part, the victims, i.e., the battered wives and children, were the ones initially studied during the 1970s and 1980s. Increasing realization that stopping or preventing these behaviors required involvement of the abusers gradually led to research and clinical programs for batterers in the 1980s.[5,6]

In 1983, Spieker[7] pointed out that while it was "common knowledge" that violence and alcohol "coexist and are exhibited" in the "all-American home," there were few studies available correlating family violence and alcohol abuse. Indeed, leafing through the articles of an issue of *Violence and Victims* recently, I found that only 2 of 150 cited references were to journals in the substance abuse field. Unfortunately, "substance abuse" and "domestic violence" still tend to remain separate conceptual entities in theory, research, and treatment. Partly this is understandable. Systematic studies of substance abuse, aggressive behavior, and family relationships are rather recent. Each

Edward Gottheil • Department of Psychiatry and Human Behavior, Thomas Jefferson University, Philadelphia, Pennsylvania 19107.   **Ellen F. Gottheil** • Department of Psychiatry and Behavioral Sciences, University of Washington Medical School, Seattle, Washington 98195.

Recent Developments in Alcoholism, Volume 13: Alcoholism and Violence, edited by Marc Galanter. Plenum Press, New York, 1997

has presented problems in definition, few practicable experimental models, and difficulty in applying controls in either community or clinical situations. Studies of interactions between substance abuse and aggression within families are even more recent and more difficult to execute.

In addition to bringing together materials from different disciplines i.e., biological, psychological, and social studies of aggressive behavior, drug use, and family interactions, with their different methodologies and terminologies, there is the need to consider the many different specific parameters within particular studies. Some of these, to note only a few examples, would include: (1) type, level, and duration of alcohol or other drug (AOD) intake, e.g., cocaine binges or chronic inebriation; (2) type, severity, and duration of domestic violence (DV) involving spouse and/or child abuse; (3) source of data from community sample, treatment group, jail, etc,; (4) relationship between perpetrator AOD intake and DV; (5) relationships among victim's AOD use, perpetrator's AOD use and DV; (6) personality factors, antisocial behavior, neurotic conflicts; and (7) history of AOD and/or DV in family of origin of the perpetrator and of the victim.

Clearly the design of relevant research, the interpretation of findings, and the integration of the data across studies are not simple tasks. A question we face in our attempt to study and treat very troubled families is: How do we appreciate the complexity without becoming overwhelmed and ineffective? One way to do this is to organize problems into unitary areas. In situations where factors coexist, however, we may be more effective if we can keep in mind and relate more than one model. As in all cases of dual diagnosis, this requires that we as researchers and clinicians maintain flexibility without losing our energy and direction. Undaunted, the authors of the following four chapters have attempted to bring together and summarize information available on selected topics relating to family violence from the perspective of the spouse, the batterer, the child, and treatment.

Theories of spouse abuse and theories of alcohol-induced aggression are reviewed in Chapter 13 by Kaufman Kantor and Asdigian in an attempt to understand the linkage between them as well as the possible contribution to the linkage, if any, of the victim's AOD use. In general, the theories have focused on male behavior and intoxication–aggression effects. There has been great sensitivity in the DV field to the problem of blaming the victim, and perhaps there has been some reluctance to study possible relationships between the victim's AOD use and her victimization out of concern that she will be blamed for "causing" her abuse. There have been suggestions, however, that intoxication–victimization effects also occur. The chapter then addresses: (1) hypothesized dimensions and mechanisms of intoxication–victimization effects; (2) whether the literature indicates that women who drink or use drugs are at greater risk for spouse abuse; (3) variation according to population sampled or type of victimization; and (4) whether such effects are mediated or confounded by other variables.

If intoxication–victimization as well as intoxication–aggression effects are to be considered, theoretical explanations of the relationship between AOD and violence will need to take into account and integrate findings about differences between men and women in their AOD effects and expectations. Actually, Kaufman Kantor and Asdigian found that the "empirical evidence supporting an association between women's intoxication and physical assaults by husbands" was mixed according to whether alcohol or other drugs were involved, whether the assaults were more severe or less severe, whether use was at the time of the assault or general usage, and whether the research was conducted with clinical samples of heavy drinking women and/or battered women.

In summing up, they suggest that while AOD use by women does, for the most part, seem to be associated with victimization, this may not be because the victim's intoxication is an immediate behavioral precedent to her victimization, but may be due to a number of possible underlying reasons. Among these could be the lower rate of self-esteem, decreased resources, and level of functioning of AOD-addicted women, making it more difficult to deal effectively with violence at home. Another could be a history of victimization in the woman's family of origin. Family violence is known to be an important factor in the history of male batterers, and assaulted women were reported to have about double the rate of growing up in a violent home as nonassaulted women. There is also a greater likelihood of having a heavy-drinking or drug-abusing partner. Finally, the occurrence of substance abuse may be a consequence of victimization rather than an antecedent.

The male who beats his wife and batters his children has long been regarded more as a repulsive criminal than as an interesting subject for study or a person in need of care and support. This view has not been especially conducive to the development of research or therapeutic programs for the batterer. Nevertheless, if we are to intervene and hope to prevent recurrences and ultimately develop preventive programs, we need to study, treat, and better understand spouse and child abusers. In their review of the literature, Lee and Weinstein, in Chapter 14, report that in recent years (over 80% of the references they cite were dated 1983 or later) a number of treatment programs for batterers have been initiated and a considerable amount of research has been done. In the first part of their chapter they examine research studies that attempt to identify the causes of partner abuse and note a number of interesting ideas and findings, but they conclude that the causes are varied and that men abuse their partners for many different reasons. A major part of their chapter is devoted to attempts that have been made to define unique characteristics of male batterers. Rather than a definition or typical profile, however, what emerges is a wide variety of background, behavioral, psychological, and social characteristics of the batterer, as well as several promising typologies, which taken together strongly suggest that batterers are heterogeneous. The importance of this concept of heterogeneity[8] is that it then behooves us to search for causes and treatment approaches rather than the cause of or the treatment for the batterer.

Lee and Weinstein describe many studies that indicate that AOD abuse is commonly found in batterers. Although neither alcohol or drug abuse are necessary or sufficient for the occurrence of domestic violence, they are often present. As more studies are being done, they are becoming increasingly more sophisticated, with some now seeking to differentiate the characteristics of spouse abusers from those of substance abusers by controlling for one or the other; for example, they describe a Jefferson Medical College study in which the characteristics of cocaine users who do and who do not batter are compared.

Regarding treatment, a variety of approaches have been employed, three of which were selected for discussion: divorce mediation, group treatment for batterers focusing on shame as a core issue and on confessions, and mandatory arrests. These were selected and their potential advantages and disadvantages described and evaluated in some detail because of their unique relationship to battering treatment. Regardless of treatment approach, however, a number of studies were reviewed indicating that alcohol and drug abuse were important contributors to recidivism in treatment for battering.

In Chapter 15, Miller, Maguin, and Downs provide us with a comprehensive review of the current state of knowledge regarding (1) the extent to which AOD use by the perpetrator is related to the perpetration of physical or sexual abuse against children and (2) the relationship between experiencing physical or sexual abuse during childhood and the subsequent development of AOD use/abuse. It may be worth noting that when the authors compare differences in findings between earlier and more recent reviews, the more recent reviews are more sophisticated in design and the earlier ones, for the most part, were done only 10 to 15 years ago. Clearly, a great deal has been accomplished during the last decade, yielding the many new findings reported in this review.

In studying relationships between AOD use and family violence, additional methodological considerations are involved when the child is the victim. For example, if the validity of the information obtained by asking patients coming to a substance abuse clinic about their substance abuse and aggressive behavior has been questioned, how questionable is the validity of the information obtained from parents when asked, no matter how gently and how indirectly, about their use/abuse of substances in relation to their physical and sexual abuse of their children? If, instead, retrospective reports are obtained regarding parental AOD use and abusive behaviors from their grown-up children, they may be overreported on the basis of false memories or fabrications, or underreported due to repression, suppression, or a simple unwillingness to reveal the information (a study is described in which one third of officially documented cases of childhood sexual abuse were not reported when the victims were later interviewed as adults). Furthermore, regarding sexual abuse, the victims may not know about the AOD usage of the perpetrators, since the majority of them are not parents but strangers.

Results of studies of the effects of experiencing childhood physical and/or sexual abuse are not always consistent and vary according to the type, severity, duration, and context of the abuse, whether the victim is male or female, and whether the perpetrator is of the same or opposite sex. In Chapter 15, several hypotheses are described by Miller and coauthors regarding the accessibility of perpetrators to the children, including whether AOD addiction decreases parental ability to protect children, framing this important topic for further research. Taking into account the complexity of the issues and methodological limitations, the authors conclude that there is suitable evidence indicating that parental AOD is related to physical and sexual abuse of their children, that parental AOD problems increase the likelihood of their children being victimized by others, and that childhood victimization is related to the later development of AOD. Nevertheless, there are many gaps and inconsistencies in the theoretical explanations and our state of knowledge, and Miller and coauthors end their chapter with a discussion of theoretical and methodological considerations, special ethical and legal issues (e.g., the duty to warn authorities about findings of abuse as well as the need to warn subjects about this duty), and clearly specified directions for future research.

In Chapter 16, the desirability and practicability of linking services for the treatment of alcoholism and domestic violence are addressed by Collins and associates. Reviewing the role of alcoholism in domestic violence, they find consistent evidence in the literature of a strong association between husband's drinking and spouse abuse. A number of studies also indicate that drinking on the part of the woman may increase the likelihood of being victimized, and that in some instances drinking by the abused spouse follows the abuse and perpetuates the cycle. It seems reasonable to expect, then, that for men who are batterers and also spouse abusers, for women who have been battered and are substance abusers, and for their families, treatment efforts would be enhanced by attending to both the substance abuse and the spouse abuse.

Nevertheless, they report that although staff of substance abuse and domestic violence programs when asked endorse the idea of treating both problems, very few programs actually do so. Few of the programs screen for the other abuse condition; even when the coexistence of these problems is recognized, the most common form of linkage is referral to another agency, which is accomplished only some of the time and often without ongoing provider interaction and cooperation.

Domestic violence programs are concerned, of course, about the safety and interests of the battered women and providing them with shelter, child care services, legal assistance, and protection from the batterer. For the batterer, they are most interested in programming to emphasize behavioral management, anger control, acceptance of personal responsibility, and meeting family responsibilities. The concept of alcoholism as a disease may be seen as an excuse for not accepting responsibility, frequent attendance at Alcoholic Anonymous (AA) meetings as an avoidance of assuming family responsibilities, and ideas regarding enabling and codependency as a means of shifting blame to the victims. Indeed, staff of substance abuse programs often view the addiction as the disease and as the primary problem, deemphasize personal accountability for past behavior during the "active" disease, encourage frequent AA attendance and sponsorship, and often consider the spouse abuse as secondary to the addiction.

Although Collins and his coauthors describe clear advantages to providing integrated services to the multiproblem families involved in domestic violence, there are impediments to developing linkages. These include different organizational placements, separate funding streams, and lack of resources, but the most important and difficult to deal with perhaps are the differences in philosophy, goals, training, and management concerns of the treatment staffs. AOD staff may assume that battering will decrease as addiction is treated, despite evidence that this will not happen unless the battering is directly addressed. DV staff may not recognize the extent to which victim's substance use or abuse makes it harder for her to deal with or leave her relationship, or the extent to which substance abuse may exacerbate the husband's battering.

The authors suggest that, "It would be premature to recommend implementation of widespread attempts at linking substance abuse and domestic violence services in the absence of well-developed and effective models for doing so." They complete the chapter by describing some examples of current linkages, the advantages of linking services, and different models for linkages and they outline research and clinical steps to be taken to further develop a better integration of effective services.

Reading these four lucidly written, comprehensive, well-referenced review chapters on substance abuse and domestic violence, one cannot help being impressed by the complexity of the conceptual and methodological issues confronting those wishing to study these conditions and their interactions. Much, of course, remains to be learned about aggressive behavior, substance abuse, and family relationships before one can hope to really understand how their interactions may culminate in abuse of the spouse or child. At the same time, one is also impressed by the clear recognition of methodological problems and limitations, the increasing sophistication of the studies, and the progress that has been made with respect to new findings, research techniques, and theoretical development. The authors of these chapters have made a significant contribution toward bringing together information and theory about aggressive behaviors, AOD, and domestic violence, which should serve to further the process of cross-fertilization.

Nevertheless, a continuing problem is insufficient communication across disciplines. There is much relevant information within the journals and expressed in the esoteric verbiage of the separate disciplines. This lack of integration is to the detriment of the disciplines as well as to our patients. For, if we treat only the problem with which we are familiar and ignore associated problems, we may unwittingly sow the seeds for relapse of the very problem we are trying to treat. While Collins and his coauthors wisely caution against leaping full-scale into linking AOD and DV services in the absence of well-developed effective models for doing so, it is clear that the development of these models is urgently needed to address these problems when they are intertwined. In addition to having caseworkers refer, manage, and integrate services, we might add that it is not too early to begin educating clinicians and researchers in training to be sensitive to other kinds of abuse than the one on which they are specifically focused, to introduce them to complexity, to expose them to additional theoretical models, and to familiarize them with chapters like the four to follow in order to keep our patients from falling through the large cracks between disciplines.

References

1. Beck AJ, Gilliard DK: Prisoners in 1994. *Bureau of Justice Statistics Bulletin*, August 1995, p 11.
2. Pizzey E: *Scream Quietly or the Neighbors Will Hear.* London, Penguin, 1974.
3. Gelles RJ: *The Violent Home.* Beverly Hills, CA, Sage, 1974.
4. Steinmetz SK, Straus M: *Violence in the Family.* New York, Harper & Row, 1974.
5. Eddy MJ, Myers T: *Helping Men Who Batter: A Profile of Programs in the US.* Arlington, TX, Texas State Department of Human Resources, 1984.
6. Roberts AR: A national survey of services for batterers, in Roy M (ed): *The Abusive Partner: An Analysis of Domestic Battering.* New York, Van Nostrand-Reinhold, 1982, pp 17–35.
7. Spieker G: What is the linkage between alcohol abuse and violence, in Gottheil E, Druley KA, Skoloda TE, Waxman HM (eds): *Alcohol, Drug Abuse and Aggression.* Springfield, IL, Charles C. Thomas, 1983, pp 125–136.
8. Institute of Medicine: *Broadening the Base of Treatment for Alcohol Problems.* Washington, DC, National Academy Press, 1990.

13

When Women Are under the Influence

Does Drinking or Drug Use by Women Provoke Beatings by Men?

Glenda Kaufman Kantor and Nancy Asdigian

Abstract. This chapter examines theoretical and empirical evidence for the existence of "intoxication–victimization" effects. Theories of victimization and theories of alcohol-induced aggression are examined for their relevance to the phenomenon of concern. The results of our examination of theory and research indicates theoretical support for an integrated theory of intoxication–victimization effects. However, we found that the temporal precedence of women's drinking related to their victimizations has not been established by prior investigations. Supporting evidence for intoxication–victimization effects is strongest among studies of rape, homicide, and studies of alcoholic women. Despite the strength of alcohol's association with wife assaults, intoxication's centrality and temporal relationship to specific wife-assault episodes is highly variable. Our review indicates that women's intoxication might be spuriously associated with victimization through its association with husband's intoxication and via the indirect effects of victimization histories in the family of origin of both partners.

1. Introduction

Most theory and research on the link between drugs, particularly alcohol, and crimes of violence have focused on male behavior and have been from the

Glenda Kaufman Kantor and Nancy Asdigian • Family Research Laboratory, University of New Hampshire, Durham, New Hampshire 03824.

Recent Developments in Alcoholism, Volume 13: Alcoholism and Violence, edited by Marc Galanter. Plenum Press, New York, 1997

perspective of "intoxication–aggressor" effects, i.e., intoxication as a precipitant of aggressive acts.[1-7] A complementary perspective suggested by Kaufman Kantor and Straus,[8] and the focus of this chapter, is that "intoxication–victim" effects may also exist. This perspective is based on the idea that women under the influence of alcohol and other drugs may become targets of male aggression (i.e., "fair game"). Many assume that intoxicated women violate the norms of appropriate female behavior, and thus lose the protection afforded by other traditional gender role norms, such as "never hit a woman,"[9-11] and a physically violent response to "provocation" is therefore legitimated. Similarly, women under the influence of drugs or alcohol are viewed as sexually available,[12] and are more likely to be victims of sexual aggression.[13] However, studies suggesting that males increase their aggression toward women who violate gender role expectations may provide only a partial explanation of why intoxicated women are at risk for victimization, and the "fair game" assumption is difficult to establish. Few studies specifically assess the vocabularies of offender motive, and more often motive is intuited as a post-hoc explanation of alcohol–victimization effects.[8] Additionally, there is a need to consider whether, in fact, women who drink heavily or use drugs are at greater risk for spouse abuse, as well as the adequacy of theory and research conducted on intoxication–victimization effects.

There are apparent limitations in generalizing from experimental studies of alcohol-induced aggression[1,5,14] to studies of alcohol and wife assault, because in the former condition most confederates are strangers. Moreover, the vast majority of alcohol and aggression studies do not take into account the mediating effects of an intoxicated partner. Experimental studies that include intoxicated dyads with real partners[15] or that examine the effects of an intoxicated female partner on male aggression are also uncommon. Although experimental analogue studies have yielded important information about alcohol-induced aggression, the experimental paradigms (e.g., the competitive reaction-time paradigm) have not been suitable for studying marital aggression.[16] Additionally, many studies of alcohol-related marital violence have failed to take into account the intoxicant usage pattern of both partners. Empirical studies documenting the incidence of victimization among heavy-drinking or alcoholic women compared to moderate-drinking counterparts are a relatively recent area of study.[17,18] The latter studies are important to consider because they suggest that female intoxication may have direct or indirect effects on women's victimization experiences.

Experts on alcohol-related wife assaults concur that alcohol–aggression relationships are complex phenomena mediated by a number of factors such as family history, personality, the drinking context, the amount drunk, and alcohol- and violence-related cognitions.[19-22] However, as Pernanen[23] observed, most theoretical approaches have been individual-based, thus minimizing the social dynamics of alcohol-related interactions. In this chapter we consider the relevance and adequacy of existing theory to explaining intoxicant–victimization effects, as well as the empirical basis for the hypothesized relationships. Specifically, we address the following questions: (1) What are the hypothesized dimensions and mechanisms of intoxication–victimization effects? (2) Does the empirical literature show that women who drink heavily or use drugs are at greater risk for abuse by spouses? (3) Does the importance of female drinking to victimization vary by the event (type of victimization) or by the population sample studied? (4) Is this a "spurious" relationship; for example, a relationship that simply reflects drug/alcohol use by the husband or reflects other confounding variables such as a history of abuse in the family of origin?

2. What Are the Theoretical Mechanisms?

Both theories of wife abuse and theories of alcohol-induced aggression must be considered in formulating an integrated conceptual framework for interpreting intoxication–victimization effects.

2.1. Theories of Victimization

A number of theoretical perspectives have been utilized to explain wife abuse. For example, Bersani and Chen[24] (1988) examine seven theoretical perspectives on family violence. Gelles and Straus[25] identify 15 theories, which they organize into three broad categories: intraindividual theory, social psychological theory, and sociocultural theory. Intraindividual theory has emphasized alcohol–drug effects and psychological traits such as self-esteem[26–28] and antisocial personality disorder.[29] Sociocultural theories such as systems theory have attempted to integrate social structural and family processes.[30,31] Feminist explanations of women's victimization also emphasize sociocultural factors, especially the male-dominated social structure and socialization practices.[32,33] Social–psychological approaches have stressed, for one, social learning through experience and exposure to violence.[34–36]

It is important to note that even though we cast the above approaches as theories of victimization, for the most part the theories pertain to explanations of the perpetrator's aggression. This theoretical emphasis on the perpetrator is supported by previous analyses finding that 14 characteristics were consistently associated with being an abuser, whereas only one factor was consistently associated with being a victim of wife abuse.[37] Furthermore, Dobash and Dobash[38] point out that blaming the victim of wife beating provides a justification for batterers' violence. When women nag, try to have an equal say in family decisions, or refuse sex, husbands may feel they are justified in using force.[39] In these cases, the woman is blamed for her own victimization. This same mechanism may apply when women are intoxicated.

Alcohol figures in only two of the many theories discussed above—intraindividual theory and social-learning theory. For example, O'Leary's[35] social-learning model of spousal aggression incorporates five major factors that predict spousal aggression: (1) violence in the family of origin; (2) aggressive personality style; (3) stress; (4) alcohol use and abuse; and (5) marital dissatisfaction. Prior research[2] on alcohol–wife assault relationships has concluded that alcohol use at the time of wife assault is far from necessary or sufficient for wife abuse to ensue, despite the stereotype that all drunks hit or all hitting involves drunks. Yet, alcohol use by the perpetrator has emerged as a major risk factor in wife assault research.[2,4,15,40–42]

2.2. Theories of Intoxicant-Induced Aggression

General theories of alcohol-induced aggression are usually advanced to explain alcohol-related wife assaults, but their ability to account for the special case of wife assault or for intoxication–victimization effects needs to be evaluated. A primary theory utilized to explain the relationship between alcohol and aggression is that alcohol has psychopharmacological effects, i.e., intoxicants affect personality and affective states.[43] Researchers employing experimental paradigms in examining alcohol effects on aggression have generally demonstrated both direct dose effects of alcohol on aggression and indirect effects mediated by social, psychological, and environmental factors. The factors include, but are not limited to, the aggressive predisposition of the individual, expectancies, and perceptions of threat or provocation.[1,3,6,14,44–48]

Alcohol is the drug most commonly associated with violence[19,43]; however, other psychoactive drugs have been associated with aggression such as barbiturates, amphetamines, opiate (withdrawal), phencyclidine, cocaine, and alcohol–cocaine combinations.[43,49] Altogether, the aggressive effects of psychoactive drugs other than alcohol have received less empirical scrutiny, and the results have been inconsistent. Taylor and Chermack's[50] review finds that drugs with depressogenic characteristics are most likely to facilitate aggression, and Fagan[43] finds solid evidence of a psychopharmacological basis only for the combined effects of an alcohol–cocaine combination. It must also be concluded that aggression is not an inevitable consequence of any intoxicant usage.

2.3. Mechanisms of Intoxicant-Induced Victimization

2.3.1. Cognitive Effects. Despite ongoing debate about the precise pharmacological effects, there is consensus that alcohol disrupts cognitive functioning by diminishing ability to reason, reducing ability to perceive or calculate consequences of aggressive behaviors, and by enhancing perception of threat.[51,50] All of the latter mechanisms bear upon the process of social interaction, and are likely mechanisms that could increase the risk of victimization. It is clear that aggression may be a consequence of alcohol's impairment of perception, judgment, and memory. Distorted perceptions increase the likelihood of miscommunications, developing resentment, and the inability to take into account the consequences of aggressive actions. A greater possibility exists for escalating verbal aggression between partners that in turn leads to physical aggression. All of the cognitive misprocessing and miscommunication may be magnified when both partners are under the influence. However, the latter assumes a certain invariance in the dynamics of the social interaction. For one, men and women may not behave similarly when under the influence.[52]

2.3.2. Expectancy Effects. Although gender differences in alcohol expectancies have been examined in a number of studies, most researchers have not systematically explored the specific alcohol-related beliefs held by males and females.[53,54] Previous assessments have been very general in scope, involving comparisons between males and females across a wide spectrum of emotional and behavioral expectancies. For example, in their analysis of the Alcohol Expectancy Questionnaire's (AEQ) six dimensions, Brown and associates[55] reported that females were more likely than males to expect alcohol to result in positive social experiences, whereas males were more likely to expect heightened arousal and aggression. Rohsenhow[56] examined gender differences on a number of alcohol expectancy dimensions in addition to those identified by the AEQ. After differences in drinking habits were controlled, women expected more cognitive and motor impairment than men did, but less positive affect, social and physical pleasure, and relaxation. Aggressive alcohol expectancies did not vary, however, as a function of gender in Rohsenhow's study or in a subsequent investigation.[57] In Kline's[58] study, gender differences were not observed on any of the five AEQ factors included in that research (the arousal/aggression dimension was not used). Critchlow-Leigh[54] administered a different expectancy measure to male and female subjects and found that women expected to suffer more cognitive and physical impairment (e.g., feeling sleepy, sick, dizzy) from drinking than men did. Expectancies regarding alcohol-induced nastiness (e.g., being mean, becoming aggressive) were, however, stronger among males even after controlling for gender differences in drinking patterns.

In a more recent study,[59] we focused specifically on gender differences in expectations concerning drinking-related aggression. The results of this study of nonabstinent couples suggested that the structure of alcohol beliefs varies by gender, and that gender differences in aggressive alcohol expectancies are highly specific. Male respondents were more likely than their female counterparts to associate drinking with heightened feelings of power and influence over others and with irritability and short-temperedness. These findings suggest that alcohol consumption, because it enhances feelings of male dominance and increases the ease with which men are provoked, may create a set of conditions conducive to male-perpetrated aggression. However, both heavy-drinking men and women had similar perceptions that drinking may make aggressive acts more forgivable.

An examination of alcohol-related violence among these couples revealed that men were twice as likely as women to be drinking at the time of a spousal assault. This study also found that alcohol-related assaults against wives were more likely when both partners were heavy drinkers. Typical consumption levels of wives were the only significant predictors of husbands' alcohol-related assaults against wives. On the other hand, drinking-related assaults perpetrated by wives against husbands were predicted from both women's typical alcohol consumption patterns as well as aggressive alcohol expectancies held by the women.

2.3.3. Family History. The results of research examining gender differences in aggressive alcohol expectancies do not preclude the possibility that intoxication–aggression and victimization effects for men and women are at least partially attributable to histories of victimization. Thus, the cultural origins of aggressive alcohol expectancies, normative approval of violence toward women, and aggressive behavior may be rooted in the family. We[20] developed a model of the socialization processes underlying alcohol-related wife assaults. Based on our evaluation of that model, we concluded that men who were abused by their parents or who witnessed violence between their parents as children are, as adults, more likely to approve of aggression against wives as well as more likely to drink heavily. As a result of their heavier drinking and beliefs regarding the appropriateness of spousal violence, men have stronger expectancies concerning the aggressive consequences of alcohol and, in turn, engage in more assaults on wives. Men who grew up with alcohol-abusing parents, although not necessarily heavier drinkers, expected alcohol use to engender violence and were themselves more likely to assault their wives. Family history of alcohol problems indirectly affected wife assaults in the next generation through their effects on aggressive expectancies. Overall, our results indicated that violent socialization in the family of origin exerts stronger effects on current intrafamily violence than does a family history of heavy drinking. Our findings suggested that heavy alcohol consumption and cognitions concerning the effects of alcohol consumption on aggression represent a major pathway through which intrafamilial violence is transmitted across generations.

Exposure to childhood abuse or marital violence in the family of origin may similarly increase women's risks of victimizations as it does for men. For example, assaulted women have at least double the rate of growing up in a violent home compared to nonassaulted women.[8] However, O'Leary[35] suggests that this relationship is less consistent for women compared to men. Where intergenerational effects exist, the mechanism may be that repeated attacks by parents can lead to damaged self-esteem and suppression of rage. These effects may be manifested differentially by gender and compounded by the current life situation. Women who were harshly punished in childhood or who witnessed parental violence are more likely to be victimized as adults because they have low self-esteem and have learned that assaults from a loved one are legitimate, or because they are more likely to engage in mutual assaults with their spouses.[60] Additionally, because alcoholism and family violence are so intertwined, both women and men exposed to violence at home also may have suffered the effects of parental alcoholism.[61] Widom's[61] review of the literature on child abuse and alcohol use concludes that while studies of female alcoholics indicate a higher incidence of child abuse history, the literature is inconsistent and methodologically flawed. There may also be effects of a family history of parental alcoholism on women's future choice of partners. For example, if daughters of alcoholics are more likely to marry alcoholics,[62] then they may also be at risk for intoxication–victimization effects via this assortative mating process.

2.3.4. Personality. Powers and Kutash[47] have emphasized the contributions of premorbid personality characteristics and the interaction between substance abuse and personality as central to substance-abuse-related aggression. They view the personality characteristics of the abuser as the primary problem, independent of the behavior of the partner. Research on maritally violent men also suggests that psychopathology and personality disorders are present among some subtypes of batterers.[29] Literature based on clinical and criminal justice samples of alcoholics or assaultive men also suggests that aggressive drinking patterns may be a reflection of the concurrence of antisocial personality disorders with alcoholism.[63,64] However, research based on community samples indicates that husband's alcohol use remains significantly related to assaults on wives even after controlling for measures of hostility, self-consciousness, and other sociodemographic risk factors.[4,40]

In sum, the diversity of opinion on personality issues is most likely due to the variability found in different types of samples. Clinical samples of battered men in treatment may differ from criminal justice samples, alcoholics in treatment, or men from community samples.

There is little research examining the contribution of women's personality disorders to their own victimization. Researchers have concluded that abusive men's characteristics are the appropriate area of inquiry.[37] However, because studies do find high rates of assaults among alcoholic women, we need to consider the possibility that personality factors among such women may play a role in the dynamics of victimization. For example, clinical data on alcoholics in treatment show that depression and low self-esteem are common among alcoholic women.[65,66] Such symptomatology may perpetuate or exacerbate marital disharmony by producing resentment and rejection on the part of the nondepressed spouse, or by serving as justification for the assaults of an abusive mate. It is also just as likely that poor self-esteem and depression are reciprocally related and worsened by the denigration and physical abuse of a partner.

2.3.5. Social Dynamics. Drinking patterns of husbands and wives tend to be highly similar.[67] It is not surprising then that a married alcoholic has a high probability of having an alcoholic partner.[68] As suggested above, assaults are more common in relationships where both partners are heavy drinkers.[59]

Furthermore, alcoholic women may be more verbally or physically aggressive toward a partner.[69] However, we also need to consider the social dynamics of relationships where only one partner (usually the male) is a heavy drinker. Conflicts may ensue over any number of issues, including the partner's drinking or drug problems. Additionally, the partner's violent acts may be unpredictable or inconsistent with episodes of intoxication.

Powers and Kutash[47] suggest that nondrinking partners may resent drinking episodes and become less nurturant and sympathetic, which, in turn, increases the abuser/drinker's rage. They allege that this dynamic is especially true in the case of the drinker with high dependency needs, who experiences frustration in response to his perception of a nonempathic partner. Some support for this description of the social dynamics of alcohol-related conflicts is found in the experimental literature as well. For example, Jacob, Ritchey, Cvitkovic, and Blane[70] report greater negativity of alcoholic couples (more disagreements by wives) on "drink night" compared to normal couples. But there may also be differences in communication patterns, depending on the drinking pattern of the husband. When binge and steady drinkers were compared, binge drinkers were found to have more negative communications when drinking, while steady drinkers had more positive communications when drinking during the experimental manipulation. Such effects may occur because partners adapt or become habituated to steady drinking behaviors or because binge drinkers may themselves have other characteristics such as greater aggressiveness that are confounded with drinking. Additionally, chronic alcohol use can create economic stresses on the family such as unemployment, which increase family conflict and the likelihood of abuse.[41] Finally, alcohol may be used to excuse the violence by the husband or wife, or by both partners.

3. How Common Is Drinking by Both Parties?

Evidence for drinking by both parties or the association of female intoxication with victimization is most apparent in studies of homicide and rape victims. Wolfgang's[71] classic study of victim-precipitated homicide carefully defines this category as one in which the victim was the first to use physical force or display a weapon. He found that alcohol was present in almost two thirds of the cases. In forty-four percent of those cases, both victim and offender were drinking. However, all of the case illustrations Wolfgang provides of victim precipitation in families are instances where the victim is a male batterer killed by his beaten wife. More recent research on the alcohol–homicide relationship indicates that between one third and two thirds of victims had positive blood alcohol levels. Consistent with the greater prevalence of heavier drinking by males, the majority of epidemiological data shows that intoxication is more common among male homicide victims compared to female homicide victims.[72–74]

Murdoch, Pihl, and Ross[75] reviewed 19 studies of homicides and 7 studies of assaults to determine who was drinking during crimes of violence. Our reinterpretation of the data presented by these authors indicates that more than half of all homicide offenders were drinking in 13 of 19 studies. It was rare for findings on victim intoxication to parallel those for offenders. For example, more than half of all victims were drinking in only 3 of the 19 homicide studies reviewed. Of the seven assault studies reviewed, more than half of all offenders were drinking in three of the seven studies, but in no cases were more than half of the victim group drinking. It should also be noted that in three of the seven assault studies the incidence of victim drinking ranged from 25 to 40% of all victims. These authors[75] conclude that the instigator of the attack is more likely to be intoxicated, but the victim is "as likely as the offender to initiate the altercation by attacking or moving in a way that can be interpreted as an attack" (p. 1070). However, gender issues are blurred in this analysis, and the fact that intoxication can distort perceptions of threat and provocation needs to be considered.

Data provided by rape victims indicate that 40% report drinking or intoxication prior to their rape.[76] Roizen's[77] analysis of data on arrested populations finds considerable variability regarding alcohol involvement by perpetrators or victims in rape cases. Roizen rejects the concept of "victim precipitation" relevant to crimes of rape, noting that intoxication is responsible for the misreading of cues by victim and offender. Women's greater vulnerability to rape when intoxicated may also occur because they are less able to escape undesirable or dangerous situations. Her comments regarding the potential mechanisms involved in the association between alcohol and rape are also relevant to alcohol's role in wife-assault victimizations. She notes the following:

> Thus drinking in rape, as in other crimes, may play any one of a number of different roles: It may be present but have no effect; it may enhance chances of victimization when the parties are strangers; it can be present in the offender alone and exert an effect only on the offender, such as misreading social cues in relation to prevailing norms; or it may begin an evening gathering of a group of men that ends in drunkenness and rape. (p. 17)

4. Empirical Studies of Wife Assault and Intoxication by Female Victims

Empirical evidence supporting an association between women's intoxication and physical assaults by husbands is mixed. In one early review of the risk markers for husband-to-wife assaults, Hotaling and Sugarman[37] examined existing case-control research on women's drug use and alcohol consumption. Drug use was declared an "inconsistent risk marker," bearing a significant relation to husband-to-wife violence in 60% of the studies reviewed. Nevertheless, the fact that three of the five studies of drug use by wives did find an association with wife abuse suggests that drug use may put women at risk of being a victim of spouse abuse. In contrast, alcohol consumption by wives was related to violence in only 17% (1 of 6) of the studies reviewed. As such, Hotaling and Sugarman concluded that women's use of alcohol does not aid in the prediction of spousal assaults and should be considered a "consistent nonrisk marker."

4.1. Evidence from General Population Surveys

Since the publication of the aforementioned review, other investigations have obtained somewhat stronger support for an intoxication–victimization effect. Based on data from the 1985 National Family Violence Survey (NFVS), Kaufman Kantor and Straus[8] found that female respondents who reported minor physical assaults by husbands during the survey year were more than three times as likely as nonvictims to have been high on drugs during the preceding year and more than twice as likely to have been drunk at least once. In addition, any prior year, drunkenness was three times as likely among victims of severe assaults compared to nonvictims and rates of drug intoxication were six times higher among the former. It should be emphasized, however, that the measures used by Kaufman Kantor and Straus[8] were limited. They only assessed the use of any prior year illicit drug use and any episodes of drunkenness by the husband or the wife.

The National Alcohol and Family Violence Survey (NAFVS)[31] also examined questions concerning substance abuse–aggression and –victimization relationships. One of the parallel purposes for both survey years (1985 and 1992) was to consider whether substance abuse by the wife or husband contributed to assaults on wives. In 1992, Kaufman Kantor and Jasinski[78] examined this association using much more precise measures of alcohol and other drug use, yet found similar results. Wives' substance abuse showed similarly strong bivariate associations to husband-to-wife violence in Kaufman Kantor and Jasinski's[78] analysis of the 1992 NAFVS. That analysis examined relations between husband-to-wife violence and both husband's and wife's use of alcohol and other illicit drugs.

As shown in Fig. 1, rates of wife assault were between two and six times higher among women who abused alcohol and/or drugs in the previous year than among women who reported no substance abuse. The highest rates of victimization were observed among women who either used both alcohol and marijuana or marijuana only. However, because relatively few women reported abusing alcohol or other drugs, some caution is needed regarding the reliability of these results. Indeed, the higher frequency of substance abuse among men may be responsible for the somewhat stronger role of husband's substance abuse in wife assaults apparent in Fig. 1. The results of the bivariate analyses for men indicate that multiple drug use patterns, i.e., the combined

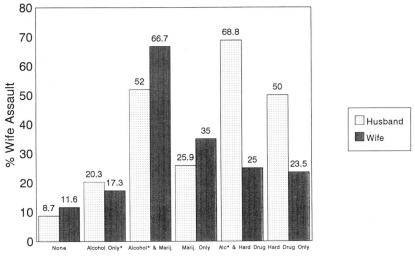

Figure 1. Rates of wife assault as a function of husband's and wife's substance use patterns.

pattern of alcohol and marijuana use and use of alcohol and hard drugs are associated with the highest rates of assaults against women.

Although impressive, the bivariate data reviewed above paints only an incomplete picture of intoxication–victimization effects in the general population. In Kaufman Kantor and Straus'[8] multivariate analysis of NFVS data, neither wife's drinking nor drug use were significantly related to severe assaults (a low-base-rate phenomenon in general population samples). However, past-year drinking and drug use by the wife did predict minor physical assaults, after controlling for husband drinking and drug use and other sociodemographic risk factors as covariates in the prediction of husband-to-wife violence. Kaufman Kantor and Jasinski[79] failed to show significant effects of wife's alcohol use on husband-to-wife violence when tested along with a similar set of covariates (see Table I).

Table I summarizes the results of comparable multivariate analyses across surveys. In 1985, the most significant predictors were husband's illicit drug use, drunkenness by husband and wife, low income, violence in the family of origin, and normative approval of violence. In 1992, the results of multivariate analysis showed that husband's illicit drug use and heavy drinking again strongly predicted wife assaults, as did family of origin violence,

Table I. Substance Abuse & Wife Assault: Significant Predictors

1985 NFVS	1992 NAFVS
Husband illicit drug use 1 or $>X$	Husband illicit drug use 1 or $>X$
Wife drunk 1 or $>X$	Problem drinking husband
Husband drunk 1 or $>X$	Wife marijuana use
Low income	Youth
Family of origin violence	Family of origin violence
Violence approval	Violence approval
	Unemployment

violence approval, youth, and unemployment. Heavy drinking by the wife did not emerge as a significant predictor.

Additional analyses of the 1992 survey data examined models of specific types of substance abuse, while controlling for important sociodemographic risk factors. The results of these analyses suggested that past-year usage of illicit hard drugs (e.g., nonprescription amphetamines, barbiturates, tranquilizers, cocaine, and heroin) by the husband and marijuana use by the wife significantly increased the odds of wife assault, net of other risk factors in the models.

4.1.1. Drinking at the Time of Wife Assault. Moreover, it is important to emphasize that the measures used by both Kaufman Kantor and Straus[8] and Kaufman Kantor and Jasinski[79] assessed prior-year drug and alcohol use rather than usage in relation to specific events, such as assaults by husbands. Given the omission of data on the temporal ordering of women's intoxication and their victimizations, no conclusions can be made about the precise role of women's intoxication in the etiology of husband-to-wife violence. When data on drinking at the time of wife assaults has been assessed, women are much less likely than men to report intoxication during violent episodes. As shown in Table II, only 10% of all wife assaults reported in the 1985 NFVS involved drinking by wives compared to the 22% that involved drinking by husbands. Likewise, wives were drinking in only 8% of the violent episodes reported in the 1992 NAFVS in contrast to 28% of those episodes in which husbands were drinking. Thus, at least part of the association between wife's intoxication patterns and histories of victimization may involve postabuse drinking or drinking unrelated to the specific episodes of assault. Overall, it is rare for women to be the sole substance abuser in intimate relationships, while this is not uncommon among husbands. The results show that drinking by the woman at the time of violence is uncommon among abused women in general population samples.

4.1.2. Drug Use at the Time of Wife Assault. One strength of the 1992 study is that data were collected on the use of drugs other than alcohol at the time of

Table II. Drinking at the Time of Violence

	1985 NFVS	1992 NAFVS
Neither drinking	76%	71%
Husband only drinking	14%	22%
Wife only drinking	2%	2%
Both drinking	8%	6%

assaults on wives. We found that alcohol is the drug most commonly associated with intoxicated aggression. Other drug use at the time of violence occurred in only 5% of all families and more often in conjunction with alcohol. Although wives infrequently used alcohol at the time of their victimizations, those who did so were significantly more likely than nondrinking abused women to be using other drugs at the time of assault.

Leonard and Senchak[80] obtained similar results to those of the two national surveys discussed above when they examined the relationship between heavy drinking among newly married women and levels of premarital aggression by husbands. At the bivariate level, frequent excessive drinking by wives was modestly correlated with husband's use of minor violence prior to marriage, as was husband's excessive use of alcohol. When the overlap between husband and wife alcohol abuse was disentangled in multivariate analyses, women's drinking no longer predicted husband-to-wife violence. As with the analyses by Kaufman Kantor and Jasinski,[79] these findings suggest that the confounding of husband and wife intoxication might underlie the apparent effects of drug or alcohol use among female victims of domestic violence.

4.2. Evidence from Clinical Populations

Unlike the analyses based on data from the two national probability surveys, most intoxication–victimization research has been conducted with clinical samples of heavy-drinking and/or battered women. For example, Frieze and Schafer's[52] report of a study of battered women suggests that alcohol use by either partner is related to marital violence in varying ways. In a primary group of families identified by factor analysis, both husband and wife were frequently intoxicated and marital violence was consistently associated with drinking. In other families, drinking was less consistently associated with fighting. Based on their sample of battered women, these authors conclude that high levels of violence in both husband and wife are more likely in families where the husband has the drinking problem and the wife does not.

Miller, Downs, and Gondoli[81] compared rates of spousal assault among women in treatment for alcoholism and nonalcoholic women in the general population. Reports of both minor and severe physical assaults were higher among alcoholic women, and husband-to-wife violence was a highly significant predictor of female alcoholism in multivariate analyses that controlled for husband drinking and family of origin alcoholism and childhood physical abuse. Miller and associates, however, did not report whether female alcoholism aided in the prediction of spousal victimization after controlling for its overlap with family of origin dysfunction and husband's alcohol problems.

Miller, Downs, Testa, and Panek[82] extended the above analysis by comparing the female alcoholics to groups of nonalcoholic women sampled from battered women's shelters, mental health centers, driving while intoxicated classes, and the general population. The alcoholics reported higher levels and more frequent verbal and physical aggression than all other groups except shelter women, who obtained the highest scores on all violence measures. Alcoholism, however, did predict high-frequency verbal and physical assaults by husbands after controlling for group differences in sociodemographic characteristics and mental health symptomatology. The results of these multivariate analyses, although more informative than the bivariate findings, are not entirely conclusive because they fail to consider the overlap between women's alcohol abuse and that of husbands.

Additional findings from Miller and associates[82] suggest that the severity of a woman's alcohol abuse may explain why intoxication–victimization effects are obtained in some investigations but not others. They failed to find a difference in husband-to-wife verbal and physical aggression between alcohol-abusing women in the mental health and shelter groups (who had been excluded from the primary analyses) and their nonabusing counterparts. It is possible that the alcohol problems of these women were not as advanced as those among the alcohol-treatment women. If so, it may be that heavy drinking is not as strong of a risk factor for spousal assaults than is the clinical syndrome of alcoholism. Such an explanation would be consistent with the tendency of researchers to observe intoxication–victimization effects in clinical samples but not in community samples.[80]

Using a different sample, Bergman, Larsson, Brismar, and Klang[83] compared the victimization experiences of hospitalized female alcoholics to those of women seeking treatment for either spousal assaults or medical conditions unrelated to domestic violence. Compared to the medical control group, alcoholics were more likely to have been battered at least once and to have had multiple experiences of battering. Moreover, assault victims in the alcoholic group were more likely than victims in both the medical control and battered group to have suffered assault-related injuries severe enough to necessitate medical treatment. In a supplementary analysis, Bergman and associates also found rates of alcohol dependency to be three times as high among women in treatment for spousal assaults than among women in treatment for medical conditions. However, it should also be noted that 70% of the women in the alcoholic and spousal assault groups had husbands who abused alcohol compared to only 14% of the husbands in the medical control group. Thus, it is unclear whether the association between alcohol abuse and victimization observed in this investigation is due to women's drinking or that of husbands.

In addition to comparing rates of wife assault among alcoholic and non-alcoholic women, researchers have also assessed levels of alcohol and/or drug use among couples in violent and nonviolent relationships. This approach was used by Barnett and Fagan,[84] who asked four groups of men to report on their own and their wife's typical pattern of drinking. Two groups included physically abusive husbands who either were or were not in treatment for wife battering. The remaining groups included maritally discordant but non-abusive husbands and maritally satisfied husbands.

Compared to the self- and partner-reports provided by men in both non-abusive groups, quantity of alcohol consumption was higher among both maritally violent men and their wives. Moreover, when asked about drinking context, violent men revealed that they were significantly more likely than their abused wives to be drinking during a violent episode. In contrast, post-abuse drinking by wives was much more common than postabuse drinking by husbands. These findings are consistent with Kaufman Kantor and Straus'[2] report that drinking at the time of husband-to-wife violence is more common among men than among women.

5. Conclusions

5.1. The Role of Women's Intoxication in Husband-to-Wife Violence

The evidence reviewed above, although suggestive of an association between women's intoxication and assaults by husbands, does not clearly indicate the nature or direction of that association. The findings, however, can be used to evaluate which of several mechanisms might underlie such an association.

5.1.1. Women's Intoxication Provokes Assaults by Husbands. Perhaps the most frequently espoused hypothesis is that drinking or drug use by women can incite their male partners to behave violently. Such attacks are presumed to stem from men's anger at their intoxicated women's violation of gender role prescriptions against female drunkenness.[8] In a similar vein, it has also been suggested that assaults on drunken wives might be precipitated by an increase in verbal aggression that often accompanies female intoxication.[59]

Support for this hypothesis is weak, if not nonexistent, because the temporal precedence of women's drinking has not been established in any intoxication–victimization investigation that we have reviewed. Most research either reports correlational data on women's typical usage patterns over a specified referent period and their victimization experiences during the same time period[8,84] or examines the relation between current alcohol status and victimization history.[81–83] When drinking at the time of the violence has been specifically assessed,[2,59,79,84] intoxication is much more common among husbands than it is among wives. Thus, as frequently as the above hypothesis is advanced, there is little evidence from the empirical literature that women's drinking provokes or even precedes aggression by husbands.

However, much of the empirical literature that specifically examines issues of temporal precedence is based on general population samples in which problem-drinking women are a low-base-rate phenomenon. Research examining clinical samples of alcoholic women does suggest that such women have high rates of victimization over multiple relationships. Such victimizations appear to be more a function of their partner's drinking and propensity to violent behavior. However, the empirical literature has rarely attended to specific motivations for assaults on wives. There is evidence that cultural norms about the appropriateness of hitting wives are associated with wife assaults. Similarly, the likelihood of victimizations may also be influenced and perpetuated by societal beliefs that denigrate alcoholic women, as well as the low self-esteem and depression characteristic of many alcoholic women. These processes may operate independently of whether the woman is consuming alcohol or other drugs at the time of an assault. Among couples where both are intoxicated at the time of a conflict situation, there is, at minimum, theoretical evidence that the psychopharmacological effects of intoxication can increase cognitive distortions, which escalate aggressive behavior in men and women. However, theory development and empirical testing are needed in regard to understanding the social dynamics of alcohol-related interactions.

5.1.2. Women's Intoxication Is a Consequence of Victimization. An alternative explanation for the intoxication–victimization relation is that women drink or use drugs as a means of coping with a violent partner. As mentioned previously, Barnett and Fagan[84] reported that postviolence drinking was more common than drinking prior to and/or during a violent incident among the wives of assaultive men. This explanation is also consistent with another body of literature showing that battered women are at particular risk for depressive symptomatology,[85,86] and thus may use alcohol and/or drugs to self-medicate their dysphoria. Analysis of hospital record data in one study revealed greater problem drug use for battered women treated for injuries than for nonbattered women.[87] This suggests that at minimum, among the subpopulation of the most severely battered and injured women seeking help, that substance abuse may be a means of coping with victimization or it may be a correlate of family life where there is limited commitment to conventional behaviors.

5.1.3. Women's Intoxication Is Indirectly Related to Victimization via Husband's Intoxication. A large body of literature has established that drinking by husbands increases a woman's risk for physical assault.[2,4,8,15,40,41,88] In addition, it is also well documented that the substance abuse patterns of wives are highly correlated with those of their husbands. Women's intoxication might then be spuriously associated with victimization through its association with husband's intoxication. Recall that the strong bivariate associations that Kaufman Kantor and Straus[8] observed between women's drinking/drug use and victimization were either eliminated or substantially weakened in multivariate analyses that statistically controlled for husband's drinking and drug use. A comparison of the bivariate and multivariate results reported by Leonard and Senchak[80] showed the identical pattern. Moreover, the strongest evidence of an intoxication–victimization effect has come from studies that failed to control for husband drinking.[82,83] Unequivocal support for a direct role of women's drinking in spousal assaults can only come from analyses that disentangle the overlap between husband and wife intoxication.

5.1.4. Women's Intoxication Is Indirectly Related to Victimization via Family of Origin Abuse. Intoxication–victimization effects might also be observed because both excess drinking among women and spousal victimization have common roots in childhood experiences of physical and sexual victimization. A host of studies[8,34,36,89] have demonstrated that victimization in one generation is often repeated in the next generation, such that childhood abuse at the hands of parents or the witnessing of parental violence significantly increases a woman's risk of spousal violence in adulthood. In addition, evidence from a number of investigations[90,91] indicates that female alcoholics experienced higher levels of verbal and physical aggression (particularly at the hands of fathers) than did nonalcoholic women. The common effects of violence in the family of origin could thus produce significant, albeit noncausal, relationships between wife's drinking and victimization by husbands.

In sum, the evidence for intoxication–victimization effects are strongest among studies of rape, homicide, and studies of alcoholic women. We conclude that the theoretical basis for intoxication–victimization effects is best exemplified in situations in which both partners are heavy drinkers and where the social dynamics of situations are taken into account. We also conclude that, in reality, women are less often intoxicated than their partner at the time of an assaultive episode. Despite the strength of alcohol's association with wife assaults, intoxication's centrality and temporal relationship to specific wife assault episodes is highly variable, regardless of whether it is a component of the husband's or wife's behavior.

Among alcoholic women, risks for victimization are greater for a number of reasons, including their violation of traditional female societal norms that stigmatize alcoholism in women more so than in men.[11] They are also at risk due to their increased use of aggression[59] and because they are more likely to have a heavy-drinking male partner. Finally, women drinking to intoxication are at risk because they are more likely to have a history of victimization in their family of origin. They may bring a low sense of self to the relationship that reinforces beliefs that they deserved to be beaten owing to their drunkenness, aggression, or unworthiness. Often, abusive men will instill or reinforce such beliefs by their own accusations and behaviors toward the woman. Women growing up in a violent home are also more likely to consider violent modes of conflict resolution as a "normal" part of intimate behavior. Outreach efforts to alcoholic women are important because women who believe they provoked the violence or were responsible for the violence may perpetuate these patterns by avoidance of help-seeking due to guilt, shame, or even denial that they have been battered. Unfortunately, similar mechanisms of denial and minimization exist for both alcoholism and battering. Treatment providers must also address the complex mechanisms of intoxication–victimization and aggression processes, rather than emphasizing simple justification explanations (e.g., drunkenness as a means of excusing the violence) or explanations of intentionality (e.g., men drink in order to beat their wives) as a means of reducing wife assaults.

ACKNOWLEDGMENTS. The research reported here was supported by research grant No. RO1AA09070 from the National Institute on Alcohol Abuse and Alcoholism. We are grateful to Kelly Foster for her assistance in manuscript preparation.

References

1. Bushman BJ, Cooper HM: Effects of alcohol on human aggression: An integrative research review. *Psychol Bull* 107(3):341–354, 1990.
2. Kaufman Kantor G, Straus MA: The "drunken bum" theory of wife beating. *Soc Prob* 34(3):213–230, 1987.
3. Lang AR, Goeckner DJ, Adesso VJ, Marlatt GA: Effects of alcohol on aggression in male social drinkers. *J Abnorm Psychol* 84:508–518, 1975.
4. Leonard KE, Bromet EJ, Parkinson DK, *et al:* Patterns of alcohol use and physically aggressive behavior in men. *J Stud Alcohol* 46(4):279–282, 1985.
5. Taylor SP, Gammon CB: Effects of type and dose of alcohol on human physical aggression. *J Personal Soc Psychol* 32(1):169–175, 1975.
6. Taylor SP, Gammon CB, Capasso DR: Aggression as a function of the interaction of alcohol and threat. *J Personal Soc Psychol* 34:938–941, 1976.
7. Taylor SP: Experimental investigation of alcohol-induced aggression in humans. *Alcohol Health Res World* 17(2):108–112, 1993.
8. Kaufman Kantor G, Straus MA: Substance abuse as a precipitant of wife abuse victimizations. *Am J Drug Alcohol Abuse* 15(2):173–189, 1989.
9. Young DM, Beier EG, Beier P, Barton C: Is chivalry dead? *J Commun* 28:57–64, 1975.
10. Frodi A, Macaulay J, Thome PR: Are women always less aggressive than men? *Psychol Bull* 84:634–660, 1977.
11. Sandmaier M: *The Invisible Alcoholics: Women and Alcohol Abuse in America.* New York, McGraw-Hill, 1980.
12. Goodchilds JD, Zellman GL: Sexual signaling and sexual aggression in adolescent relationships, in Malamuth NM, Donnerstein E (eds): *Pornography and Sexual Aggression.* Orlando, FL, Academic Press, 1984, pp 233–243.
13. Koss MP, Dinero TE: Discriminant analysis of risk factors for sexual victimization among a national sample of college women. *J Consult Clin Psychol* 57:242–250, 1989.
14. Taylor SP, Leonard KE: Alcohol and human physical aggression, in Geen RG, Donnerstein EI (eds): *Aggression: Theoretical and Empirical Reviews,* vol 2, *Issues in Research.* New York, Academic Press, 1983, pp 77–101.
15. Leonard KE: Alcohol consumption and escalatory aggression in intoxicated and sober dyads. *J Stud Alcohol* 45:75–80, 1984.
16. Leonard KE: Drinking patterns and intoxication in marital violence: Review, critique, and

future directions for research, in National Institute on Alcohol Abuse and Alcoholism Research Monograph-24 (ed): *Alcohol and Interpersonal Violence: Fostering Multidisciplinary Perspectives*. NIH Publication No. 93-3496. Rockville, MD, NIAAA, pp 253–280.

17. Miller BA, Downs WR: The impact of family violence on the use of alcohol by women. *Alcohol Health Res World* 17(2):137–143, 1993.

18. Miller BA, Downs WR, Testa M: Relationship between women's alcohol problems and experiences of childhood violence. Paper presented at the annual convention of the American Psychological Association, Boston, MA, 1990.

19. Fagan J: Set and setting revisited: Influences of alcohol and illicit drugs on the social context of violent events, in National Institute on Alcohol Abuse and Alcoholism Research Monograph-24 (ed): *Alcohol and Interpersonal Violence: Fostering Multidisciplinary Perspectives*. NIH Publication No. 93-3496. Rockville, MD, NIAAA, 1993, pp 161–191.

20. Kaufman Kantor G, Asdigian N: Socialization to alcohol-related family violence: Disentangling the effects of family history on current violence. Paper presented at the Annual Meetings of the American Society of Criminology, Phoenix, AZ, 1993.

21. Pernanen K: Theoretical aspects of the relationship between alcohol and crime, in Collins JJ (ed): *Drinking and Crime: Perspectives on the Relationship between Alcohol and Consumption and Criminal Behavior*. New York, Guilford Press, 1981, pp 1–69.

22. Pernanen K: *Alcohol and Human Violence*. New York, Guilford Press, 1991.

23. Pernanen K: Research approaches in the study of alcohol-related violence. *Alcohol Health Res World* 17(2):101–107, 1993.

24. Bersani CA, Chen H: Sociological perspectives in family violence, in Van Hasselt VB, Morrison RL, Bellack AS, Hersen M (eds): *Handbook of Family Violence*. New York, Plenum Press, 1988, pp 57–86.

25. Gelles RJ, Straus MA: Determinants of violence in the family: Towards a theoretical integration, in Burr WR, Hill R, Nye FI, Reiss IL (eds): *Contemporary Theories About the Family*. New York, Free Press, 1979, chap 21.

26. Hamburger LK, Hastings JE: Personality correlates of men who abuse their partners: A cross validation study. *J Fam Viol* 1(4):323–341, 1986.

27. Hudson WW, McIntosh SR: The assessment of spouse abuse: Two quantifiable dimensions. *J Marriage Fam* 43:873–885, 1981.

28. Roy M: A current study of 150 cases, in Roy M (ed): *Battered Women: A Psychosocial Study of Domestic Violence*. New York, Van Nostrand Reinhold, 1977, pp 25–44.

29. Holtzworth-Munroe A, Stuart GL: Typologies of male batterers: Three subtypes and the differences among them. *Psychol Bull* 116:476–497, 1994.

30. Straus MA: A general systems theory approach to a theory of violence between family members. *Soc Sci Info* 12:105–125, 1973.

31. Kaufman Kantor G, Jasinski JL, Aldarondo E: Socioeconomic status and incidence of marital violence in Hispanic families. *Violence Vict* 9(3):207–222, 1994.

32. Pagelow MD: *Family Violence*. New York, Praeger, 1984.

33. Yllo KA, Straus MA: Patriarchy and violence against wives: The impact of structural and normative factors. *J Int Comp Soc Welf* 1:16–29, 1984.

34. Kalmus D: The intergenerational transmission of marital aggression. *J Marriage Fam* 46:11–19, 1984.

35. O'Leary KD: Physical aggression between spouses: A social learning theory perspective, in Van Hasselt VB, Morrison RL, Bellack AS, Hersen M (eds): *The Handbook of Family Violence*. New York, Plenum Press, 1988, pp 31–56.

36. Straus MA, Gelles RJ, Steinmetz SK: *Behind Closed Doors: Violence in the American Family*. Newbury Park, CA, Sage, 1980.

37. Hotaling G, Sugarman D: An analysis of risk markers in husband to wife violence: The current state of knowledge. *Violence Vict* 1(2):101–124, 1986.

38. Dobash RE, Dobash RP: Wives: The appropriate victims of marital violence. *Victimology* 1:416–441, 1978.

39. LaRossa R: And we haven't had any problems since: Conjugal violence and the politics of marriage, in Straus MA, Hotaling GT (eds): *The Social Causes of Husband–Wife Violence*. Minneapolis, University of Minnesota Press, 1980, pp 157–175.
40. Leonard KE, Blane HT: Alcohol and marital aggression in a national sample of young men. *J Interpers Violence* 7(1):19–30, 1992.
41. Leonard KE, Jacob T: Alcohol, alcoholism, and family violence, in Van Hasselt VB, Morrison RL, Bellack AS, Hersen M (eds): *Handbook of Family Violence*. New York, Plenum Press, 1988, pp 383–406.
42. Kaufman Kantor G: Parental drinking, violence and child aggression. Paper presented at the American Psychological Association Annual Meetings: Mini-Conference on Substance Abuse and Violence, Boston, 1990.
43. Fagan J: Intoxication and aggression, in Tonry M, Wilson JQ (eds): *Drugs and Crime*. Chicago, University of Chicago Press, 1990, pp 241–320.
44. Gustafson R: Threat as a determinant of alcohol-related aggression. *Psychol Rep* 58:287–297, 1986.
45. Pihl RO, Zeichner A, Niuara R, *et al:* Attribution and alcohol-mediated aggression. *J Abnorm Psychol* 90(5):468–475, 1981.
46. Schmutte GT, Leonard KE, Taylor SP: Alcohol and expectation of attack. *Psychol Rep* 45:163–167, 1979.
47. Powers RJ, Kutash IL: Alcohol, drugs, and partner abuse, in Roy M (ed): *The Abusive Partner*. New York, Van Nostrand Reinhold, 1982, pp 39–75.
48. Zeichner A, Pihl RO: Effects of alcohol and behavior contingencies on human aggression. *J Abnorm Psychol* 88:153–160, 1979.
49. Goldstein PJ, Belluci PA, Spunt BJ, Miller T: *Frequency of Cocaine Use and Violence: A Comparison between Men and Women*. Unpublished, New York, Narcotic and Drug Research, 1988.
50. Taylor SP, Chermack ST: Alcohol, drugs and human physical aggression. *J Stud Alcohol* 11:78–88, 1993.
51. Pihl RO, Peterson JB, Lau MA: A biosocial model of the alcohol–aggression relationship. *J Stud Alcohol* 11:128–139, 1993.
52. Frieze IH, Schafer PC: Alcohol use and marital violence: Female and male differences in reactions to alcohol, in Wilsnack SC, Beckman LJ (eds): *Alcohol Problems in Women*. New York, Guilford Press, 1984, pp 260–279.
53. Critchlow-Leigh BC: The powers of John Barleycorn: Beliefs about the effects of alcohol on social behavior. *Am Psychol* 41(7):751–764, 1986.
54. Critchlow-Leigh BC: Beliefs about the effects of alcohol on self and others. *J Stud Alcohol* 48(5):467–475, 1987.
55. Brown SA, Goldman MS, Inn A, Anderson LR: Expectations of reinforcement from alcohol: Their domain and relation to drinking patterns. *J Consult Clin Psychol* 48:419–426, 1980.
56. Rohsenhow DJ: Drinking habits and expectancies about alcohol's effects for self versus others. *J Consult Clin Psychol* 51(5):752–756, 1983.
57. Rohsenhow DJ, Bachorowski JA: Effects of alcohol and expectancies on verbal aggression in men and women. *J Abnorm Psychol* 93:418–432, 1984.
58. Kline RB: The relation of alcohol expectancies to drinking patterns among alcoholics: Generalization across gender and race. *J Stud Alcohol* 51:175–182, 1990.
59. Kaufman Kantor G, Asdigian N: Gender differences in alcohol-related spousal aggression, in Wilsnack RW, Wilsnack SC (eds): *Gender and Alcohol*. New Brunswick, NJ: Rutgers University Press, 1995, in press.
60. Straus MA, Kaufman Kantor G: Corporal punishment of adolescents by parents: A risk factor in the epidemiology of depression, suicide, alcohol abuse, child abuse, and wife beating. *Adolescence* 29(115):543–562, 1994.
61. Widom CS: Child abuse and alcohol use and abuse, in National Institute on Alcohol Abuse and Alcoholism Research Monograph-24 (ed): *Alcohol and Interpersonal Violence: Fostering Multidisciplinary Perspectives*. NIH Publication No. 93-3496. Rockville, MD, 1993, pp 291–314.

62. Schuckit MA, Tipp JE, Kelner E: Are daughters of alcoholics more likely to marry alcoholics? *Am J Drug Alcohol Abuse* 20(2):237–245, 1994.
63. Abram KM, Teplin LA, McClelland GM: The effects of co-occurring disorders on the relationship between alcoholism and violent crime: A 3-year followup of male jail detainees, in National Institute on Alcohol Abuse and Alcoholism Research Monograph-24 (ed): *Alcohol and Interpersonal Violence: Fostering Multidisciplinary Perspectives.* NIH Publication No. 93-3496. Rockville, MD, 1993, pp 237–251.
64. Collins JJ: Drinking and violence: An individual offender focus, in National Institute on Alcohol Abuse and Alcoholism Research Monograph-24 (ed): *Alcohol and Interpersonal Violence: Fostering Multidisciplinary Perspectives.* NIH Publication No. 93-3496. Rockville, MD, 1993, pp 221–235.
65. Kaufman E: *Psychotherapy of Addicted Persons.* New York, Guilford Press, 1994.
66. Wilsnack SC: Patterns and trends in women's drinking: Recent findings and some implications for prevention. Paper presented to the Working Group for Prevention Research on Women and Alcohol, Bethesda, MD, 1993.
67. Wilsnack RW, Wilsnack SC: Husbands and wives as drinking partners. Paper presented at the 16th Annual Alcohol Epidemiology Symposium of the Kettil Bruun Society for Social and Epidemiological Research on Alcohol, Budapest, Hungary, 1990.
68. Jacob T, Bremer DA: Assortative mating among men and women alcoholics. *J Stud Alcohol* 47:219–222, 1986.
69. Miller BA, Downs WR, Testa M, Keil A: Thematic analyses of severe spousal violence incidents: Women's perceptions of their victimization. Paper presented at the Annual Meeting of the American Society of Criminology, San Francisco, CA, 1991.
70. Jacob T, Ritchey D, Cvitkovic J, Blane H: Communication styles of alcoholic and nonalcoholic families when drinking and not drinking. *J Stud Alcohol* 42:466–482, 1981.
71. Wolfgang ME: *Patterns in Criminal Homicide.* New York, John Wiley, 1958.
72. Goodman RA, Mercy JA, Loya F, *et al:* Alcohol use and interpersonal violence–alcohol detected in homicide victims. *Am J Public Health* 76(2):144–149, 1986.
73. Haberman PW, Baden MM: *Alcohol, Other Drugs, and Violent Death.* New York, Oxford University Press, 1978.
74. Vikkunen M: Alcohol as a factor precipitating aggression and conflict behavior leading too homicide. *Br J Addict* 69:149–154, 1974.
75. Murdoch D, Pihl RO, Ross D: Alcohol and crimes of violence: Present issues. *Int J Addict* 25(9):1065–1081, 1990.
76. Koss MP, Dinero TE: Predictors of sexual aggression among a national sample of male college students. *Ann NY Acad Sci* 528:1133–1147, 1988.
77. Roizen J: Issues in epidemiology of alcohol and violence, in National Institute on Alcohol Abuse and Alcoholism Research Monograph-24 (ed): *Alcohol and Interpersonal Violence: Fostering Multidisciplinary Perspectives.* NIH Publication No. 93-3496. Rockville, MD, 1993, pp 3–36.
78. Kaufman Kantor G, Jasinski J: Prevention of teen violence: Evaluation of a multidimensional model. Paper presented at the 4th International Family Violence Conference, Durham, NH, 1995.
79. Kaufman Kantor G, Jasinski J: Family members polydrug use as a risk factor in family violence. Paper presented at the Research Institute on Additions, Fall Seminar Series, Buffalo, NY, 1994.
80. Leonard KE, Senchak M: Alcohol and premarital aggression among newlywed couples. *J Stud Alcohol* 11:96–108, 1993.
81. Miller BA, Downs WR, Gondoli DM: Spousal violence among alcoholic women as compared to a random household sample of women. *J Stud Alcohol* 50(6):533–540, 1989.
82. Miller BA, Downs WR, Testa M, Panek D: The relationship between victim's perpetrators alcohol use and spousal violence. Paper presented at the Annual Meeting of the American Society of Criminology, Baltimore, MD, 1990.

83. Bergman B, Larsson G, Brismar B, Klang M: Battered wives and female alcoholics: A comparitive social and psychiatricc study. *J Adv Nurs* 14:727–734, 1989.

84. Barnett OW, Fagan RW: Alcohol use in male spouse abusers and their female partners. *J Fam Violence* 8(1):1–25, 1993.

85. Gelles RJ, Harrop JW: Violence, battering, and psychological distress among women. *J Interpers Violence* 4:400–420, 1989.

86. Hilberman E, Munson K: Sixty battered women. *Victimology* 2:460–470, 1977.

87. Stark E, Flitcraft A, Zuckerman D, *et al:* Wife abuse in the medical setting: An introduction for health personnel, in: *Domestic Violence Monograph Series No. 7.* Rockville, MD, National Clearinghouse on Domestic Violence, 1981.

88. Kaufman Kantor G: Refining the brushstrokes in portraits of alcohol and wife assaults, in National Institute on Alcohol Abuse and Alcoholism Research Monograph-24 (ed): *Alcohol and Interpersonal Violence: Fostering Multidisciplinary Perspectives.* NIH Publication No. 93-3496. Rockville, MD, 1993, pp 281–290.

89. Arias I: *A Social Learning Theory Explication of the Intergenerational Transmission of Physical Aggression in Intimate Heterosexual Relationships.* Unpublished doctoral dissertation. Stony Brook, State University of New York, 1984.

90. Downs WR, Miller BA, Gondoli DM: Childhood experiences of parental physical violence for alcoholic women as compared with a randomly selected household sample of women. *Violence Vict* 2(4):225–240, 1987.

91. Downs WR, Miller BA, Testa M, Panek D: Long-term effects of parent-to-child violence for women. *J Interpers Violence* 7(3):365–382, 1992.

14

How Far Have We Come?

A Critical Review of the Research on Men Who Batter

W. Vernon Lee and Stephen P. Weinstein

Abstract. Although the effects of domestic violence and partner abuse have been known throughout history, the topic has recently begun to receive attention in the research literature. Indeed, it was not until 1986 that two interdisciplinary journals were dedicated exclusively to the study of family violence. Popular lore has frequently cited a connection between substance use (particularly alcohol) and domestic violence; however, this interaction has now begun to be formally recognized and addressed in research and treatment paradigms. This chapter presents some of the research findings regarding the multidimensional relationship between family violence and alcohol and/or drug abuse. Theories and data about the causes of family violence and characteristics of the male batterer and of the substance-abusing men who batter are offered. The final section examines several current models of treatment and their outcome.

1. Introduction

The study of male batterers and their response to treatment interventions is a relatively new area of exploration. With stories of murder and abuse filling the pages of our newspapers, the problem of partner abuse has catapulted into national prominence. Section 2 of this chapter examines research that attempts to identify the causes of partner abuse and to define what leads

W. Vernon Lee • Penn Recovery Systems, Philadelphia, Pennsylvania 19104-1953.   **Stephen P. Weinstein** • Department of Psychiatry and Human Behavior, Thomas Jefferson University, Philadelphia, Pennsylvania 19107.

Recent Developments in Alcoholism, Volume 13: Alcoholism and Violence, edited by Marc Galanter. Plenum Press, New York, 1997

some men to batter their partners while others do not. Section 3 focuses on current research regarding characteristics of men who batter and identifying psychological and behavioral characteristics of batterers. Section 4 examines some of the characteristics of substance-abusing men who batter, while seeking a connection between battering and chemical abuse. These two disorders challenge the clinician to find new strategies for working with the male batterer. With the spread of batterers' programs and mandated treatment for batterers, the final section examines current methods of treatment and their outcomes in an effort to determine if anything has worked to turn the tide of male violence against intimate partners.

2. Causes of Domestic Violence

Society has frequently been accused of being the source of male violence against their intimate partners.[1,2] Some feminists consider aggression toward women to be a manifestation of a patriarchal social system that seeks to discriminate against women and perpetuates the myth that men are superior to women. They maintain that the belief structure used to repress women is conveyed in attitudes such as sexual conservatism, adversarial sexual beliefs, and acceptance of interpersonal violence. While sexist attitudes are themselves not purported to be a sufficient condition for the occurrence of aggression against women, their presence increases the likelihood of women being victimized.[3,4]

Another point of view is offered by supporters of the psychodynamic perspective who contend that personality factors specific to the individual facilitate the commission of aggressive acts. The batterer utilizes violence as a means to deal with deep-seated resentments and fears that may or may not be available to the batterer's conscious thought processes. Gondolf[5] summarized this perspective by stating that men act aggressively against women in order to express infantile hostility and womb envy; such men simultaneously hate and fear women.

Although feminist and psychodynamic theorists recognize hostility as a central aspect of aggression against women by men, in isolation each theoretical perspective fails to address critical aspects of the issue.[6] On the one hand, feminist theory does not address why two men from similar environments do not both offend, while on the other hand the psychodynamic approach is insufficient to explain why two men with roughly similar personality traits do not both abuse women. Further, neither theory adequately accounts for the individual man's choice of offense style, i.e., battering or verbal or sexual abuse. Dewhurst et al.[6] suggested that aggression against women by men may be facilitated by the misogynist values of a male-dominated culture, as feminists would argue. But the dynamics that influence an individual's choice of abuse style may be more related to the personality characteristics of the offender.

In addition to theories that suggest that it is the culture and/or personality characteristics of the batterer that cause abuse, it has also been suggested that men may become batterers after witnessing abuse in their family of origin.[7] Still another more controversial position is that a man abuses because his partner pressures him into hitting her. This perspective has not been validated by experimental study. A most controversial position is taken by proponents of what has come to be called "the battered-husband syndrome." These theorists contend that men are frequently victims in their homes and view the women as wielding power over them, which leads the men to act out abusively.[8]

This entire issue of a reversal of the classic male dominance (i.e., role reversal) has been studied. Some experimental research has indicated that when the traditional power hierarchy of husband being in the one-up position over his wife is challenged in a marriage, abuse is more likely to occur. This is particularly true when a woman appears to have more status than her partner because of a higher educational level or occupation.[9] This perspective is in direct contrast with the "battered-woman syndrome," which attributes abuse to a woman's lack of power and her role as a "victim" in the home.[10–12] These and other studies are inconclusive and leave many questions unanswered regarding the relationship of power in battering relationships.

Given the relative paucity of research on men identified as batterers and the controversy regarding power in abusive relationships, Claes and Rosenthal[9] examined the conflict tactics used by men arrested for domestic assault and their perception of their partner's power. The results of their study indicated that the severity of abuse toward a female partner is related to the batterer's perception of the partner's power to reward. Men who used the most severe violent tactics perceived their partners as having high rewarding power. Claes and Rosenthal's explanation of this result is that battering males look to their partners in a dependent fashion to provide their primary personal support, and therefore perceive their partner as having high rewarding power or a level of control that they cannot accept, leading to an abusive cycle.

In summary, this section explored some of the possible causes of partner abuse. Feminist and psychodynamic theoretical perspectives as well as the sociocultural and personality researchers each contribute valuable information to this ongoing debate. No one theory has fully explained the causes of male violence against intimate partners. Men do it for different reasons, and some whom you might expect to abuse, because of criminal history or family background, do not abuse at all.

3. Characteristics of Male Batterers

The efforts to define the characteristics unique to male batterers have produced somewhat inconclusive and often contradictory results.[13–15] Much of the literature directed at describing the batterer has been derived from three theoretical models or approaches designed to facilitate an understanding of battering. Broadly defined, these are personality–behavioral models, social learning approaches, and psychodynamic explanations. The personality–behavioral depictions of battering are generally based on empirical assessments, behavioral observations, and reports or combinations of the two. Social learning approaches are primarily presented as observations fitting a social learning model of behavior. Psychodynamic explanations of battering are presented in a framework of modified Freudian theory.

3.1. Personality Behavioral Models

Wodarski[11] reports that batterers in an abusive family system tend to have the following general personality and behavioral characteristics: (1) their behavior was learned from the family of origin, and violence occurs in the family of origin among batterers much more frequently than among nonbatterers; (2) they project blame for the abuse onto their victim, i.e., batterers externalize the blame; (3) they are highly possessive of their victim, creating problems around jealousy and control; (4) the violence directed at an intimate partner can represent an attempt to displace anger meant for authority figures; (5) they have inappropriate expectations around their partners' role in the relationship and a distorted perception of their victims' behavior toward them; and (6) they often cannot recall details surrounding abuse incidents.[11] Among the more specific personality characteristics of batterers most frequently cited in the research are indications that batterers are less assertive, more hostile, more abusive of alcohol, lower in self-esteem, and more likely to show identifiable personality disorder than their nonbatterer counterparts.[7,9,16]

Researchers have begun to develop multiple-category typologies designed to tease out and explain characteristics of batterers, based either on the batterer's personality or behavior. Several of the current existing typologies based on the batterer's personality/behavioral style have evolved from both clinical and empirical assessments of batterers in treatment. Utilizing clinical observations to define batterer's emotional needs, Elbow[17] described four types of batterers: (1) the "controller," who views his wife as an object to control; (2) the "defender," who believes he must overprotect his wife; (3) the "approval seeker," who makes excessive demands in order to reinforce his self-image; and (4) the "incorporator," a type of batterer who needs his partner to validate and define himself. Ceasar,[18] in an effort to empirically discriminate the batter from the nonviolent therapy patient, found no differences on the Minnesota Multiphasic Personality Inventory (MMPI). However, she was able to develop a four-category typology of batterers based on extensive clinical interviews. Ceasar[18] titled them the "tyrant," the "exposed rescuer," the "nonexposed altruist," and the "psychotic wife assaulter." The tyrant subgroup was described as self-centered, hostile, and paranoid and less likely to be arrested than other wife-abuser subgroups. The exposed rescuers were described as having hysterical personalities and alternating between sociability and hostility. The nonexposed altruists were unassertive and constantly trying to please their wives; consequently, they felt unappreciated and victimized. The psychotic wife assaulter's anger does not stem from any rationally defineable source and appears erratic.

Hamberger and Hastings[19] and Hastings and Hamberger[20] attempted to formulate an empirically based typology of batterers. Male batterers ($N = 99$) were recruited from a treatment program, along with 71 help-seeking nonbatterers recruited from local marriage and family therapy clinics. All subjects were tested with the Millon Clinical Multiaxial Inventory-I.[21] Factor analyses indicated three major personality "factors" common to the partner abusers: factor 1, borderline/schizoidal; factor 2, histrionic/narcissistic; and, factor 3, antisocial/narcissistic. There was very little overlap in the factor structure of the batterers and nonbatterers, suggesting that qualitatively they represent largely different populations of men.

Saunders[22] used a combination of attitude and behavior measures in a cluster analysis to study batterers. Scores for depression, anger toward partner, and attitudes toward women were derived, along with measures of generalized violence, severity of partner abuse, and alcohol use. One cluster ($N = 31$) was characterized as being "emotionally volatile," scoring higher on measures of anger, depression, and jealousy, while demonstrating moderate levels of violence and alcohol use. The batterers in the second cluster ($N = 48$) were more likely to score low on the anger and depression measures and were the most likely to be violent outside the home. A third cluster ($N = 86$) appeared to be composed largely of batterers who suppressed their feelings, while confining their violence primarily to home; that is, they scored low on anger and depression measures but the highest on a scale for social desirability. Gondolf[13] points out that it is still unclear whether the "feelings" of anger and depression are merely associated with different levels of expression of violence or are in themselves causative of the violence. It is also unclear if the "types" as empirically assessed actually describe men in different phases of abuse.

Gondolf[13] indicated that the previous research attempting to demonstrate either behavioral or personality typologies had too many methodological (sampling, instrumentation) problems and lacked a theoretical frame of reference. He believed that the shortcomings of the empirically based personality typologies outweighed those of the more descriptive behavioral typologies. Assessed attitudinal or personality characteristics are insufficient to explain or predict violent behavior. In his view, behavioral patterns are well established and less varied than the complex personality attributes associated with batterers. Therefore, Gondolf argues, because of their destructive impact, it is the behavior of batterers that is of more immediate concern. Behavior is more likely to be predictive of future violence, and thus has direct implications for the victims and for the extent and effectiveness of interventions.

As a result, Gondolf[13] attempted to establish a behavioral typology of batterers by focusing on the descriptions offered by the victims of abuse. His typology was based on the self-report of battered women admitted to Texas shelters during an 18-month period, from 1984–1985 ($N = 6000$). The typology he developed does not represent diagnostic categories but rather an interpretable summary of cluster findings. The batterer "types" include two highly antisocial and severely abusive types, one of which is typified by an unusually high number of arrests for general violence and substance abuse, and a third less antisocial and less abusive type. He labeled the most antisocial as "sociopathic," given the extreme criminal nature of the behaviors. The sociopathic batterer type is most likely to have been previously arrested for property, violent, and drug- or alcohol-related crime. The second antisocial type was labeled the "antisocial" batterer. This type of batterer is also extremely abusive physically and verbally. While he is likely to have been generally violent, he is less likely to have been arrested than the sociopathic batterer. The third less severe type was referred to as the "typical" batterer, who may exhibit either chronic or sporadic patterns of abuse. The typical batterer conforms more to the prevailing clinical profiles of batterers. He is particularly less likely to have used weapons than the other types of batterers. These findings substantiate earlier studies based on victims' reports, which point to the presence of a "violence-prone" personality and an association between the severity of partner abuse and general violence. This also confirms recent research on personality types that include a sociopathic/narcissistic type of batterer, whose abuse is not anger driven.[13,20]

Notwithstanding Gondolf's criticism of personality typologies, research in the 1990s continues to search for typologies that characterize personality traits and psychological and cognitive characteristics of men who batter women in order to distinguish them from nonbattering men. Else et al.[16] compared a group of 21 batterers with a comparable group of nonbatterers recruited as a control group from the local community. Utilizing the MMPI and its personality disorder scales (MMPI-PDS) as well as the Hostility and Direction of Hostility Questionnaire, Else's results showed that batterers score higher on the borderline and antisocial MMPI-PDS and on the acting-out hostility and self-criticism scales of the hostility questionnaire. No significant differences were found between the groups' performances on cognitive measures, depression scale scores, or overall scores on the MMPI. While finding very few differences on the MMPI, he did find that child abuse was a common experience among batterers.

Murphy et al.[23] examined associations between family of origin violence, self-reports of psychopathology on the Millon Clinical Multiaxial Inventory-II,[21] and current spouse abuse among partner assaultive men. Compared to nonviolent men in discordant ($N = 24$) and well-adjusted ($N = 24$) relationships, partner-assaultive men ($N = 24$) were significantly more likely to report childhood histories of physical abuse and physical abuse of the mother in the family of origin. The partner-assaultive men also reported significantly higher scores on a variety of Millon Clinical Multiaxial Inventory-II personality disorder and Axis I disorder scales.

Also in search of an explanation for violence in relationships, Wesner *et al.*[24] examined "explosive rage" in 51 cases of troubled marriages. Physical violence not involving direct partner abuse (i.e., violence against inanimate objects not causing injury to persons) had received little attention in the research literature. However, Wesner *et al.*[24] were impressed with the frequent appearance of several common features to this reaction. Explosive rage seemed to occur most often in the presence of a female friend or spouse, with alcohol being consumed, and in the absence of another person other than a child (family member or male friend). The study strongly suggested a role for alcohol in sensitizing trigger conditions (it was present in 82% of the sample), and that the presence of another person not a spouse or girlfriend may exert an inhibiting effect. In this study, 24% of the sample who engaged in explosive rage involved actual battering at some point in the history of the relationship.

Taking a different route toward attempting to develop an understanding of the characteristics of the male batterer, Bergman and Brismar[25] hypothesized that the same background and precipitating factors would be found in both male victims and male assailants, and that these factors could predetermine the social career for selected males: that of assailant, victim, or both. The researchers chose two highly selected and not necessarily representative groups of assailants and victims. Batterers (MB) included men sent to prison for wife abuse, a group that constitutes only a limited proportion of all men who beat their wives or partners. The men identified as "victim" (BM) had such severe injuries from battering that they required inpatient care; however, they represent only a small portion of all men who are injured in fights. Bergman and Brismar's[25] study groups consisted of 18 male batterers and 19 battered males and two control groups selected from the general population of Stockholm. The control groups, one for the MB group and one for the BM group, also comprised 18 and 19 men, respectively. The authors believed that the strength of studying these highly selected groups was that any specific characteristics, either social or psychological, would probably be more easily identifiable in these extreme groups.

Although the sample sizes were relatively small, results showed that a large majority of the MB group (15 of 18) and nearly half (9 of 19) of the BM group had been abused as a child. Half of the men (9) in the MB group and 7 of the 19 men in the BM group reported that they were alcohol-dependent. Both the victims and the batterers had a higher proportion of divorces and a smaller proportion of being married than the controls.

Dutton and Hart[26] assessed the prevalence of risk markers for partner abuse in federal offenders. Evidence suggested that this population may demonstrate high rates of family violence, since demographic and psychological factors commonly found in incarcerated populations are also mentioned in most of the literature describing assaultive males. Their study found evidence of high risk for wife assault in this incarcerated population. Specific risk markers included abuse in the family of origin, personality disorders, and prior record of violence.

Bersani et al.[27] also studied offenders convicted of partner abuse to determine if specific psychological variables could be used to create a personal profile. The revised Taylor-Johnson Temperament Analysis (T-JTA) was used. This 180-item inventory is divided equally among nine bipolar traits. Based on these traits, a constellation of behavior patterns were derived. Two factors were identified for the offenders studied: internal or emotional balance and social interaction. Under factor 1—internal or emotional balance—batterers registered high on the Nervous, Depressive, Indifferent, Subjective, Hostile, and Impulsive subscales. This profile represents men, who as a group, are conflicted internally. However, it was the negative implications of four of the six subscale measures that Bersani et al.[27] believed to be most significant for this population: Indifferent—referring to the incapacity to see another's point of view or identify with another's feelings; Subjective—indicating internal turmoil over unresolved difficulties; Hostile—indicating outwardly expressed anger; and Impulsive—indicating the tendency to react without reason.

For factor 2, social interaction, the batterers registered high on the Active/Social, Expressive/Responsive, and Dominant subscales. This profile represents a picture of social attributes that are acceptable (even rewarded) in our society. The T-JTA indicated that these men, as a group, prefer social interaction (Active/Social) and are highly outgoing (Expressive/Responsive). The added measure of Dominance, or assertiveness, completes a combined profile of social interaction that is both admired and required in many occupational contexts. While this extroverted profile seems inconsistent with the notion that abusing men are isolated or introverted, it may be characteristic of the educated, professional, socially successful batterer not frequently studied in research situations.

Pistole and Tarrant[28] also studied men convicted of partner abuse. As part of his probation, each male participated in a psychoeducational group designed to improve anger management skills. They examined the relationship between self-reported attachment styles and hostility in intimate relationships. Attachment styles defined as dismissing, fearful, preoccupied, and secure were represented in proportions that were similar to those found in nonviolent samples. Multivariate analysis of variance revealed significant differences among the attachment styles displaying resentment, suspiciousness, and guilt. Attachment and aggression have also been linked to shame. Future research might explore the empirical relationship of shame and attachment in male batterers. In addition, measurement at the time of the violence might reveal differences in attachment behavior and aggression that were not elicited in this study.

Dewhurst et al.[6] compared the personality traits, attitudes, and beliefs of men who batter, men who perpetrate sexual assault, and nonabusive men in an effort to facilitate the development of a clearer picture of the abusive males choice process. They found that the attitudes and personality characteristics of men identified as batterers and men who perpetrate sexual assaults against adult women were similar and that they differed from a community sample of men who did not self-disclose violence against women. The attitudes and personality characteristics of men from the community who voluntarily self-disclosed physical or sexually assaultive behavior toward women and men who have been formally identified as perpetrators were similar; however, they, too, differed from nondisclosing community men.

Davidovich[29] explored psychological variables that have been identified as characteristic of males who physically abuse their partners in an attempt to determine which psychological variables could explain the actions of male batterers in the context of broader theories of behavior. Her most cogent explanation of battering behavior was drawn from social learning theory.

3.2. Social Learning Approaches

Reviewing earlier research on the interaction of multiple stressors and social learning theory offered by Hofeller,[30] Hotaling and Sugarman,[14] MacEwen and Barling,[31] and Hastings and Hamberger,[20] Davidovich[29] noted that most of the reports were inconclusive. However, two important findings did emerge from the Hotaling and Sugarman[14] study. Witnessing parental violence as a child or adolescent was found to be a consistent risk marker for adult violence, while personally experiencing physical abuse as a child showed inconsistency as a risk marker.

Hastings and Hamberger,[20] confirming Hotaling and Sugarmans'[14] results, also found that males who witnessed abuse as children were more likely to engage in partner abuse. They found, however, that personally experiencing abuse as a child also led to a greater likelihood of becoming an adult abuser. In addition, these researchers noted that children who either witnessed or experienced abuse and who later became adult batterers were also more likely to have a concurrent alcohol problem. These abusers tend to come from dysfunctional families, often from alcoholic and/or drug-abusing parents.

In Davidovich's[29] discussion of violence against women, she describes batterers as young, generally between the ages of 18 and 34 years old; 54% are white, 44% are African American, 47% are unemployed, 40% have some prior criminal record; 60% being intoxicated during the attack on their wives, and 70% are under the influence of drugs and–or alcohol during their violent episode. Her application of social learning theory to the batterer and to spouse abuse begins with an individual who learns to respond violently to stressful situations through modeling of the behavior of family members, peers, and significant others. When, as an adult, he is confronted with stressor stimuli, he becomes frustrated and resorts to violence as an appropriate and justified action. Although this theory seems to present a compelling argument for generational patterns of family violence, Davidovich notes that the process of translating life events and stressors into violence is not yet known. Davidovich[29] argues that knowledge of the "psychology of the individual and personality variables might serve to fill the gap between situational factors and differential responses" (p. 36).

Davidovich[29] concluded that the weight of the evidence seems to suggest that either witnessing and/or experiencing violence in one's family of origin strongly increased the likelihood that an individual would engage in spouse abuse. Furthermore, dysfunctional families of origin, particularly those in which alcoholism and/or drug addiction were prevalent, play an important role in the intergenerational transmission of violence.

3.3. Psychodynamic Explanations

Although Davidovich[29] indicated that another approach to understanding abusive behavior could be derived from psychoanalytic theory, her psychodynamic explanations were more descriptive of the psychosocial dimensions defining the males who batter. Guerney et al.[32] offered a psychodynamic theoretical construct to explain the development and maintenance of wife battering and provided a rationale for the type of therapy deemed most likely to be effective with wife batterers. Their constructs are tied to research evidence along with clinical observations. Although psychodynamic in nature, the explanation was conceived in terms of Dollard and Miller's[33] integration of Freudian concepts with learning theory.

In their theoretical approach, being abused as a child gives rise to feelings of rage, but to express this rage to the abuser is dangerous, and the rage is suppressed or repressed. As is the case with any extremely strong feeling denied full expression at the time of its occurrence, the individual seeks ways to express the rage in ways that are relatively safe (e.g., dreams). The inability to escape from the abuse in childhood leads to a deep sense of powerlessness that the individual seeks to overcome, often through the artificial sense of power derived from alcohol or by attempting to exert power/control over others. However, because of the fear of authority figures that generalizes from fear of an abusing parent, the attempt to gain power and control over others is directed mainly toward those who are physically weaker than the self (e.g., a child and/or wife).

At the same time the individual is attempting to overcome the powerlessness and express rage, there is a conflict between fear of one's rage and the fear of loss of affection from a loved one. Therefore, the effort to control others and/or to express rage against others is likely to be inconsistent and sporadic, often alternating with genuine expressions of concern and affection. Within this context, while seeking an outlet for the feelings of rage, the batterer can readily interpret or engineer events in his marital relationship in such a way as to provide an excuse for expressing his anger. And finally, since the feelings of rage frequently need to be repressed and repression requires significant psychological effort, any general disinhibitor (such as alcohol) strongly increases the probability that control will be lost and rage overtly expressed.

It appears that personality, behavioral, social learning, and psychodynamic perspectives provide valuable information on characteristics of the male batterer, and perhaps they should be seen as complementary rather than mutually exclusive and exhaustive. In order to understand battering, it is necessary to look at the batterers themselves to comprehend the process of translating stressors and life events into acts of violence within the sociocultural context in which the batterer lives.

In conclusion, research in the 1990s continues to demonstrate that although partner abuse is not strictly limited to men with personality problems or other identifiable psychological problems, such men do seem to constitute a larger proportion of the identified treatment population, especially those with concurrent substance abuse problems. It is clear from the above-cited studies that men who seek or are forced into treatment as batterers are likely to have psychological problems that can affect their treatment. The role that drugs and alcohol play in the mix with personality, sociocultural, and behavioral factors needs further exploration. The influence of substance of abuse also requires further clarification because presumably nonalcoholic or nonsubstance-abusing battering samples may be confounded by the presence of undetected alcohol or drug problems.

The evidence presented thus far strongly suggests heterogeneity of characteristics of men who batter. Because of this heterogeneity, many researchers have identified different specific clusters of psychological and/or behavioral characteristics that they believe identify male batterers. Such analyses may be helpful if they lead to theoretical formulations, provided they also recognize the importance of the sociocultural context of violence. Physical abuse directed at women has only recently begun to be been addressed in national policy and legislation. There is still relatively little concrete knowledge about the batterer and little real information about the prevalence, severity, and outcome of violence perpetrated by men against female partners. The above-cited research describing a variety of background, behavioral, psychological, and social characteristics of the batterer and suggesting that no one pathology can be linked to battering is a beginning in the effort to address this scarcity of information.

4. Substance Abuse and Battering

Although many batterers are alcoholic and/or substance abusers, the role of alcohol and other substances in domestic violence remains controversial. At present, neither alcohol nor other drugs are considered necessary or sufficient for the occurrence of domestic violence. However, alcohol and/or drugs have been found to be present in many domestic violence cases. Estimates of the percentage of batterers who assault their partners while intoxicated range from 60 to 70% for alcohol abuse and 13 to 20% for drug abuse.[34,35] Alcohol and drug use are often invoked by batterers to excuse or explain their abusive behavior. In fact, these substances may well serve a disinhibiting or releasing function, which may be associated with violence.[36]

There is a general consensus that alcohol is the drug that is most often associated with violence.[37] According to Miller et al.,[38] this is probably due to the high base rate of alcohol use in the population rather than to anger-inducing effects of ethanol. Alcohol use can trigger aggression during either intoxication or withdrawal. The linkage is best viewed as a mixture of personality, social, and physiological causes.[39-42] Alcohol consumption under some circumstances may be associated with an increase in aggressive behavior,[42-47] acts of criminal violence,[48,49] and assaultive behaviors.[50,51] Other studies have reported a more specific association between drinking and marital violence. Between 30 and 70% of battered wives report problem drinking or alcoholic husbands.[52-54] Eberle[55] reported that victims of alcohol-abusing batterers were themselves more likely to abuse alcohol than were victims of batterers who did not use alcohol. Byles[56] noted a significant association between alcohol abuse and spouse battering in 139 people appearing in Family Court. In studying causes of divorce, Cleek and Pearson[57] found a strong association between alcohol abuse and spouse battering.

Other substances of abuse have also been studied in relation to their propensity to lead to violence. These have included amphetamines, PCP, barbiturates, heroin, and most recently crack cocaine.[58-63]

Roberts[64] reported the results of an exploratory study into the relationship between battering and substance abuse. This research was important since little had been done on the incidence of combined drug and alcohol abuse among men who batter. Studying the intake records of 234 male batterers who had charges filed against them, Roberts found that men who committed more serious battery offenses (i.e., an attack resulting in bodily injury) were significantly more likely than those who committed lesser battery offenses (i.e., slapping, pushing, etc.) to have either a drug problem or a dual problem with alcohol and drugs. Almost one half (49.9%) of the serious offenders abused drugs either alone or in combination with alcohol, while under one fourth (22.4%) of the lesser offenders had this problem. One surprising finding was that the results did not support previous research that suggested that more severe violence is associated with the batterer's abuse of alcohol.[12,34,35] In the Roberts[,64] study, the number of alcohol abusers in the two groups was almost equal: 28 were charged with serious battering and 29 were charged with the lesser offense. However, severe physical abuse was found to be associated with drug abuse and the dual problem of alcohol and drug abuse, not solely with alcohol use. This finding suggests the need to establish specific criteria and assessment methods for determining the nature and extent of a substance abuse problem that could be "predictive" of ones' battering behavior.

Miller[34] also reported that a combination of drug and alcohol abuse is more predictive of domestic violence than is alcohol use alone. The subjects ($N = 82$) were selected from all male parolees in western New York who were convicted of either nonviolent or violent offenses. They were given the Diagnostic Interview Schedule[65] and a modified version of the Conflict Tactics Scale.[66] Alcohol problems were present in 76% of the parolees and 73% of the parolees reported using some type of illegal drug on a regular basis. Rates of spousal violence were also high for this sample. During 3 months preceding the interview, 78% of the parolees committed acts of moderate violence, while 33% of the parolees committed acts of severe violence (some committed both moderate and severe acts of violence). Examining the contribution of the parolees' alcohol and drug problems to their violence toward a spouse revealed that neither drug abuse nor alcohol problems independently contributed significantly to the degree of violence, but the interaction effect (alcohol × drugs) contributed significantly to the level of parolee-to-spouse violence.

However, some of their results appear to contradict popular conceptions of the impact of substance use. For example, alcohol abuse increased the risk of parolee-to-spouse violence in the absence of drug abuse, but there was a tendency for alcohol abuse to decrease violence when there was drug abuse. One possible explanation for this contradictory finding is that the type of drug use may lessen the violence that was associated with alcohol problems. The psychopharmacological effects of marijuana and heroin, for instance, have been attributed to "mellowing out" or causing individuals to "nod out," respectively, conditions that are likely to lessen violent tendencies. In addition, considering the popular notion that cocaine use increases the violence rate, the researchers expected that cocaine users would have an elevated level of violence or a level of violence at least similar to that for alcohol abusers only. However, there were more violent activities (parolee-to-spouse) reported for barbiturate and marijuana users compared to cocaine users.

Our own inner city, publicly funded, intensive cocaine treatment program at Thomas Jefferson University has produced some interesting data about cocaine users who do and do not batter. A battery of standard psychometric instruments and a brief battering questionnaire were administered to cocaine-dependent men entering the treatment program that identified those who were partner batters and those who were not. The partner batterers did not differ significantly from the nonbatterers on demographic measures. Results showed a longer history of regular weekly drinking reported by the batterers and a greater number of years of drinking to intoxication by this same group. Differences were found on the Addiction Severity Index Family and Psychological composite scores where the batterers scored significantly higher than the nonbatterers. Eighty-nine percent of the batterers reported a history of serious conflict with their sexual partners as compared to 62% of the nonbatterers, and 79% of the batterers reported that they had experienced trouble controlling violent behavior as compared to 49% of the nonbatterers. Regarding psychiatric symptomatology, a comparison of SCL-90-R scores indicated that on four of the nine clinical scales, the partner batterers reported significantly greater disturbance than the nonbatterers. Specifically, the batterers received higher scores on depression, paranoid ideation, psychoticism, and interpersonal sensitivity. In our clinical–research setting, efforts are now being directed at developing and evaluating a treatment approach that may be effective in dealing with the combined problems of cocaine use and partner abuse.[67]

Although the connection between substances of abuse and family violence has been receiving increased public as well as professional attention,[43,60,62] little has been done or written about the treatment of individuals who are both chemically dependent and partner abusers and guidelines for their clinical management are yet to be developed.

5. Treatment Interventions

Social workers, psychiatrists, psychologists, and other mental health workers are increasingly being asked and funded to offer treatment services to men who batter their partners, even though the causes of this violence, the motivations for participation in treatment, and the most effective treatments are not significantly understood. In addition to avoiding prison, a real incentive for men to enter treatment was reported by Gondolf[13] who found that women were more than twice as likely to return to their relationship after leaving a shelter if their partner was in counseling. This can be a positive incentive and should be an excellent initiation to treatment, but do efforts aimed at treating batterers really work? And if they do work, are the effects sustained over time?

Tolman and Bennett[7] reviewed the literature on interventions directed at helping men who batter become nonabusive. The studies reviewed employed follow-up periods ranging from a few weeks to several years. Several methodological concerns were raised, including (1) definitions of successful outcome, (2) data sources, (3) length of the follow-up period, and (4) percentage of participants actually contacted for follow-up. The 16 studies reviewed consistently indicated that the majority of men stopped their physical abuse subsequent to intervention. Percentages of successful outcome ranged from 53 to 85%. Lower percentages of success tended to occur (1) in programs with lengthier follow-up, indicating that effects may dissipate over time, and (2) when successful outcomes were based on spouses' reports rather than on arrests or self-reports.

Unfortunately, few investigators have examined the impact of treatment beyond a 12-month period. For example, of the 16 evaluations reviewed by Tolman and Bennett,[7] only three reported follow-up data collected more than 12 months after treatment. Edleson and Syers[68] went beyond the 12-month period with their study of the long-term effects of group treatment on men who batter. They compared three types of brief treatment groups: (1) a self-help model, (2) an educational model, and (3) a combined model that integrated the other two. Of 283 men randomly assigned to one of the treatment conditions, 153 completed 80% or more of the assigned sessions. Eighteen-month follow-up interviews were conducted with 70 program completers or their partners. Almost two thirds of the men who completed education and combined groups were reported to be nonviolent at the 18-month follow-up. The results indicated that short-term, relatively structured group treatment tended to produce the most consistent successful results. However, there was no control group and follow-ups were conducted with only a minority (approximately 25%) of the original sample of men in the study. No information was available on the large number of missing subjects.

Additional support for the positive outcome cited by Edleson and Syers[68] came from Palmer et al.,[69] who examined long-term outcomes of a short-term treatment program for abusive husbands. Recidivism rates, based on police reports, were found to be lower than those for a control group of untreated abusive husbands. The researchers also believe that the results contribute to a relatively unstudied area by empirically attempting to evaluate an unstructured treatment program. However, the researchers qualify their results by indicating that the reliability of self-reports given by the batterers did not always match police reports, and police reports are considered to be a conservative measure of recidivism. The Palmer et al.[69] study did not include an interview with the victimized partner.

Shepard[70] designed a study to address batterer recidivism in relation to community intervention (law enforcement, criminal justice system, and mandated counseling programs). This study was unique in that it followed up men 5 years after they had completed a treatment program in an effort to discover background and intervention variables that discriminated batterers who were recidivists from those who were not. A total of 100 men were included in the study sample. The sample was drawn from the Duluth Domestic Abuse Intervention Project, which was one of the first community intervention programs in the country. Results showed that 40% of the men fell into the category of recidivists. Twenty-two percent had been convicted for domestic assault, 15% had been the subject of a protection order, and 33% had been police suspects for domestic assault.[70]

The long-term study also found that alcohol and drug abuse were important contributors to recidivism, results reported previously by Eberle[55] and DeMaris and Jackson.[71] Batterers who were abused as children also appeared to be somewhat more likely to be recividists, replicating results reported by Grusznski.[72] Shepard's[70] work reflected the need for a stronger emphasis on preventive measures in the areas of child abuse and chemical dependency.

The above studies were conducted to evaluate predominantly cognitive–behavioral counseling programs that have reported lower rates of physical abuse for treated groups, although most were not able to control for other variables that may have influenced outcome.[70] Such issues as severity and type of abuse may need to be addressed in future studies.[73]

In addition to evaluating outcomes, researchers and treatment professionals are also designing new ways of working with the batterer. Three studies warrant examination because of their unique approaches to battering treatment.

Geffner[74] argues for the use of divorce mediation with abusive couples. Because of the inherent dangerousness of working with abusers and their partners, he suggested that a thorough assessment be completed prior to the mediation to ascertain the extent of the abuse. The counselor then must determine if the couple needs or requires individual counseling, reconciliation, or mediation–divorce counseling. If batterer and victim have independently stated that they desire mediation (or that it is court mandated), if the abused partner is willing and able to participate, and if it appears that any attempts at intimidation would be manageable, then mediation may be an appropriate approach.[74] He offers guidelines for the counselor in the use of mediation with a discussion of power and control issues (of the batterer) that may undermine the mediation attempt as well as put the partner in danger. However, no information is presented on the efficacy of working with the batterer in couples' sessions or on the outcomes associated with this counseling approach. Within this context the capacity to "mediate" with a woman who may be suffering symptoms of battered women's syndrome, a type of posttraumatic stress disorder where the victim exhibits many symptoms of fear and intimidation, should be further researched. Mediation may do more harm than good. The rational, goal-directed thinking necessary for mediation is also suspect in a man who has demonstrated difficulty with his own dependency needs and the sharing of power and control in his relationships. Geffner indicates that if mediation is to be used with couples when abuse has occurred in the marriage, then it is important to overcome the intimidation and to balance the power.

Wallace and Nosko[75] offer treatment guidelines for working with another central issue when treating abusive men. They believe that shame associated with their abuse is the core issue for many men who assault their partners and that these feelings can best be addressed and resolved in group treatment approaches. However, its immediate impact on the abusive male may be the reverse. The requirement of having to attend a batterers' group through informal or formal coercion can be a shame-inducing experience. Furthermore, the group norms, necessary to achieve safety and deal with feelings, may be contrary to traditional masculine norms. Group members are required to disclose their worst incident of violence toward their partner. This intervention becomes the "confession." No empirical data are offered to substantiate the efficacy of this treatment intervention, except for transcripts from treatment sessions. Research utilizing control groups that examines how shame is elicited and how the shame is negotiated through the various stages of group development is needed.

A third treatment intervention that has gained considerable attention in the 1990s is the mandatory arrest of batterers. Although there are no studies in the literature examining its efficacy, this approach has received widespread criticism. Stark[2] defines the debate that has ensued over the past 10 years with a summary of the interpretations of the proponents' positions. The critics who are against mandatory arrest make their case through three points: (1) mandatory arrest does not work; (2) mandatory arrest is inhumane; and (3) the very people we are trying to protect do not want it. Stark argues against these three points. He believes mandatory arrest helps to control behavior: There is less opportunity for disregarding the battering, minimizing its consequences, and blaming the victims of abuse. Mandatory arrest offers immediate protection from current violence. Furthermore, Stark believes that arrest provides a meaningful opportunity for battered women to consider their options and give those women ready to end their relationship time to go elsewhere or to obtain a protection order. Stark further argues that arrest might deter recidivism and send a clear message that battery is unacceptable.

Mandatory arrest, like other approaches to treating the batterer, is in its infancy. With the majority of the women returning to their abusive partners, there is little doubt that mediation and mandatory arrest will gain in popularity. Only the future will tell how effective these efforts have been. The debate has begun and it is a lively and necessary debate.

6. Conclusions

In this chapter we have attempted to present a distillation of theory and research regarding the causes of domestic abuse, the identification of the psychological and behavioral characteristics of batterers in general, and more specifically the characteristics of substance abusers who batter their partners. We have also reviewed some of the more traditional as well as the newer innovative approaches to treating batterers. None of the findings are convincingly conclusive in either defining the full range of dynamics, behaviors, and characteristics that describe the population of batterers or in accurately predicting a clear at-risk battering group. However, these research efforts have been highly productive in helping to develop a better understanding of the complex, sometimes violent, tapestry that characterizes human relationships. Additional research and continuing debate and discussion are needed as increasingly we recognize the degree to which domestic violence permeates our society.

References

1. Browne A: Violence against women by male partners: Prevalence, outcomes, and policy implications. *Am Psychol* 48(10):1077–1087, 1993.
2. Stark E: Mandatory arrest of batterers. *Am Behav Sci* 36(5):651–680, 1993.
3. Scott R, Tetreault L: Attitudes of rapists and other violent offenders toward women. *J Soc Psychol* 127(4):375–380, 1986.
4. Koss M, Gidyez C, Wisniewski N: The scope of rape: Incidence and prevalence of sexual

aggression an victimization in a national sample of higher education students. *J Consult Clin Psychol* 55(2):162–170, 1987.

5. Gondolf E: Fighting for control: A clinical assessment of men who batter. *Soc Casework* 66(1):48–54, 1985.

6. Dewhurst A, Moore R, Alfano D: Aggression against women by men: Sexual and spousal assault. *J Offender Rehab* 18(3/4):39–47, 1992.

7. Tolman R, Bennett L: A review of quantitative research on men who batter. *J Interpers Violence* 5(1):87–118, 1990.

8. Steinmetz S: The battered husband syndrome. *Victimology* 2(3–4):499–509, 1978.

9. Claes J, Rosenthal D: Men who batter women: A study in power. *J Fam Violence* 5(3):309–322, 1990.

10. Margolin G, Burman B: Wife abuse versus marital violence: Different terminologies, explanations, and solutions. *Clin Psychol Rev* 13:59–73, 1993.

11. Wodarski J: An examination of spouse abuse: Practice issues for the profession. *Clin Soc Work J* 15(2):172–187, 1987.

12. Walker L: *The Battered Woman.* New York, Harper & Row, 1979.

13. Gondolf E: Who are those guys? Toward a behavioral typology of batterers. *Violence Vict* 3(3):187–203, 1988.

14. Hotaling G, Sugarman D: An analysis of risk markers in husband to wife violence: The current state of knowledge. *Violence Vict* 1(2):101–124, 1986.

15. Edleson J, Eisikovits I, Guttman E: Men who batter women: A critical review of the evidence. *J Fam Issues* 6(2):229–247, 1985.

16. Else L, Wonderlich S, Beatty W, Christie D, Staton R: Personality characteristics of men who physically abuse women. *Hosp Commun Psychiatry* 44(1):54–58, 1993.

17. Elbow M: Theoretical considerations of violent marriage, *Soc Casework* 58:515–526, 1977.

18. Ceasar P: Men who batter: A heterogeneous group. Presented at the American Psychological Association, Washington, DC, 1986.

19. Hamberger K, Hastings JE: Personality correlates of men who abuse their partners: A cross validation study. *J Fam Violence* 1(4):323–341, 1986.

20. Hastings J, Hamberger K: Personality correlates of spouse abusers: A controlled comparison. *Violence Vict* 3(1):31–48, 1988.

21. Millon T: Millon Clinical Multiaxial Inventory Manual. Minneapolis, Interpretive Scoring Systems, 1983.

22. Saunders D: Are there different types of men who batter? An empirical study with possible implication for treatment. Presented at the Third National Family Violence Research Conference, Durham, NH, 1987.

23. Murphy C, Meyer S, O'Leary D: Family of origin violence and millon clinical multiaxial inventory. II. Psychopathology among partner assaultive men. *Violence Vict* 8(2):165–176, 1993.

24. Wesner D, Patel C, Allen J: A study of explosive rage in male spouses counseled in an Appalachian mental health clinic. *J Counsel Dev* 70:235–241, 1991.

25. Bergman B, Brismar B: Assailants and victims: A comparative study of male wife-beaters and battered males. *J Addict Dis* 12(4):1–10, 1993.

26. Dutton D, Hart S: Risk markers for family violence in a federally incarcerated population. *Int J Law Psychiatry* 15:101–112, 1992.

27. Bersani C, Chen H, Pendelton B, Denton R: Personality traits of convicted male batterers. *J Fam Violence* 7(2):123–134, 1992.

28. Pistole M, Tarrant N: Attachment style and aggression in male batterers. *Fam Ther* 20(3):165–173, 1993.

29. Davidovich J: Men who abuse their spouse: Social and psychological supports. *J Offender Counsel Serv Rehab* 15(1):27–44, 1990.

30. Hofeller KH: *Battered Women, Shattered Lives.* CA, R & E Research Associates, 1983.

31. MacEwen K, Barling J: Multiple stressors, violence in the family of origin and marital aggression: A longitudinal investigation. *J Fam Violence* 3(1):73–87, 1988.

32. Guerney B, Waldo M, Firestone L: Wife-battering: A theoretical construct and case report. *Am J Fam Ther* 15(1):34–43, 1987.
33. Dollard J, Miller NE: *Personality and Psychotherapy.* New York, McGraw-Hill, 1950.
34. Miller B: The interrelationships between alcohol and drugs and family violence, in De LaRosa M, Lambert Y, Gropper B, (eds): *Drugs and Violence: Causes, Correlates, and Consequences.* NIDA Research Monograph 103. Rockville, MD, US Department of Health and Human Services, National Institute on Drug Abuse, 1990, pp 177–207.
35. Gorney B: Domestic violence and chemical dependency: Dual problems, dual interventions. *J Psychoact Drugs* 21(2):229–238, 1989.
36. Geffner R, Rosenbaum A: Characteristics and treatment of batterers. *Behav Sci Law* 8:131–140, 1990.
37. Cohen S: Aggression: The role of drugs, in *The Substance Abuse Problems*, vol 2. New York, Haworth Press, 1985, pp 358–363.
38. Miller N, Millman R, Keskinen S: Outcome at six and twelve months post inpatient treatment for cocaine and alcohol dependence. *Adv Alcohol Subst Abuse* 9(3/4):101–120, 1990.
39. Cloninger D: Neurogenic adaptive mechanisms in alcoholism. *Science* 236:410–416, 1987.
40. Van Hasselt VB, Morrison RL, Bellock AS: Alcohol use in wife abusers and their spouses. *Addict Behav* 10:127–135, 1985.
41. Schukit J, Russell J: An evaluation of primary alcoholics with histories of violence. *J Clin Psychiatry* 14:3–6, 1984.
42. Taylor S, Leonard K: Alcohol and human physical aggression, in Green RG, Donnerstein EI (eds): *Aggression: Theoretical and Empirical Reviews.* New York, Academic Press, 1983, pp 77–111.
43. Leonard K, Blane E: Alcohol and marital aggression in a national sample of young men. *J Interpers Violence* 7(1):19–30, 1992.
44. Pihl R, Zacchia C: Alcohol and aggression: A test of the affect–arousal hypothesis. *Aggressive Behav* 12:367–375, 1986.
45. Cherek D, Steinberg J, Manno B: Effects of alcohol on human aggressive behavior. *J Stud Alcohol* 46:321–328, 1985.
46. Leonard K: Alcohol consumption and escalatory aggression in dyads. *J Stud Alcohol* 45:75–80, 1984.
47. Zeichner R, Phil R: Effects of alcohol and behavior contingencies on human aggression. *J Abnorm Psychol* 88:153–160, 1979.
48. Voss H, Hepburn J: Patterns in criminal homicide in Chicago. *J Crim Law Criminol Pol Sci* 59:499–508, 1969.
49. Wolfgang M, Strohm R: The relationship between alcohol and criminal homicide. *Q J Stud Alcohol* 17:411–425, 1956.
50. Leonard K, Bromet E, Parkinson D, *et al:* Patterns of alcohol use and physically aggressive behavior in men. *J Stud Alcohol* 46:279–282, 1985.
51. Pernanen K: Alcohol and crimes of violence, in Kissin B, Begleiter H (eds): *The Biology of Alcoholism: Social Aspects of Alcoholism,* vol 4. New York, Plenum Press, 1976, pp 351–444.
52. Fagan J, Stewart D, Hansen K: Violent men or violent husbands: Background factors and situational correlates, in Finkelhor D, Gelles RJ, Hotaling GT, Straus MA (eds): *The Dark Side of Families.* Beverly Hills, CA, Sage, 1983, pp 49–67.
53. Roy M: Four thousand partners in violence: A trend analysis, in *The Abusive Partner: An Analysis of Domestic Battering.* New York, Van Nostrand-Reinhold, 1982, pp 17–35.
54. Labell L: Wife abuse: A sociological study of battered women and their mates. *Victimology* 4:258–267, 1979.
55. Eberle P: Alcohol abusers and non-abusers: A discriminant analysis of differences between two subgroups of batterers. *J Health Soc Behav* 23:260–271, 1982.
56. Byles J: Violence, alcohol problems and other problems in disintegrating families, *J Stud Alcohol* 39:551–553, 1978.
57. Cleek M, Pearson T: Perceived causes of divorce: An analysis of interrelationships. *J Marriage Fam* 47:179–183, 1985.

58. Sterling RC, Weinstein SP, Gottheil E, Shannon D: Psychiatric symptomatology of crack cocaine abusers. *J Nerv Ment Dis* 182:564–569, 1995, in press.
59. Honer W, Gewirtz G, Turey M: Psychosis and violence in cocaine smokers. *Lancet* 451, 1987.
60. Sanchez J, Johnson B: Women and the drugs-crime connection: Crime rates among drug abusing women at Rikers Island. *J Psychoact Drugs* 19:2, 1987.
61. Grinspoon L, Bakalar J: Drug dependence: Non-narcotic agents, in Kaplan HI, Sadock BS (eds): *Comprehensive Textbook of Psychiatry/IV.* Baltimore, Williams & Williams, 1985, pp 1003–1015.
62. Cohen S: The cocaine problems. *Drug Abuse Alcohol Newslett* 12(10): 1983.
63. Allen L: PCP: A schizophrenomimetic. *US Pharm* 60–66, 1980.
64. Roberts A: Substance abuse among men who batter their mates: The dangerous mix. *J Subst Abuse Treat* 5:83–87, 1988.
65. Robins LN, Helzer JE, Croughan J, Ratcliff KS: National Institute of Mental Health: Diagnostic Interview Schedule. *Arch Gen Psychiatry* 38:381–389, 1989.
66. Straus M: Measuring intrafamily conflicts and violence: The Conflicts Tactics (CT) Scale. *J Marriage Fam* 41:75–88, 1979.
67. Lee V, Gottheil E, Weinstein SP: Personality characteristics of cocaine users who batter. Paper presented at the American Society of Addictive Medicine, Chicago, 1995.
68. Edleson J, Syers M: The effects of group treatment for men who batter: An 18-month follow-up study. *Res Soc Work Pract* 1(3):227–243, 1991.
69. Palmer S, Brown R, Barrera M: Group treatment program for abusive husbands. *Am J Orthopsychiatry* 62(2):276–283, 1992.
70. Shepard M: Predicting batterer recidivism five years after community intervention. *J Fam Violence* 7(3):167–178, 1992.
71. DeMaris A, Jackson J: Batterer's report of recidivism after counseling. *Soc Casework* 68:458–465, 1987.
72. Grusznski RJ, Carrillo, TP: Who completes batterer's treatment groups? *J Fam Violence* 3(2):141–150, 1988.
73. O'Leary KD: Assessment and treatment of partner abuse. *Clin Res Dig Suppl Bull 12.* American Psychological Association, 1995.
74. Geffner R: Guidelines for using mediation with abusive couples. *Psychother Individ Pract,* 1992.
75. Wallace B, Nosko A: Working with shame in the group treatment of male batterers. *Int J Group Psychother* 43(1):45–61, 1993.

Alcohol, Drugs, and Violence in Children's Lives

Brenda A. Miller, Eugene Maguin, and William R. Downs

Abstract. This chapter reviews the current state of knowledge concerning the interrelationship between the cycle of alcohol and other drugs (AOD) use and the cycle of violence. This issue is framed in terms of two questions. The first is the extent to which AOD use by the perpetrator is related to the perpetration of violence toward children, defined here as including both physical and sexual abuse. The second question is whether the experience of abuse during childhood is related to the subsequent development of the abuse of alcohol and other drugs. The review indicates that parental AOD abuse is related to physical and sexual abuse. However, because most perpetrators are not parents, the relationship is not yet clear. The data do support the link between experiencing childhood violence and the development of later AOD abuse. Theoretical explanations for each link are reviewed and mediating variables are identified. The review concludes with a presentation of methodological issues and the directions for future research.

1. Introduction

This chapter addresses the current state of knowledge about the interrelationship between the cycle of alcohol and other drugs (AOD) and the cycle of violence[1] by focusing on two questions. First, to what extent is AOD use* by

---

* While much of the work covered addresses these relationships for alcohol use/abuse, there is some evidence that these relationships exist with other types of drugs, particularly illegal or nonmedical use of drugs. Some cautions are needed in examining the relationships for drugs other than alcohol. First, the psychopharmacological effects of other substances vary widely.

Brenda A. Miller and Eugene Maguin • Research Institute on Addictions, Buffalo, New York 14203.   **William R. Downs** • Center for the Study of Adolescence, University of Northern Iowa, Cedar Falls, Iowa 50614.

Recent Developments in Alcoholism, Volume 13: Alcoholism and Violence, edited by Marc Galanter. Plenum Press, New York, 1997.

the perpetrator related to the perpetration of physical or sexual abuse against children?[†] Second, is the experience of physical or sexual abuse during childhood related to the subsequent development of AOD use/abuse? However, this chapter does not address the important question of whether AOD use by children is related to the perpetration of violence toward other children or adults (see Miczek et al.[2] review for a current review of this topic).

Studies pertaining to each question are covered first and are then followed by possible theoretical explanations for the links between these phenomena. The chapter next presents a discussion of the methodological considerations for researchers interested in pursuing these lines of inquiry and concludes with our recommendations for future research directions.

2. Perpetrator's Substance Use/Abuse and Physical and Sexual Abuse of Children

2.1. Parental Substance Problems and Perpetration of Child Physical Abuse

Early reviews concluded that, at most, only a modest association existed between parental alcohol problems and the perpetration of child physical abuse by the parents.[3,4] More recent reviews have concluded that either no relationship exists,[5] or that the association is limited to certain (unidentified) subgroups of those with alcohol problems.[6] However, all of these reviews have also acknowledged that the research testing these relationships had serious methodological shortcomings, including a lack of standardized instruments for the two main concepts of child abuse and parental alcohol problems, and an overrepresentation of minority and poor subgroups in the selection of samples.[3] Another concern was the inclusion of samples based on identified cases of child maltreatment, which limited the findings to children officially investigated. Thus, self-report cases that were never investigated were not represented in early studies. Where clinical samples of alcoholics were used without adequate comparison groups, it was difficult to separate the effects of treatment seeking from the effects of parental alcohol problems.

More recent studies that have used stronger methodological approaches support the association between parental AOD problems and experiences of physical abuse by the child.[7,8] Smyth et al.[8] compared 102 mothers with and

---

Different substances may play different roles. Second, the illegal nature of other drugs complicates the examination of the roles; relationships may exist more as a result of the illegal nature of the substance rather than the substance itself.

[†] Describing adolescents and teenagers as children in this chapter is meant to simplify the presentation but not meant as an oversight of the different developmental issues for the different age ranges. For an excellent review of the developmental issues as they relate to childhood victimization, see Finkelhor.[118]

66 mothers without lifetime histories of alcohol problems on their reported levels of harsh punishment as measured by the Conflict Tactics Scale (CTS)[9,10] and the Child Abuse Potential Scale.[11] Smyth et al.[8] found that mothers with histories of alcohol problems were more likely to use harsh punishments on their children. Furthermore, mothers with histories of alcohol problems were more likely to report that their partner was verbally aggressive toward their children, suggesting that mothers with alcohol problems may be less capable of shielding their children from victimization from others. In the Reider et al.[7] study, mothers and fathers in alcoholic families and nonalcoholic families completed the CTS and measures of lifetime alcohol problems. Reider et al.[7] found the same relationship for both parents: a higher level of lifetime alcohol problems was associated with a higher level of parent-to-child violence for that parent. Thus, there is evidence that the association holds in samples with clinically significant levels of alcohol problems.

Other recent studies that have used samples drawn from the general population have also supported a link between parental AOD problems and perpetration of violence toward children. For instance, Holmes and Robins[12] used the Ecological Catchment Area (ECA) study sample, which was designed to determine the general population prevalence and incidence rates of psychiatric disorders across five different sites in the nation. They found that parents with diagnoses of alcohol abuse/dependence (primarily fathers) or with diagnoses of depression (primarily mothers) reported higher levels of harsh, unfair discipline and parent-to-child violence than parents with neither diagnoses. However, given that the levels of harsh, unfair discipline and violence were similar for parents who had either an alcohol or a depression diagnosis, it would appear that psychiatric diagnoses in parents may raise the level of risk for violence toward children, rather than specifically alcohol problems. Thus, the study provides support for a link between alcohol problems and child maltreatment in the general population. However, given the relationship between parental depression and child physical abuse and the high concordance between depression and alcoholism,[13] the link between parental alcoholism and child physical abuse may be due to the common association with depression specifically or parent psychiatric disorders generally.

Because parents may be biased against reporting their own use of harsh punishment or severe violence toward their children, some researchers have asked adults to retrospectively report on use of physical violence and their parents' AOD use. In one such study, Radomsky[14] separated 120 consecutive female patients from a general medical practice into one of three groups according to whether they described their parents as (1) alcohol dependent; (2) harsh, rigid, or difficult but not alcohol dependent; or (3) neither alcohol dependent nor harsh, rigid, or difficult. Physical or sexual abuse levels were similar for the women who described their parents as either alcohol dependent or harsh, rigid, or difficult, and these levels were significantly higher than for women whose parents had neither of these problems. In another study,[15] women's reports of maternal and paternal alcohol problems (assessed by questions from the Research Diagnostic Criteria[16]) and both maternal and paternal child violence (assessed by the CTS) were collected from 472 women.* After controlling for race, number of changes in childhood family structure, and childhood socioeconomic status (SES) each parents' alcohol problems was found to be related to that parents' violence toward the respondent. Thus, there is evidence from several recent studies of a relationship between parental alcohol use and child physical abuse.

Most, if not all previous studies, have assumed that both parents in a family with an alcoholic or drug-abusing parent would report elevated levels of child physical abuse. To our knowledge only two studies have examined this question. Two different studies, one for male parolees[17] and one for women in treatment settings and the community,[15] found that parent-to-child violence was related to the parent with alcohol problems but not to the parent without the alcohol problems. Furthermore, Downs and Miller[15] found that these relationships remained after controlling for race, SES, and number of changes in the family structure. While these studies need to be replicated, the methodological precision of assessing both alcohol dependence and perpetration of violence for the same parent to correctly estimate the association between parent AOD and perpetration of violence toward children should not be overlooked.

In summary, the methodological shortcomings of the early literature may have led researchers to conclude that no relationship between parental AOD use and child physical abuse existed. Although more recent studies, using more representative samples, as well as a variety of types of samples and comparison groups and better assessments of the constructs, have found parental AOD use to be related to child physical abuse, further studies are needed to build confidence in this tentative conclusion.

2.2. Perpetrator AOD Problems and the Sexual Abuse of Children

Unlike child physical abuse, which implies a custodial relationship between the perpetrator and the child, child sexual abuse (CSA) does not necessarily imply such a relationship with the perpetrator. This definitional difference has a significant consequence for the types of questions that have been addressed. The question of the relationship between AOD problems and CSA requires that CSA perpetrators be studied or that CSA victims be able to accurately describe their assailant's level of substance use problems. If, instead, victims describe their parents' levels of AOD problems, the resulting association is a combination of the association between perpetrator AOD

---

* This study included samples of women in treatment for alcoholism ($n = 98$), mandatory education programs for driving while intoxicated ($n = 100$), in a shelter for battered women or in groups for battered women from an agency affiliated with the shelter ($n = 97$), in outpatient treatment for mental health issues ($n = 77$), and selected from the community using random digit dialing ($n = 82$).[82]

problems and CSA, given that their parent was the perpetrator, and the association between parent AOD problems and being assaulted by a non-parental adult, given that their parent was not the perpetrator. Thus, two distinct questions are blurred together.

Early studies of the relationship between substance use problems and CSA were primarily single-sample designs with subjects drawn from clinical or correctional populations of males convicted of sexual offenses. An early review of this literature concluded that alcohol use was involved in a substantial minority (approximately 40%) of sexual abuse incidents and that approximately half of all offenders had histories of alcohol problems.[18] However, because these early studies included no control or comparison group, it was difficult to definitively conclude that alcohol problems are related to CSA.

More recent studies have incorporated a number of methodological improvements to remedy the weaknesses of previous studies. However, these more recent studies have also approached this question from the perspective of the victims of CSA rather than that of the perpetrator. For example, Yama et al.[19] studied a convenience sample of 364 female college students who were asked to retrospectively describe their histories of CSA according to Finkelhor's[20] protocol and their parents' alcohol problems. The results showed a significant relationship between parental alcoholism and CSA. In a second study, Windle et al.[21] assessed the presence of a family history of alcoholism and the presence of physical and sexual abuse in a group of male and female alcoholic inpatients. Exactly 72% of men who had experienced both childhood physical and sexual abuse had a positive family history of alcoholism compared to about 39% of men who had experienced sexual abuse only and about 32% of the men who had neither physical nor sexual abuse during their childhoods. For women in the study, about 40% of women who had experienced neither form of abuse had a positive family history of alcoholism compared to 53% who had experienced sexual abuse and about 60% who had experienced both forms of abuse. Thus, experiences of CSA were associated with a family history of alcoholism for both males and females. Finally, Downs and Miller[15] examined the association between CSA and parental alcoholism in a sample of 472 women.* A significant bivariate relationship was found and the relationship remained after controlling for race of respondent, number of changes in childhood family, and childhood SES. In conclusion, more recent studies incorporating methodologically improved assessments of CSA and alcohol problems have consistently found a relationship between parental alcoholism and CSA.

Because more recent studies have used standardized assessments of CSA, some data, although sparse, are available on the relationship of the victim and the perpetrator. Yama et al.[19] found that 18% of their subjects had been sexually abused by a father or stepfather, 33% by another relative, and the remainder by strangers. Downs and Miller[15] reported that only 4% of women had been abused by the biological father or adoptive father. Although neither of these studies provide data on the magnitude of the association between perpetrator AOD problems and CSA (since victims could not report on the AOD problems of perpetrators who were not their parent), Downs and Miller[15] reported that a significantly higher percentage of women in the alcoholism treatment sample (37%) had been assaulted by a male family friend than in either the driving while intoxicated (DWI) sample (12%) or the household sample (16%).

Although many of the early studies on the parental AOD problems and CSA relationship suffer from a number of methodological weaknesses, current studies have used much improved and standardized methods of assessing CSA and parental alcoholism and substance use. While two recent studies have reported a significant association between parental AOD use and CSA, the fact that these studies also indicate that the majority of CSA is perpetrated by persons who are not the victim's parents means that very little is known about the magnitude of the association between CSA and the perpetrator's substance use. As a result, it seems advisable to study the CSA–parental substance use relationship in the context of the type of perpetrator (e.g., parent versus nonparent). These studies also highlight the importance of identifying how nonparental perpetrators gain access to their victims.

2.3. Explanations for the Link between Perpetrators' Substance Problems and Violence toward Children

Various hypotheses have been proposed to account for the link between perpetrator's alcohol use and his or her violence. One of the more promising is the cognitive disorganization hypothesis, which proposes that alcohol use results in the narrowing of attention to some social cues but not others.[22] Intoxication results in a "myopic" view of the world and only the most salient cues are acknowledged.[23] This narrowing of focus limits the abilities of the individual to process information to appropriately avoid behavioral consequences.[24] As applied to family violence, alcohol use results in miscommunication between family members, a focus on some cues but not others, overestimation of present threat, underestimation of consequences for aggression, and ultimately an increase in the likelihood of violence.

Collins[25] has pointed out the need to distinguish between acute and chronic effects of alcohol. For example, over a period of many years, chronic heavy alcohol use results in a number of cognitive impairments that are evident whether or not the person is currently drinking. Thus, alcohol use can have both acute effects on cognition (i.e., while drinking) and chronic cumulative effects on cognition. These possibilities help explain certain data regarding patterns of drinking and alcohol use. For example, Kantor and

---

* This study included samples of women in treatment for alcoholism ($n = 98$), mandatory education programs for driving while intoxicated ($n = 100$), in a shelter for battered women or in groups for battered women from an agency affiliated with the shelter ($n = 97$), in outpatient treatment for mental health issues ($n = 77$), and selected from the community using random digit dialing ($n = 82$).[82]

Straus[26] found parents with the highest levels of abuse to be mothers with binge-drinking patterns (reflecting perhaps acute effects of alcohol on cognition) and fathers with high daily alcohol consumption patterns (perhaps reflecting chronic alcohol effects).

A second promising explanation is the deviance disavowal hypothesis. According to this hypothesis, alcohol use allows the perpetrator to attribute the violence to the alcohol use, thereby avoiding or minimizing personal responsibility for the violence.[27–30] Thus, rather than creating a pharmacological effect, alcohol use is connected to cultural expectancies, and it is these cultural expectancies that create a greater likelihood of deviant, aggressive, or violent behavior. This hypothesis explains why alcohol use might be related to aggression in some settings but not others and why the cultural expectations about alcohol use may be important to explaining the behaviors exhibited when drinking.

A third hypothesis that has been advanced is the disinhibition hypothesis, which posits a direct pharmacological link between alcohol use and aggression such that alcohol anesthetizes brain centers that control inhibitions.[22,31–33] However, there has been little direct empirical support for the hypothesis.[34–37] In particular, the disinhibition hypothesis cannot explain why alcohol increases aggression in some experimental paradigms but not others.[38] Finally, cultural norms approve the use of corporal punishment (i.e., violence) against children,[39] and thus it might be argued that there are fewer inhibitions against harsh or punitive punishments of children.

The finding that an apparent majority of the perpetrators of child sexual abuse are not the child's parents or surrogates requires that the mechanism by which adults outside the nuclear family gain access to the child be identified. Parental unavailability is one construct that has been found to be associated with childhood sexual abuse.[40] Substance-abusing parents would be presumed to be less available to protect children from extrafamilial sexual abuse than nonsubstance-abusing parents. For example, Downs and Miller[15] found that the lack of paternal protection due to father's alcohol problems may have contributed to other males known to the family perpetrating sexual abuse against daughters, and formulated two hypotheses to account for these findings. First, daughters growing up in homes with an alcoholic father may not receive the typical emotional support, nurturance, and sustenance from their fathers. As a result, these girls may be more vulnerable to the manipulations of adult males outside the nuclear family who provide that support and nurturance, but at the cost of sexually abusing the girl. Second, daughters in homes with an alcoholic father may be more likely to be placed temporarily with relatives as the parents attempt to cope with the problems of alcohol dependence. These girls may then be more likely to be abused at the homes of these relatives. However, no studies of either theorized linkage have been conducted.

A second hypothesized explanatory construct is parental protectiveness. Most of our understanding about parental protectiveness comes from studies that have examined what mothers do in response to their children's victimization. Faller[41] reports a range of maternal responses toward children victimized by violence. Protective responses for children victimized by CSA include calling the police or protective services, leaving the house with the children, making the perpetrator leave, and/or initiating divorce proceedings when the perpetrator is a partner/spouse, placing the child where the alleged perpetrator cannot have access to the child, and insisting the perpetrator get treatment. Nonprotective responses include blaming or disbelieving the child, or allowing the child to remain in the risky environment.

Mothers may have difficulty making protective responses because of their substance abuse, as well as their own history of physical violence.[42,43] In addition, women with a history of CSA may be unable to protect their children from dangerous persons in the child's environment.[44–46] In particular, women who have been sexually victimized as children are frequently revictimized as adults,[47,48] an experience that may make it more difficult for these women to protect their children.[49] For instance, if mothers develop relationships with abusive partners, not only are they in danger, but their children may be in danger also. In their review of long-term effects of child sexual abuse, Beitchman and colleagues[47] suggest several explanations for this pattern, including: victimized children are forced out of the family and into high-risk situations; the impact on self-esteem may make mothers conspicuous targets for sexually exploitive men who may also abuse their children; women may idealize abusive men, seeking to reestablish the special relationship with their father (when father was the source of abuse); and impaired ability to identify correctly untrustworthy persons who may abuse their children.

Mothers' ability to maintain a quality parent–child relationship, in an environment conducive to skilled parenting, is limited by coexisting comorbidity problems.[46] A review by Finkelhor and Browne[50] report that sexually abused women in the general population displayed more mental health problems compared to nonvictims. Furthermore, women who abuse alcohol and other drugs show a similar high comorbidity of mental health problems when compared to the general population.[51] Jumper's[52] meta-analysis confirms the relationship between childhood sexual abuse and impaired adult psychological adjustment, typically resulting in depression, low self-esteem, childhood psychopathology, and adult emotional and behavioral problems. Together, these factors place women at greater risk to abuse their children.[53,54]

Although these explanations may prove to account for the direct links between AOD use and the perpetration of physical or sexual abuse against children, it may also be that the bivariate relationship is completely accounted for by variables that are strongly correlated with both substance use and physical or sexual abuse (i.e., third variables). In their review, West and Prinz[55] suggested a number of possible third variables including SES, maternal psychiatric illness, parental discord, divorce, financial problems, parental imprisonment, and reporting bias. In addition to these variables, it is critical that comorbid antisocial personality disorder (ASP) be tested as well, since it is well known that ASP is related to the early onset of alcohol problems, referred to as primary ASP and secondary alcoholism,[56–58] type II alcoholism,[59] or as type B alcoholism.[60] Also, DiLalla and Gottesman[61] have suggested that children of ASP-positive parents are more likely to be physically abused than children of ASP-negative parents. Thus, the association between parental alcohol problems and physical child abuse may be due to their common link with ASP or with other variables such as those suggested by West and Prinz.[55] Furthermore, these same relationships may also be true for CSA.

A few studies have controlled for third variables including a variable conceptually related to ASP. Among the variables included as possible third variables include antisocial behavior, depression, and marital aggression[7]; social support, stress, and SES[62]; and race, number of changes in childhood family structure, and childhood SES.[15] In each study cited, the association between parent alcohol problems and child physical abuse remained significant.

Downs et al.[63] have argued that there are serious empirical and definitional problems with the ASP construct such as low interrater reliability, low diagnostic stability, and conceptual ambiguity, which limits its usefulness as an explanatory construct. Although more work is needed, the results to date suggest the relationship is not due to a third variable. More research is needed to unravel additional factors that may be related to both parental alcohol problems and childhood maltreatment.

The existing body of literature pertaining to perpetrator AOD use and the perpetration of abusive behavior toward children needs to be enlarged. However, more than simple bivariate studies are needed. Future studies need to measure and control for possible third variables as well as include measures of theoretical constructs suggested by the several theories proposed as explanations of the substance use and violence toward children relationship.

3. Childhood Victimization as Antecedent to Later Substance Use

3.1 Childhood Physical Abuse Prior to Substance Use

Several studies using retrospective reports for adults suggest that individuals with AOD problems are more likely to report histories of physical abuse. Straus and Kantor[64] found that retrospectively measured severe parent-to-child violence during adolescence was related to increased drinking as adults in a national probability sample of adults. Holmes and Robins[65] found that alcoholic subjects (males and females) were significantly more likely to report that their parents had used severe forms of violence than controls. Brown and Anderson[66] found that among a sample of males and females receiving care at a military psychiatric hospital, physically abused patients were more likely to receive a alcohol disorder diagnosis than control patients who reported neither physical nor sexual abuse. In another study, Blane et al.[67] found that a greater exposure to childhood victimization led to an increased likelihood of an alcohol-dependence diagnosis in adulthood for a sample of male offenders on parole. Finally, Windle *et al.*[21] found that the prevalence of child physical abuse histories for both male and female inpatients in alcohol treatment facilities were considerably higher than rates for community-based studies, although the rates did not differ significantly for males and females. Thus, in samples of adults using retrospective recall, the evidence indicates a relationship between experiences of childhood physical abuse and the subsequent development of adult substance use problems.

While this evidence is compelling, neither of the two longitudinal studies that examined this question were able to find a link between experiences of childhood physical abuse and the development of later alcohol problems. Widom *et al.*[68] matched adults who had an official record of physical or sexual abuse or neglect from juvenile or adult court records as children to adults without such records as children on age, sex, and race, residence, and family economic status. Because Widom *et al.*[68] used only official records, it is likely that the comparison group contained an unknown percentage of cases with a history of unreported abuse or neglect. As adults, subjects completed an extensive assessment including diagnostic interview protocols. They found no relationships between physical abuse and measures of current or lifetime alcohol symptoms or diagnoses for either males or females. McCord[69] followed a group of 232 males originally assigned to the control group of the Cambridge–Somerville Study and interviewed them as adults. In 1957, the males were divided into four groups (abused, neglected, rejected, or loved) based on nearly 6 years of case records of interviews with the boys and their parents conducted by project social workers when the boys were from 5 to 9 years of age. McCord[69] found that the proportion of males who later became alcoholics in adulthood was not related to whether or not they had been abused, neglected, rejected, or "loved" as children. Further analyses of longitudinal datasets are needed to provide additional clarity on this question.

The few studies of adolescents using retrospective recall of physical abuse have yielded inconsistent results. A series of studies by Dembo and associates[70–72] of several different samples of adolescents in detention facilities found significant bivariate relationships for males and females separately and in combined samples between physical abuse and lifetime drug use. However, physical abuse failed to predict either adverse alcohol or marijuana consequences after controlling for background characteristics, self-reported delinquency, referral history, and psychological functioning in either cross-sectional analyses or in longitudinal analyses.[73] Although Dembo and associates used several different samples, other studies are needed to address this question with different types of samples. Even so, it may be that effect of physical abuse on the development of AOD problems becomes distinguishable only in adulthood.

Most studies have simply examined the effect of parental violence on children. The question these studies cannot address is whether father-to-child violence, for example, has different effects than mother-to-child violence for female children. In two separate samples of women, Downs et al.[74] and Miller et al.[43] found that alcoholic women in treatment reported significantly higher levels of verbal aggression, moderate violence, and severe violence from their father but not their mother than did nonalcoholic women. Although the Miller et al.[43] study found that alcoholic women also reported higher levels of verbal aggression, moderate violence, and severe violence from their mother, these differences disappeared once background characteristics including parental alcoholism were controlled. Furthermore, these relationships also held when involvement in treatment was controlled.[43]

Overall, the data indicate that the relationship between child physical abuse and later AOD problems is stronger for adult samples than for adolescent samples. However, further studies using adolescent samples are needed, since the current database consists of only two samples from a single source. Furthermore, there is some evidence that the effects of severe violence in the family depend, at least for female children, on whether paternal or maternal violence is examined.

3.2. Child Sexual Abuse Prior to Substance Use

Although early reviews of the consequences of CSA[47,75,76] did not consider substance abuse, a more recent review did do so. Polusny and Follette[77] identified a number of studies, using both community and clinical samples, that reported significantly higher rates of AOD diagnoses (either alcohol or drugs) for women who had been CSA victims. Their summary shows that the prevalence of lifetime AOD diagnoses in community samples ranged from 13.7 to 31.0% among female CSA victims compared to 3.1 to 12.0% among non-CSA females. In clinical samples the prevalence ranged from 20.9 to 57.0% among female CSA victims compared to 2.3 to 27.0% among non-CSA females. Polusny and Follette[77] included studies that defined CSA as any forced or coerced sexual behavior imposed on a child and sexual activity between a child and a much older person, whether or not coercion was involved. However, because many studies relied on single-item assessments or other nonstandardized assessments, there was likely some degree of variability in the prevalence data attributable to methods.

More recent studies also generally support the relationship between CSA and AOD problems for adult women; however, much less is known about adolescent women. For example, Wilsnack et al.[78] found that CSA, as measured by the Russell[79] and the Wyatt[80] methodology, was related to an increased prevalence of alcohol problems over the past 12 months, including dependence symptoms, problem drinking, and heavy drinking, as well as lifetime substance use in a large national probability sample of US women. Also, Mullen et al.[81] found that CSA involving intercourse was related to both heavy drinking and drug dependence in an enriched probability sample of Dunedin, New Zealand adult women. In this study, sexual abuse was measured by self-report followed by an interview to confirm the self-reported experiences. Only one study, that of Dembo et al.,[70] was found that studied adolescent females. This study, which measured CSA by the Finkelhor[20] criteria, found that CSA was related to lifetime drug use for a sample of adolescent females in detention facilities. Thus, these three studies support the CSA–substance abuse relationship for both adult and adolescent women.

Widom et al.[68] also studied this question with their sample of adults with officially recorded sexual abuse and matched adults. They found that officially recorded CSA was associated with a higher level of current alcohol symptoms for females. However, no difference was noted for the lifetime alcohol symptoms, current alcoholism diagnosis, and lifetime alcoholism diagnosis.

Since the mid-1980s, Miller and associates have studied the links between early childhood victimization and the later development of alcohol and other drug problems in women (see Miller and Downs[82] for a review). In an early study,[42] which compared 45 women who either had previously received treatment or were currently in treatment to 40 women without alcohol problems recruited from the community, women with alcohol problems were found to be 2.5 times more likely to have been CSA victims. In a later study, Miller et al.[43] found that alcoholic women were significantly more likely to have experienced all forms of sexual abuse (exposure, touching, and penetration) than were women in either the DWI or community samples. In a second analysis, women in treatment settings with and without alcohol problems and women in the community were compared to assess the effects of treatment involvement. Women in treatment with alcohol problems were significantly more likely to have CSA histories compared to women in treatment without alcohol problems after controlling for parental alcohol problems.

Taken together, the evidence from a number of retrospective studies of adults, a study of adolescents, and a prospective cohort study indicates that females who have been sexually abused as children are more likely to have AOD problems later in life. The evidence is clearer for adult women than for adolescent women by virtue of the fact that more studies have been conducted for adults. Thus, further work is needed with adolescent samples.

By comparison, few studies have included samples of males, regardless of the source.[21] In fact, Polusny and Follette's[77] review included only one study of males[83] and only a few others were located in a literature search. Stein et al.,[83] who used the Los Angeles ECA sample, found that significantly more males who had been sexually assaulted as children (44.9%) had received an abuse or dependence diagnosis for drugs as adults than did males who had not been assaulted (7.8%). However, no difference in the rates of an alcoholism abuse or dependence diagnosis was found between the two groups. In a prospective cohort study of adults, Widom et al.[68] did not find any association between CSA and either current or lifetime alcohol symptoms, or between CSA and either lifetime or current diagnosis for males. In a third study, Harrison et al.[84] found that sexually abused male adolescent patients in a substance abuse treatment program were more likely to report daily drinking than nonabused male patients. Finally, Dembo et al.[70] found that CSA was related to lifetime drug use for male adolescents in a detention facility. Thus, the data for males is mixed as some studies have found significant results, while others using different designs have not.

Overall, the data indicate that CSA is related to later AOD problems in adulthood for women, irrespective of whether the women are drawn from clinical samples or community samples when retrospective measures of CSA are used. Although there have been considerably fewer studies of males, CSA may also be related to later AOD problems. Furthermore, the relationship between CSA and alcohol problems, at least for women, has remained when personal and family background characteristics, including the presence of parental alcoholism, were controlled. Similar analyses are needed for males.

The literature suggests that one of the consequences for children who are either physically or sexually abused is a greater likelihood of AOD problems in adulthood and possibly in adolescence. At present, the data are not sufficient to determine whether one type of abuse is associated with a greater likelihood of AOD problems or whether males or females, given the experience of abuse, are more prone later AOD problems. Further work is needed on these points.

3.3. Explanations of the Linkage from CSA and Parent-to-Child Violence to AOD Problems

Although the explanations of the linkage from CSA and parent-to-child violence to AOD problems are not well understood, Miller and Downs[82] proposed three possibilities for women. In this chapter, these explanations will be expanded to include men (see also Downs and Miller,[15] Downs et al.[63]).

3.3.1. Substance Use as a Coping Mechanism. Reviews of both CSA and child physical abuse consequences have concluded that depression, suicidal ideation, and low self-esteem are among the sequela of CSA and child physical abuse in adult samples.[77,85] And, subsequent studies reaffirm these conclusions.[64,78] Although these data point to depression as a mediating variable between victimization and subsequent substance use, the comorbidity data for alcoholism and depression do not completely support this view. Results from the ECA studies indicate that for males the observed comorbidity of depression and alcoholism abuse or dependence is usually—in about 78% of the cases—due to the secondary depression; that is, depression which follows the onset of alcoholism.[13] However, Hesselbrock et al.[57] found the converse for females: that a diagnosis of major depression preceded a diagnosis of alcohol dependence. Thus, the role of depression as a mediating variable may depend on gender.

Another perspective is offered by studies of the effects of childhood abuse for adolescent samples. Reviews of the effects of CSA and physical abuse on children[85,86] have also found elevated levels of depression, withdrawal, and anxiety. More recently, Boney-McCoy and Finkelhor[87] found that 10- to 16-year-old males from a community sample who have experienced

CSA, but not similar females, reported increased sadness. They also noted no relationship between parental violence and sadness for either males or females. However, McCloskey et al.[88] found that, after controlling for all forms of family violence, a canonical correlation analysis revealed associations between both father-to-child violence and severe father-to-child violence by both maternal and child report and depression by maternal report in their community sample of 6- to 12-year-old children. Furthermore, CSA was not related to depression by either maternal or child report. Studies of clinical samples of adolescents who had experienced either physical or sexual abuse have also found increased depression and self-destructive behavior for both males and females.[84,89,90] Thus, it does appear that on the whole depression is also a consequence of abuse for adolescents, just as it is for adults. However, further studies are clearly needed to reinforce this conclusion and to examine whether gender differences also exist for adolescents.

Kaplan's[91] theory of low self-esteem (i.e., self-derogation), although developed to explain adolescent drug abuse, provides a cogent theoretical linkage between depression and low self-esteem reported by children and adolescents who have experienced CSA and physical abuse and the development of substance abuse problems. Briefly (see Miller and Downs[82]), CSA and physical abuse are posited to lead to self-devaluation and a loss of self-esteem when the emotional impact of the abusive events overwhelm the coping abilities of the child victim. Ultimately, depression and possible self-destructive behavior may result. Substance use is viewed as a method for keeping both the short-term and long-term emotional consequences at bay.

The empirical model implied by these data and Kaplan's[91] theory has not been completely tested with either child or adolescent samples. However, Dembo et al.[70] was able to test a portion of the model in a cross-sectional analysis of data from a sample of male and female juveniles in detention facilities. They found that both CSA and child physical abuse predicted increased self-derogation, and that self-derogation subsequently predicted lifetime drug use. However, their data also showed that self-derogation did not fully mediate the bivariate relationship between either CSA or child physical abuse and lifetime drug use. Thus, their results indicate that additional variables may be needed to account for the bivariate relationships.

3.3.2. Externalizing Behavior. Although reviews of studies using adult samples have not reported any evidence of a possible relationship between CSA and externalizing behaviors (i.e., aggression, violence, hyperactivity, and delinquency) either during adolescence or adulthood, reviews focusing on child and adolescent samples have done so. Kendall-Tackett et al.[86] concluded that increased aggression, delinquency, and cruel or antisocial behavior was a consequence of CSA. Malinosky-Rummell and Hansen's[85] review of the consequences of physical abuse also reached similar conclusions. In addition, Malinosky-Rummell and Hansen[85] concluded that physical abuse is associated with an increased frequency of noncompliance, nonaggressive conduct disorders in children, and possibly nonviolent delinquency (i.e., property crimes). Recent studies have also generally supported these conclusions. Boney-McCoy and Finkelhor[87] found that CSA was associated with increased "teacher trouble" for both males and females. Contact CSA, a more severe form of CSA, was also associated with teacher trouble for female adolescents (the parallel analysis was not done for males due to insufficient sample size). They also found that parental violence was associated with teacher trouble for female adolescents but not for males. Although McCloskey et al.[88] did not find any evidence that CSA was associated with increased oppositional behavior in their sample of preadolescent children, they did find that moderate mother–child and father–child violence but not severe father–child violence was associated with oppositional behavior, after controlling for the global level of family violence for their sample of preadolescent children.

Aggression and other forms of externalizing behavior, particularly when it appears at a young age and persists, has been repeatedly found to be a strong predictor of substance use problems (see Hawkins et al.[92] for a review). Involvement in deviant peer groups whose activities are organized around delinquency or substance use has been posited by several investigators as the key mediating variable between aggression and substance use.[91,93] Another hypothesis, advanced by Miller and Brown,[94] proposes that antisocial or aggressive behavior in childhood underlies delayed skills in self-regulation that lead to the development of alcohol and drug problems by young adulthood. In addition to the role of aggressive behavior, Kaplan[91] also proposes that children with low self-esteem and poor coping and social interaction skills may lose the motivation to conform to more prosocial peer groups, and thus join with peers involved in deviant peer groups. However, no studies were located that tested models such as these.

3.3.3. Posttraumatic Stress Disorder Related Symptoms.

Along with depression, posttraumatic stress disorder (PTSD)* is one of the more commonly occurring consequences of CSA or parent-to-child violence.[47,76,77,85,86] More recently, Boney-McCoy and Finkelhor[87] found a significant association between the presence of CSA and parent-to-child violence and increased PTSD symptoms for both male and female samples.

Currently, only one study has examined the relationship between victim-

---

* The *Diagnostic and Statistical Manual of Disorders* (DSM), 4th ed, states that this disorder occurs after exposure to extreme traumatic stressors such as: (1) personal experiences that threaten death, serious injury, or personal integrity in some other manner, or (2) witnessing or learning about another family member's or close associate's unexpected death, serious injury, or threat to personal integrity. The individual's response to the event must involve intense fear, helplessness, or horror. Such experiences can trigger symptoms characteristic of PTSD: (1) a persistent reexperiencing of the trauma (e.g., recurrent distressing dreams of the event); (2) avoidance of the associated stimuli (e.g., efforts to avoid activities, places, or people that arouse recollections of the trauma), as well as a numbing of the general responsiveness (e.g., feelings of detachment or estrangement from others); and (3) persistent symptoms of increased arousal (e.g., hypervigilance, startle response). These symptoms must be present for more than 1 month and create significant distress or impairment in social, occupational, or other important areas of functioning for a diagnosis of PTSD.

ization, PTSD symptoms, and alcohol problems. The prevalence of two or more alcohol problems among women participating in the National Women's Study[95] was 1.5% of those who had not been victimized, 3.9% among women who had been victimized but experienced no PTSD symptoms, and 14.5% among women who had been victimized and experienced PTSD symptoms. Theoretical underpinnings of these data are not clear. However, it may be that alcohol, and possibly drugs as well, may facilitate the disassociation needed to gain relief from the memories of the experience. Support for this view comes from women's own stated motives for drinking.[96–98]

Empirically, the association between CSA and parent-to-child violence and AOD problems may be due to a variable that is associated with both physical and sexual abuse and the later development of AOD problems. Parental alcoholism is one variable that has been advanced for this role.

Parental alcoholism has been linked to the perpetration of physical abuse and CSA. It has also been found to be consistently and strongly linked to the development of alcoholism in the biological offspring.[60,99,100] Although these data suggest that parental alcoholism may account for the association between child physical and sexual abuse and later alcoholism, few studies have examined this issue. However, in two separate studies, Miller et al.[42,43] found that while parental alcohol problems did predict later alcohol problems for women, CSA also predicted later alcohol problems. In addition, Miller et al.[43] also found that father-to-child severe violence but not mother-to-child severe violence also predicted later alcohol problems. Thus, there are some data to indicate that parental alcoholism does not account for the association between abuse during childhood and later substance use problems. Whether these same relationships would also hold for males is a question in need of investigation.

4. Methodological Considerations

Recent reviews on the connections either between perpetrators' alcohol problems and their victimization of children or between childhood victimization and the development of alcohol problems identify the need for improvements in research design (e.g., better control groups, multivariate rather than bivariate analyses).[5,101] This section covers three additional issues that need to be carefully considered in future studies: definitions and measurement of violence toward children, controversies regarding childhood memories of violence, and ethical and legal concerns.

4.1. Definitions and Measurement of Violence toward Children

There is great variation in how violence is defined. On one end of the continuum are studies that rely on official records of founded cases to define violence.[5] Strict definitions of physical and sexual abuse are used to identify cases, evidence verifies existence of abuse, and authorities investigate each case to ensure that legal criteria for physical or sexual abuse are met. Samples based on these official records contain few false-positive cases. For official data on incidence and prevalence of child abuse cases brought to the attention of Child Protective Service agencies, the National Center on Child Abuse and Neglect has established a national data collection and analysis program (National Child Abuse and Neglect Data System).[102] This program is authorized under Public Law 102-295, the Child Abuse, Domestic Violence, Adoption and Family Services Act of 1992.[102]

However, most incidents of physical and/or sexual abuse are not officially investigated, and thus officially identified cases are not representative of all victimized children. In 1991, states received reports on 2.7 million children,[102] but estimates of the amount of parent-to-child violence are much higher. Straus and Gelles[103] report from their National Family Violence resurvey of 1985 that an estimated 6.9 million children are severely assaulted each year and an unknown number of children are sexually abused each year. In particular, there may be a class bias as to which children will be reported and found to be a physically or sexually abused child. Given that states have different laws defining child abuse and childhood sexual abuse, there will be differences in definitions across states. Furthermore, official records are often incomplete reports and missing data can pose problems.

At the other end of the continuum are the studies that have chosen a more inclusive range of experiences to represent violence. Gelles and Straus[104] propose that violence be viewed as "an act carried out with the intention or perceived intention of physically hurting another person." Because corporal punishment is carried out with the intent to cause physical pain, Straus[105] identifies corporal punishment as a form of parent-to-child violence. To provide information for these more inclusive definitions of physical and sexual abuse of children, data from self-reports are gathered. For self-reports, measurement tools require specificity regarding types of behaviors that are considered violent. This specificity is preferable to global questions or questions that label behavior as "physical abuse" or "sexual abuse."[20,43,106] Also, global questions concerning physical or sexual abuse may result in underestimates of these events, especially if respondents are asked to label their own experiences as abuse. For this reason, researchers have constructed instruments that identify a range of specific behaviors for identifying physical and sexual abuse.

For measures of physical (nonsexual) violence, the CTS[107,108] continues to be widely accepted for measuring parent-to-child violence.* Three general sections are included in the CTS: rational discussion, termed Reasoning; verbal or nonverbal acts that symbolically hurt the other, termed Verbal Aggression; and use of physical aggression, termed Violence.[109] The Violence subscale is further divided into Minor and Severe Violence. The CTS captures frequency of the behavior within a year's time frame (although this time frame is often altered to meet the needs of the research project). Perhaps

---

* For further information, contact Family Research Laboratory, University of New Hampshire, Durham, NH 03824.

because of its wide adoption in many different contexts, there are criticisms of the CTS, including: its framing of violence in response to conflicts, limitations in the set of violent acts, assessing threats as forms of violence, inaccuracies of self-reports over a 1-year period, equating acts that differ greatly in seriousness, failure to consider context and who initiates violence, distinctions made between minor and severe violence, how gender differences for specific behaviors impact outcomes, and inability of the CTS to determine the process and sequence of violence.[109] In addition, the CTS is not designed to determine short- or long-term effects of child abuse. Despite these limitations, the CTS has been one of the most widely used measures of family violence, and data from two national studies (1975 and 1985) provide an excellent opportunity for comparing rates in specific samples with the general population.[110] Recently, the authors have created a revised version of the parent–child CTS (PCCTS), which provides more appropriate reasoning and psychological abuse scales for parent–child relationships. The PCCTS also has three supplemental scales: Neglect, Sexual Abuse, and Injury.

Researchers may choose to avoid knowing about actual parent-to-child violence in order to avoid having to report this violence to legal authorities, thereby violating the promise of confidentiality to respondents (see Section 4.3). Other measures can be considered when measures of potential for violence, rather than actual violence, are appropriate. For example, the Child Abuse Potential scale[11] provides a measure of parental propensity for violence toward children, based on parent characteristics. The Parental Punitiveness Scale[111] identifies a number of punitive responses toward hypothetical situations involving children's misbehavior and has been revised to include more severe forms of punishment.[67]

Measures of childhood sexual abuse have largely been developed for the retrospective assessment of victimization.[20,43,112] As with physical abuse, there is great variation in the definition of sexual abuse. Defining the relationship of perpetrators and victims, requiring age differences between the perpetrators and the victims (e.g., 5-year age differences), and whether to include perceived consensual events (e.g., boyfriends who are more than 5 years older) are crucial to establishing a definition of childhood sexual abuse. As with childhood physical abuse, measuring childhood sexual abuse requires careful specification of behaviors, including suggestions of sexual activity, touching, as well as penetration, without defining such behaviors as sexual abuse. In addition, the operational definitions of sexual abuse will differ between boys and girls. Identifying specific behaviors that have occurred produce higher prevalence rates than do single screening questions.[20,113]

During the research process, sensitivity must be given to the impact of respondent's having revealed traumatic events. In interview settings, individuals may reveal experiences that have not been previously shared and may display emotions (e.g., crying, anger) that require sensitive handling. Recalling experiences may exacerbate posttraumatic stress symptoms, and a list of community resources that provide counseling may be appropriate for all participants, regardless of whether they report histories of violence or not. The research staff must be carefully trained to address these situations to minimize harm to individuals and to maintain integrity of the research process.

Comparisons of self-administered questionnaires and face-to-face interviews in a retrospective survey of childhood sexual abuse suggest that interviews are not necessarily superior to self-administered formats in assisting in disclosure of childhood sexual abuse.[113] A small group of women (10%) reported childhood sexual abuse during a self-administered questionnaire but not during the face-to-face interviews. Similarly, 12.4% of the women reported childhood sexual abuse during the face-to-face interviews but not during the self-administered questionnaire. However, interviews assist in clarifying different behaviors and provide better detail regarding the incidents of childhood sexual abuse.[113] Childhood sexual abuse is perpetrated under a veil of secrecy. Even after the child becomes an adult, talking about these secrets may be difficult. Thus, individuals who have abuse histories may assess more carefully who they tell and whether there is a compelling reason to tell the person asking about the experience. Researchers need to create an atmosphere of respect and privacy to provide a safe setting where these secrets can be shared discreetly. Furthermore, respondents may question why the researcher needs to know this intimate and private information and the research team should be prepared to respond to these questions.

In this chapter, our definition of violence toward children focuses on acts of both physical and sexual abuse; we have not reviewed neglect, psychological abuse, or the impact of witnessing violence. These additional acts of commission or omission are also important potential impacts on children's lives that are interwoven with physical and sexual abuse. Furthermore, studies on violence toward children should consider the impact of multiple forms of victimization from different perpetrators, over extended periods of time.

4.2. Controversies Regarding Childhood Memories of Violence

Much of what is known about the connections between substance problems and childhood victimization is based on retrospective reports from adults. Three major concerns have emerged for such retrospective data. First, there is a concern that adults do not necessarily remember or accurately remember their experiences in childhood.[5] There is some indication that the failure to remember is specifically connected to traumatic events; individuals repress painful memories as a coping mechanism.[114] Empirical evidence exists that demonstrates that adults do fail to report their childhood victimization experiences. In a sample of women substance abusers ($n = 105$) in outpatient treatment who reported histories of CSA, 19% stated that they had forgotten the abuse at some point in their lives.[112] In a recent study of officially reported cases of CSA, reinterviewed 17 years later as adults, Williams[115] found that a large proportion of women (38%) did not recall or chose not to report the index case of sexual abuse.* Even among the women who did remember the index incident, 16% reported that there was some period of time in the past when they did not remember the incident. Being younger in age at the time of abuse and having a greater level of force used in the assault were positively related to failure to remember. Failure to recall victimization experiences will result in false-negative cases within the control group, thereby attenuating differences between groups.

Another concern is that memories that are retrieved may be false or constructed. Loftus[116] proposes that both popular writings and therapists' suggestions can create false memories. The basis for her argument is largely anecdotal evidence. Although "false recall" has been raised largely within therapeutic settings, careful consideration should be given to prevent such concerns from emerging within research settings. Questions concerning childhood sexual abuse, asked after rapport has been established but early in the questionnaire/interview, may avoid opportunities for "created memories" during the research process, particularly in studies that involve multiple follow-ups. Providing interviewers with training to ensure that they impart empathy without suggesting or leading respondents is another important concern, particularly when open-ended questions are used to probe for more detailed information. Careful selection of the research team to avoid potential assistants who may be overzealous in finding reported cases of child victimization is essential.

The final concern is that subjects may refuse to tell researchers about their victimization. Koss[106] suggests that matching sex and ethnicity may improve willingness to divulge information about prior sexual victimization. Providing confidential settings that are comfortable and safe may also promote willingness to report victimization. Concerns about adequacy of recall are important for any research project relying on self-report data. Such concerns should not devalue the importance of individual reports about their life experiences. Especially with regard to long-term consequences, memories that are recalled may have more relevance to later impact on other life events than does a "factual" accounting of the event.[1]

4.3. Ethical and Legal Issues

A number of ethical and legal issues are involved in conducting research with or about children who may be experiencing or have experienced violent victimization. For instance, asking parents or other adult figures to report on their use of violence toward children presents a dilemma when these respondents report violence. According to Socolar and Amaya-Jackson,[117] health care professionals, teachers, and other child care professionals are required

---

* Williams did not reveal the true purpose of the follow-up interview and some of the failure to report may not be due to lack of memory but rather a conscious choice not to report.

by law to report suspected maltreatment disclosed by subjects in all states, and in nearly half of the states anyone suspecting child maltreatment is required to report. Socolar and Amaya-Jackson[117] report different techniques used to avoid such dilemmas, including pursuing anonymous data. Use of anonymous data precludes the possibility of follow-up research designs or matching individuals with official data sources. Regardless of the legal requirements, researchers have ethical responsibilities for reporting suspected child abuse, and some would argue that researchers have an ethical responsibility to find out about abuse.

Institutional Review Boards require that subjects be informed of risks that may result from participation in the research project. Parents or other adult figures, once informed that their answers to questions concerning violence could potentially result in official action against them, may refuse to participate. Another research concern is the bias that occurs if individuals who perpetrate violence against children disproportionately refuse to participate. Even among participants who choose to participate, a chilling effect on the research process may be expected as participants weigh their answers for the possible actions that might be taken. If a researcher informs parents that children who participate in a research project may be at risk for intervention by the authorities in cases where there is a suspicion of child abuse, children who are victims of parental violence may not be allowed to participate.

Researchers have used various techniques to avoid such dilemmas, such as limiting questions asked. As mentioned earlier, measurements can be used that provide information about punishments for hypothetical situations involving children's misbehavior. Hypothetical situations can include responses that are both appropriate and abusive. Answers that parents give to hypothetical situations represent parental attitudes regarding what is socially acceptable, but may not measure propensity for violence adequately. Researchers may ask about punishments, excluding punishments that would be defined legally as child abuse, but that includes corporal punishment. Finally, subjects may be warned not to divert from answering the specific questions asked. Interviewers can be trained to warn or "head off" any divergence from the established questions that might lead to potential conflicts between confidentiality and protection of children.

Another difficulty for researchers involved in prospective designs is that identification of children who are suspected cases of child abuse will result in some type of intervention. Any intervention may impact the long-term outcomes under investigation. The specific issue of whether substance problems are one of the consequences of untreated childhood victimization is difficult to address in prospective designs that identify children who experience abuse. Identifying samples of official cases of child abuse avoids some of the problems of other approaches in so far as the researcher does not have to report the case. However, children may reveal additional abuse not known to authorities.

5. Future Directions

5.1. Considerations for Research Designs and Data Analyses

5.1.1. Developmental Victimology. Child development has received relatively little attention in the study of childhood victimization. Recently, a framework for examining "developmental victimology" has been proposed with two separate domains.[118] First, there are developmental aspects of risk, which are typified by the changing risks children encounter as a result of their age and level of development. Second, there are developmental aspects of impact, which identify variation in responses to victimization dependent on the developmental stage. Children at different stages of development have differing capacities for resiliency and differing vulnerabilities.[119,120] The role of alcohol or drugs in perpetrating childhood violence and the role of childhood violence in developing alcohol or drug abuse problems may operate differentially, depending on the developmental stage of the child at the time of the event. Thus, future studies should consider how risks for violence might be assessed in view of the child's age. Furthermore, to assess developmental aspects of consequences, age of the child at the time of victimization and duration of victimization across developmental stages need to be considered. Males and females may respond differently to victimization experiences at the same developmental stage. Finally, children at different developmental stages will report on victimization experiences differently. Assessments of violence that are appropriate for different stages of development are needed.

5.1.2. Examination of Mother and Father Violence Separately. Results from studies[7,43] indicate differences in impact between mother and father violence toward children. Collecting data to allow for separate analyses would benefit and further our understanding of this issue. There are several possible explanations for why this difference may exist. Mother and father violence are qualitatively different both in terms of threat and harm caused. Mother violence may occur in the context of numerous mother–child interactions, while father violence may occur within the context of fewer total interactions. Mothers may not be able to protect children from father violence, but fathers can protect children from mother violence, subsequently affecting the long-term impact of violence on children's lives. Finally, parent violence from the same-sex parent may have different meanings than parent violence from the opposite-sex parent.

5.1.3. Inclusion of Multiple Forms of Victimization. Investigations of the relationships between childhood violence and alcohol or drugs have often focused on only one form of victimization. However, research indicates that multiple forms of violent victimization often occur in children's lives.[43,21] More research is needed that includes both physical abuse and sexual abuse histories. Consideration needs to be given to the number of different types of perpetrators that may victimize children. Children may have multiple parent figures during their lives and multiple primary caregivers. Exposure to mother's boyfriends and extended families including siblings of different ages can also broaden the range of risk to children. As discussed earlier, parental alcohol and drug problems can impact the protection of children from violent victimization. Further investigation of this parental role omission should consider the vulnerability to different types of perpetrators for these children. In addition, impact of violent victimization from multiple perpetrators may have differential impact on the long-term consequences, including drug or alcohol abuse, for children.

5.1.4. Contexts and the Meanings Associated with the Victimization. One of the least developed areas of this research has been the contexts of experiences and meanings associated with victimization. For example, assumptions are sometimes made that physically invasive sexual acts (e.g., sexual intercourse) are more harmful than less invasive sexual acts (e.g., showing sexual parts of the body). Yet, when asked to choose the most traumatic or upsetting sexual experience (when multiple experiences are present), women have reported that the context of the experience can make the less physically intrusive experience more traumatic. Research that provides in-depth exploration of the meanings of these events is needed. This type of research is often avoided because of the lengthy process of analyzing and coding open-ended data. However, understanding the meanings of these events to people's lives can provide a better understanding of connections between alcohol, drugs, and childhood violence.

5.2. Summary

Our understanding of the relationships between alcohol, drugs, and childhood victimization has been aided by the growth of studies on family violence and child maltreatment and the development of alcohol and drug research in general. Combining these two major arenas into a research agenda requires a comprehensive understanding of both fields of research and how they overlap as well as differ. The prospect of pursuing research on these questions can seem overwhelmingly difficult because of the complexity of the issues and the diversity of subjects who are affected by these issues. Yet, a careful review of people's lives and the problems that they present indicates the relevance of this research. Histories of childhood violence and substance abuse problems overlap within generations and reappear in subsequent generations. Investigations that examine either cycles of violence or cycles of addiction do not provide adequate understanding of synergistic effects. There is a need to study these problems in combination and across generations.

Although our knowledge about the relationships between AOD problems and violence toward children is far from adequate, there is evidence that perpetration of violence toward children may be related to the perpetrator's AOD problems, and that parental AOD problems may increase the vulnerability of children for victimization from others. More recently, studies have focused on the relationships between victimization experiences and the development of AOD problems in subsequent years, and results indicate support for this relationship, as well. Given these results, intergenerational studies of AOD problems may also want to include investigation of inter-generational patterns of violence. Furthermore, treatment programs may need to consider the impact of victimization experiences on initiation and maintenance of dependence on alcohol and drugs. Finally, preventing violence may help prevent future AOD problems.

References

1. Miller BA: Investigating links between childhood victimization and alcohol problems, in Martin SE (ed): *Alcohol and Interpersonal Violence: Fostering Multidisciplinary Perspectives,* Monograph 24. 1993, pp 315–323. Rockville, MD: US Government Printing Office.
2. Miczek KA, DeBold JF, Haney M, *et al:* Alcohol, drugs, and violence, in Reiss AJ, Roth JA (eds): *Understanding and Preventing Violence:* vol 3: *Social and Psychological Perspectives on Violence.* Washington, DC, National Academy Press, 1993, pp 377–570.
3. Orme TC, Rimmer J: Alcoholism and child abuse: A review. *J Stud Alcohol* 42:273–287, 1981.
4. Black R, Mayer J: Parents with special problems: Alcoholism and opiate addiction. *Child Abuse Negl* 4:45–54, 1980.
5. Widom CS: *Child Abuse and Alcohol Use and Abuse: Alcohol and Interpersonal Violence: Fostering Multidisciplinary Perspectives* (Research Monograph Series 24). Rockville, MD, NIAAA US Department of Health and Human Services, 1992, pp 291–314.
6. Leonard KE, Jacob T: Alcohol, alcoholism, and family violence, in Van Hasselt VB, Morrison RL, Bellack AS, Hersen J (eds): *Handbook of Family Violence.* New York, Plenum Press, 1988, pp 383–406.
7. Reider E, Zucker RA, Maguin ET, *et al:* Alcohol involvement and violence towards children among high risk families. Paper presented at the 97th Annual Meeting of the American Psychological Association, New Orleans, LA, August 1989.
8. Smyth NJ, Miller BA, Janicki PI, *et al:* Mothers' protectiveness and child abuse: The impact of her history of childhood sexual abuse and an alcohol diagnosis. Paper presented at the American Society of Criminology Conference, Boston, MA, November 1995.
9. Straus MA, Gelles RJ, Steinmetz SK: *Behind Closed Doors: Violence in the American Family.* Garden City, NJ, Anchor Books, 1980.
10. Miller BA, Downs WR, Testa M: The relationship between women's alcohol problems and experiences of childhood violence. Paper presented at the Annual Meeting of the American Psychological Association, Boston, MA, 1990.
11. Milner JS, Wimberly RC: An inventory for the identification of child abusers. *J Clin Psychol* 35:95–100, 1979.
12. Holmes SJ, Robins LN: The role of parental disciplinary practices in the development of depression and alcoholism. *Psychiatry* 51:24–36, 1988.
13. Helzer JE, Pryzbeck TR: The co-occurrence of alcoholism with other psychiatric disorders in the general population and its impact on treatment. *J Stud Alcohol* 49:219–224, 1988.
14. Radomsky NA: The association of parental alcoholism and rigidity with chronic illness and abuse among women. *J Fam Prac* 35:54–60, 1992.
15. Downs WR, Miller BA: Intergenerational links between childhood abuse and alcohol-related problems, in Harrison L (ed): *Alcohol Problems in the Community.* London, Routledge Press, 1995, pp 14–51.
16. Andreasen NC, Endicott J, Spitzer RL, Winokur G: The family history method using diagnostic criteria. *Arch Gen Psychiatry* 34:1229–1235, 1977.

17. Miller BA: The interrelationships between alcohol and drugs and family violence, in De La Rosa M, Lambert EY, Gropper B (eds): *Drugs and Violence: Causes, Correlates, and Consequences*, Monograph 103 (DHHS Publication No. ADM-90-1721), Rockville, MD, National Institute on Drug Abuse, 1990, pp 177–207.
18. Aarens M, Cameron T, Roizen J, *et al*: *Alcohol, Casualties and Crime*. Berkeley, CA, Social Research Group, 1978.
19. Yama MF, Fogas BS, Teegarden LA, Hastings B: Childhood sexual abuse and parental alcoholism: Interactive effects in adult women. *Am J Orthopsychiatry* 63:300–305, 1993.
20. Finkelhor D: *Sexually Victimized Children*. New York, Free Press, 1979.
21. Windle M, Windle RC, Scheidt DM, *et al*: Physical and sexual abuse and associated mental disorders among alcoholic inpatients. *Am J Psychiatry* 152:1322–1328, 1995.
22. Pernanen, K: Alcohol and crimes of violence, in Kissin B, Begleiter H (eds): *Social Aspects of Alcoholism*. New York, Plenum Press, 1976, pp 351–444.
23. Steele CM, Josephs RA: Alcohol myopia: Its prized and dangerous effects. *J Stud Alcohol* 45:921–933, 1990.
24. Zeichner A, Pihl RR: Effects of alcohol and instigator intent on human aggression. *J Stud Alcohol* 41:265–276, 1980.
25. Collins JJ: Drinking and violations of the criminal law, in Pittman DJ, White HR (eds): *Society, Culture, and Drinking Patterns Reexamined*. New Brunswick, NJ, Rutgers Center of Alcohol Studies, 1991, pp 650–660.
26. Kantor GK, Straus MA: Parental drinking and violence and child aggression. Paper presented at the Annual Meeting of the American Psychological Association, Boston, MA, August 1990.
27. Coleman DH, Strauss MA: Alcohol abuse and family violence, in Gottheil E, Druley KA, Skoloda TE, Waxman HM (eds): *Alcohol Abuse and Family Violence*. Springfield, IL, Thomas, 1983, pp 104–124.
28. Gelles RJ: *The Violent Home*. Beverly Hills, CA, Sage, 1972.
29. Lang AR, Goeckner DJ, Adesso VJ, Marlatt GA: Effects of alcohol on aggression in male social drinkers. *J Abnorm Psychol*, 84:508–518, 1975.
30. MacAndrew C, Edgerton RB: *Drunken Comportment: A Social Explanation*. Chicago, IL, Aldine, 1969.
31. Wikler A: Mechanisms of action of drugs that modify personality function. *Am J Psychiatry* 108:590–599, 1952.
32. Shuntich RJ, Taylor SP: The effects of alcohol on human physical aggression. *J Exp Res Personal* 6:34–38, 1972.
33. Fitzpatrick JP: Drugs, alcohol and violent crime. *Addict Dis* 1:353–357, 1974.
34. Fagan J: Interactions among drugs, alcohol, and violence. *Violence Public Health* 12:65–79, 1993.
35. Gelles RJ: Alcohol and other drugs are associated with violence—They are not its cause, in Gelles RJ, Loseke DR (eds): *Current Controversies on Family Violence*. Newbury Park, CA, Sage, 1993, pp 182–196.
36. White HR: The drug use–delinquency connection in adolescence, in Weisheit R (ed): *Drugs, Crime, and the Criminal Justice System*. Cincinnati, OH, Anderson, 1990, pp 215–256.
37. Pernanen K: Theoretical aspects of the relationship between alcohol use and crime, in Collins JJ (ed): *Drinking and Crime*. New York, Guilford Press, 1981, pp 1–69.
38. Graham K: Theories of intoxicated aggression. *Can J Behav Sci* 12:141–158, 1980.
39. Straus MA: Discipline and deviance: Physical punishment of children and violence and other crime in adulthood. *Soc Problems* 38:133–152, 1991.
40. Finkelhor D, Baron L: High-risk children, in Finkelhor D (ed): *Sourcebook on Child Sexual Abuse*. Newbury Park, CA, Sage, 1986, pp 60–88.
41. Faller CK: *Child Sexual Abuse: An Interdisciplinary Manual for Diagnosis, Case Management, and Treatment*. New York, Columbia University Press, 1988.
42. Miller BA, Downs WR, Gondoli DM, Keil A: The role of childhood sexual abuse in the development of alcoholism in women. *Violence Vict* 2:157–172, 1987.

43. Miller BA, Downs WR, Testa M: Interrelationships between victimization experiences and women's alcohol use. *J Stud Alcohol Suppl* 11:109–117, 1993.

44. Cole PM, Woolger C, Power TG, Smith KD: Parenting difficulties among adult survivors of father–daughter incest. *Child Abuse Negl* 16:239–249, 1992.

45. Mian M, Maron P, LeBaron D, Birtwistle D: Familial risk factors associated with intrafamilial and extrafamilial sexual abuse of three- to five-year-old girls. *Can J Psychiatry* 39:348–353, 1994.

46. Davis SK: Chemical dependency in women: A description of its effects and outcomes on adequate parenting. *J Subst Abuse Treat* 7:225–232, 1990.

47. Beitchman JH, Zucker KJ, Hood JE, *et al*: A review of the long-term effects of child sexual abuse. *Child Abuse Negl* 16:101–118, 1992.

48. Wyatt GE, Guthrie D, Notgrass CM: Differential effects of women's child sexual abuse and subsequential sexual revictimization. *J Consult Clin Psychol* 60:167–173, 1992.

49. Miller BA, Downs WR, Gondoli DM: Spousal violence among alcoholic women as compared to a random household sample of women. *J Stud Alcohol* 50:533–540, 1989.

50. Finkelhor D, Browne A: *Assessing the Long-Term Impact of Child Sexual Abuse: A Review and Conceptualization.* Newbury Park, CA, Sage, 1988.

51. Regier DA, Farmer ME, Rae DS, *et al*: Comorbidity of mental disorders with alcohol and other drug abuse. *J Am Med Assoc* 264:2511–2517, 1990.

52. Jumper SA: A meta-analysis of the relationship of child sexual abuse to adult psychological adjustment. *Child Abuse Negl* 19:715–728, 1995.

53. Silber S, Bermann E, Henderson M, Lehman A: Patterns of influence and response in abusing and nonabusing families. *J Fam Violence* 8:27–38, 1993.

54. Newberger CM, Gremy IM, Waternaux CM, Newberger EH: Mothers of sexually abused children: Trauma and repair in longitudinal perspective. *Am J Orthopsychiatry* 63:92–102, 1993.

55. West MO, Prinz RJ: Parental alcoholism and childhood psychopathology. *Psychol Bull* 102:204–218, 1987.

56. Liskow B, Powell BJ, Nickel E, Penick E: Antisocial alcoholics: Are they clinically significant diagnostic subtypes? *J Stud Alcohol* 52:62–69, 1991.

57. Hesselbrock VM, Meyer RE, Keener RE: Psychopathology in hospitalized alcoholics. *Arch Gen Psychiatry* 42:1050–1055, 1985.

58. Schuckit MA: Alcoholism and sociopathy: Diagnostic confusion. *J Stud Alcohol* 34:157–164, 1973.

59. Cloninger CR: Neurogenetic adaptive mechanisms in alcoholism. *Science* 236:410–416, 1987.

60. Babor TF, Hofmann M, DelBoca FK, *et al*: Types of alcoholics, I. Evidence for an empirically derived typology based on indicators of vulnerability and severity. *Arch Gen Psychiatry* 49:599–608, 1992.

61. DiLalla LF, Gottesman II: Biological and genetic contributions to violence: Widom's untold tale. *Psychol Bull* 109:125–129, 1991.

62. Muller RT, Fitzgerald HE, Sullivan LA, Zucker RA: Social support and stress factors in child maltreatment among alcoholic families. *Can J Behav Sci* 26:438–446, 1994.

63. Downs WR, Smyth NJ, Miller BA: The relationship between childhood violence and alcohol problems among men who batter: An empirical review and synthesis. Review of Aggression and Violent Behavior, in press.

64. Straus MA, Kantor GK: Corporal punishment of adolescents by parents: A risk factor in the epidemiology of depression, suicide, alcohol abuse, child abuse, and wife beating. *Adolescence* 29:543–561, 1994.

65. Holmes SJ, Robins LN: The role of parental disciplinary practices in the development of depression and alcoholism. *Psychiatry* 51:24–36, 1988.

66. Brown GR, Anderson B: Psychiatric morbidity in adult inpatients with childhood histories of sexual and physical abuse. *Am J Psychiatry* 148:55–61, 1991.

67. Blane HT, Miller BA, Leonard KE *et al*: *Intra- and Intergenerational Aspects of Serious Domestic Violence and Alcohol and Drugs.* Buffalo, NY, Research Institute on Alcoholism, 1988.

68. Widom CS, Ireland T, Glynn PJ: Alcohol abuse in abused and neglected children followed-up: Are they at increased risk? *J Stud Alcohol* 56:207–217, 1995.

69. McCord J: A forty-year perspective on effects of child abuse and neglect. *Child Abuse Negl* 7:265–270, 1983.

70. Dembo R, Dertke M, La Voie L, *et al:* Further examination of the association between heavy marijuana use and crime among youths entering a juvenile detention center. *J Psychoactive Drugs* 19:361–373, 1987.

71. Dembo R, Dertke M, Borders S, *et al:* The relationship between physical and sexual abuse and tobacco, alcohol, and illicit drug use among youths in a juvenile detention center. *Int J Addict* 23:351–378, 1988.

72. Dembo R, Williams L, Wish ED, *et al:* The relationship between physical and sexual abuse and illicit drug use: A replication among a new sample of youths entering a juvenile detention center. *Int J Addict* 23:1101–1123, 1988.

73. Dembo R, Williams L, Schmeidler J, Wothke W: A longitudinal study of the predictors of the adverse effects of alcohol and marijuana/hashish use among a cohort of high risk youths. *Int J Addict* 28:1045–1083, 1993.

74. Downs WR, Miller BA, Gondoli DM: Childhood experiences of parental physical violence for alcoholic women as compared with a randomly selected household sample of women. *Violence Vict* 2:225–240, 1987.

75. Browne A, Finkelhor D: Impact of child sexual abuse: A review of the literature. *Psychol Bull* 99:66–77, 1986.

76. Beitchman JH, Zucker KJ, Hood JE, *et al:* A review of the short-term effects of child sexual abuse. *Child Abuse Negl* 15:537–556, 1991.

77. Polusny MA, Follette VM: Long-term correlates of child sexual abuse: Theory and review of the empirical literature. *Appl Prevent Psychol* 4:143–166, 1995.

78. Wilsnack SC, Klassen AD, Vogeltanz ND: Childhood sexual abuse and women's substance abuse: National survey findings. Paper presented at the American Psychological Association Conference, Psychosocial and Behavioral Factors in Women's Health: Creating an Agenda for the 21st Century. Washington, DC, May 1994.

79. Russell DEH: The prevalence and seriousness of incestuous abuse: Stepfathers vs. biological fathers. *Child Abuse Negl* 8:15–22, 1984.

80. Wyatt GE: The sexual abuse of Afro-American and white American women in childhood. *Child Abuse Negl* 9:507–519, 1985.

81. Mullen PE, Martin JL, Anderson JC, *et al:* Childhood sexual abuse and mental health in adult life. *Br J Psychiatry* 163:721–732, 1993.

82. Miller BA, Downs WR: Violent victimization among women with alcohol problems, in Galanter M (ed): *Recent Developments in Alcoholism,* vol 12: *Women and Alcoholism.* New York, Plenum Press, 1995, pp 81–101.

83. Stein JA, Golding JM, *et al:* Long-term psychological sequelae of child sexual abuse: The Los Angeles epidemiologic catchment area study, in Wyatt GE, Powell GJ (eds): *Lasting Effects of Child Sexual Abuse.* Newbury Park, CA, Sage, 1988, pp 135–154.

84. Harrison PA, Hoffman NG, Edwall GE: Differential drug use patterns among sexually abused adolescent girls in treatment for chemical dependency. *Int J Addict* 24:499–514, 1989.

85. Malinosky-Rummell R, Hansen DJ: Long-term consequences of childhood physical abuse. *Psychol Bull* 114:68–79, 1993.

86. Kendall-Tackett KA, Meyer Williams L, Finkelhor D: Impact of sexual abuse on children: A review and synthesis of recent empirical studies. *Psychol Bull* 113:164–180, 1993.

87. Boney-McCoy S, Finkelhor D: Psychosocial sequelae of violent victimization in a national youth sample. *J Consult Clin Psychol* 63:726–736, 1995.

88. McCloskey LA, Figueredo AJ, Koss MP: The effects of systemic family violence on children's mental health. *Child Dev* 66:1239–1261, 1995.

89. Lanktree C, Briere J, Zaidi L: Incidence and impact of sexual abuse in a child outpatient sample: The role of direct inquiry. *Child Abuse Negl* 15:447–453, 1991.

90. Becker JV, Kaplan MS, Tenke CE, Tartaglini A: The incidence of depressive symptomatology in juvenile sex offenders with a history of abuse. *Child Abuse Negl* 15:531–536, 1991.

91. Kaplan HB: Self-esteem and self-derogation theory of drug abuse, in Lettieri DJ, Sayers M, Wallenstein Pearson H (eds): *Theories on Drug Abuse* (Research Monograph Series 30). Rockville, MD, NIDA US Department of Health and Human Services, 1980, pp 128–131.

92. Hawkins JD, Catalano RF, Miller JY: Risk and protective factors for alcohol and other drug problems in adolescence and early adulthood: Implications for substance abuse prevention. *Psychol Bull* 112:64–105, 1992.

93. Dishion TJ, Capaldi D, Spracklen KM, *et al:* Peer ecology of male adolescent drug use. *Dev Psychopathol* 7(4):803–824, 1995.

94. Miller WR, Brown JM: Self-regulation as a conceptual basis for the prevention and treatment of addictive behaviors, in Heather N, Miller WR, Greeley J (eds): *Self-Control and the Addictive Behaviors.* Sydney, Australia, Macmillan, 1991, pp 3–79.

95. Crime Victims Research and Treatment Center: *A Report to the Nation.* Arlington, VA, National Victim Center, 1992.

96. Edwards G, Hensman C, Peto J: A comparison of female and male motivation for drinking. *Int J Addict* 8:577–587, 1973.

97. Fillmore KM: Drinking and problem drinking in early adulthood and middle age. *Q J Stud Alcohol* 35:819–840, 1974.

98. Fillmore KM: Relationships between specific drinking problems in early adulthood and middle age. *J Stud Alcohol* 36:882–907, 1975.

99. Chassin L, Rogosch F, Barrera M: Substance use and symptomatology among adolescent children of alcoholics. *J Abnorm Psychol* 100:449–463, 1991.

100. Lewis CE, Bucholz KK: Alcoholism, antisocial behavior and family history. *Br J Addict* 86:177–194, 1991.

101. Leonard KE, Jacob T: Alcohol, alcoholism, and family violence, in VanHasselt V, Morrison RL, Bellack AS, Hersen M (eds): *Handbook of Family Violence.* New York, Plenum Press, 1988, pp 383–406.

102. National Center on Child Abuse and Neglect: *National Child Abuse and Neglect Data System: Working Paper 2—1991 Summary Data Component.* Washington, DC: US Government Printing Office, 1992.

103. Straus MA, Gelles RJ: *Physical Violence in American Families: Risk Factors and Adaptations to Violence in 8,145 Families.* New Brunswick, NJ, Transaction Publishers, 1990.

104. Gelles RJ, Straus MA: Determinants of violence in the family: Toward a theoretical integration, in Burr WR, Hill R, Nye FI, Reiss IL (eds): *Contemporary Theories about the Family,* vol 1. New York, Free Press, 1979, pp 549–581.

105. Straus MA: *Beating the Devil Out of Them: Corporal Punishment in American Families.* New York, Lexington Books, 1994.

106. Koss MP: Detecting the scope of rape: A review of prevalence research methods. *J Interper Violence* 8:198–222, 1993.

107. Straus MA: Measuring intrafamily conflict and violence: The conflict tactics (CT) scales. *J Marriage Fam* 41:75–88, 1979.

108. Straus MA: The national family violence surveys, in Straus MA, Gelles RJ (eds): *Physical Violence in American Families: Risk Factors and Adaptations to Violence in 8,145 Families.* New Brunswick, Transaction Publishers, 1990, pp 3–16.

109. Straus MA: The Conflict Tactics scales and its critics: An evaluation and new data on validity and reliability, in Straus MA, Gelles RJ (eds): *Physical Violence in American Families: Risk Factors and Adaptions to Violence in 8,145 Families.* New Brunswick, Transaction Publishers, 1990, pp 49–74.

110. Straus MA, Gelles RJ (eds): *Physical Violence in American Families: Risk Factors and Adaptions to Violence in 8,145 Families.* New Brunswick, Transaction Publishers, 1990.

111. Epstein R, Komorita SS: The development of a scale of parental punitiveness toward aggression. *Child Dev* 36:129–142, 1965.

112. Loftus EF, Polonsky S, Fullilove MT: Memories of childhood sexual abuse: Remembering and repressing. *Psychol Women Q* 18:67–84, 1994.

113. Martin J, Anderson J, Romans S, *et al:* Asking about child sexual abuse: Methodological implications of a two stage survey. *Child Abuse Negl* 17:383–392, 1993.

114. Herman JL: *Trauma and Recovery.* New York, Basic Books, 1992.

115. Williams LM: What does it mean to forget child sexual abuse? A reply to Loftus, Garry, and Feldman (1994). *J. Consult Clin Psychol* 62:1182–1186, 1994.

116. Loftus EF: The reality of repressed memories. *Am Psychol* 48:518–537, 1993.

117. Socolar RRS, Amaya-Jackson L: Methodological and ethical issues related to studying child maltreatment. *J Fam Issues* 16:565–586, 1995.

118. Finkelhor D: The victimization of children: A developmental perspective. *Am J Orthopsychiatry* 65:177–193, 1995.

119. Cicchetti D, Toth SL: A developmental psychopathology perspective on child abuse and neglect. *J Am Acad Child Adolesc Psychiatry* 34:541–565, 1995.

120. Newberger CM, DeVos E: Abuse and victimization: A lifespan perspective. *Am J Orthopsychiatry* 58:505–511, 1988.

16

Issues in the Linkage of Alcohol and Domestic Violence Services

James J. Collins, Larry A. Kroutil, E. Joyce Roland, and Marlee Moore-Gurrera

Abstract. It is well established that alcohol is a risk factor for male against female domestic violence. Some evidence also suggests that some women victims of domestic violence develop substance abuse problems in response to their victimization. Although interpretations vary regarding the exact nature of the relationship of substance abuse and domestic violence offending and victimization, there is evidence that linking substance abuse and domestic violence services could have a positive impact on batterer cessation and victim support services. Currently, however, service linkage for the two problems is rare. There are major barriers to linkage of substance abuse and domestic violence services, including philosophical differences of treatment perspective between program types and structural impediments that make linkage difficult. The chapter discusses the barriers to linkage, examines potentially useful linkage models, and suggests the next steps to examine the feasibility of linking services for the two problems.

1. Introduction

Violence within the family is an ancient problem, but one that was largely viewed as a private problem until the past 20 or 25 years. Particularly important to the increased visibility of domestic violence was the first nationally representative survey of violence in the American family conducted in the mid-1970s. The survey found that 16% of those surveyed reported some kind

James J. Collins, Larry A. Kroutil, E. Joyce Roland, and Marlee Moore-Gurrera • Health and Social Policy Division, Research Triangle Institute, Research Triangle Park, North Carolina 27709-2194.

Recent Developments in Alcoholism, Volume 13: Alcoholism and Violence, edited by Marc Galanter. Plenum Press, New York, 1997

of violence between spouses in the year of the survey, while 28% reported marital violence at some time during the marriage.[1] This survey and numerous subsequent national and less comprehensive studies have focused attention on the family violence problem and have provided data to study its characteristics.

The reduction of violence against women by their male partners is a priority health objective for the United States[2] and was a major focus of the 1994 federal crime legislation. Violence against women is believed to affect approximately 4 million women annually in the United States.[3] Violence against women is considered to be the leading cause of nonfatal injury for women, and an estimated 1 million women each year seek emergency treatment for injuries sustained during battering.[4] This figure probably underestimates the number of women with battering-related treatment needs because battering goes largely undiagnosed as a potential cause of women's injuries or health problems.[5-9] National victimization data indicate that only 56% of incidents where women are attacked by an intimate are reported to police.[10] Research also indicates that sustained exposure to violence leads to the development of chronic and acute health problems, including chronic pain,[8,9,11-13] miscarriage,[14,15] irritable bowel syndrome,[16] depression and anxiety,[17-20] and suicide.[5,8,21] Too often, battering culminates in homicide.[22,23] In addition, and of significant importance, battered women are at higher risk for inappropriate use of prescription drugs, illicit drugs, and alcohol.[8,12,21] In fact, battering is recognized as a major risk factor for substance abuse and mental illness among women in the United States.[2]

In this chapter, we discuss the role of substance abuse in domestic violence and the implications that the association between substance abuse and domestic violence have for programs that deal with these problems. There are good reasons to think that a substance abuse–domestic violence program service linkage would be beneficial to clients. Such linkage is infrequent, however, and there are significant impediments to linkage. The chapter addresses these issues based on a review of the literature in the substance abuse and domestic violence fields and on interviews conducted with service providers in these fields.

2. Role of Alcohol in Domestic Violence

One of the aspects of domestic violence receiving attention has been the relationship of drinking to its occurrence. Three studies using data from two national domestic violence surveys found that the frequency of the husband's drinking was associated with wife abuse.[24-26] Evidence of the magnitude of the relationship between alcohol use and domestic violence varies widely, with statistics ranging from as low as 25% to as high as 80%.[24-31]

Studies of battered women indicate that their partner's alcohol use plays a role in domestic violence. In a study by Rounsaville,[32] 29% of the battered women reported that their partners were drinking when the violent episode occurred. Similarly, Gayford[33] reported that the male partner was intoxicated at the time of the abuse 44% of the time; and Carlson[34] found that alcohol was involved in 67% of abusive incidents. Roy[35] also found that more than 80% of the men who were occasional drinkers were inclined to abuse their partners, but only when they had been drinking. Several studies of women who were in shelters or used crisis hotlines indicate that there is an association between alcohol and domestic violence.[36] For example, data from New York's Abused Women's Aid in Crisis indicate that alcohol abuse by the husband is an underlying factor in over 80% of domestic violence cases. Similarly, a study in a Michigan emergency shelter indicates that over 66% of the assaults were associated with alcohol use. Furthermore, data from a Philadelphia community hotline for abused women were examined, and 55% of the callers said that their partners had become abusive when the latter had been drinking.

There is some evidence that drinking on the part of women increases the likelihood of domestic violence victimization. In a multivariate analysis of national survey data, Kantor and Straus[26] found that women who drink heavily have a higher risk of being the victim of minor (but not severe) violence by their partners. However, the bulk of empirical research indicates that only a small percentage of domestic violence events involve situations in which the woman was the sole drinker. The most common patterns are both partners drinking, no drinking, and only male partner drinking (see review by Hamilton and Collins,[28] pp. 261–275).

Substance use by domestic violence victims has been suggested to be a response to the violence they suffer. The substance use may be used to cope with the physical and emotional pain after abuse.[37,38] As stated previously, there is evidence that women who are the victims of domestic violence are at increased risk of abusing alcohol, illicit drugs, and prescription medication.[2] However, limited research is available documenting the prevalence of alcohol and drug use among battered women. In one review of the literature, 7 to 21% of female battering victims reported alcohol abuse or alcoholism.[28] Furthermore, recent literature compared with older literature suggests that the proportion of battered women engaging in the use of alcohol and other drugs may be increasing.[8,9,39–43] In support of this hypothesis, a recent survey of North Carolina's domestic violence programs found that 85% of domestic violence shelter providers believed that the number of battered women with substance abuse problems is growing, and 97.5% believed that substance-abusing battered women are an underserved population in their counties.[44]

One explanation for the increased risk of substance abuse among domestic violence victims is that battered women may suffer from posttraumatic stress disorder (PTSD). Women who suffer from PTSD and battered women in general may turn to alcohol and drugs to cope with the physical pain, emotional pain, and fears associated with being in a battering relationship.[37,38,45] Consequently, both substance abuse and traumatic stress disorders must be addressed in order to adequately serve this population.

Regardless of etiology, substance abuse by battered women is associated with and exacerbates a range of problems.[4] Substance abuse is likely to make it even more difficult for battered women to manage the complicated and dangerous process of leaving violent relationships and maintaining violence-free lives.[35] These factors, in turn, are likely to increase the morbidity and injury associated with battering,[41] contribute to increased use of health care services,[46] enhance the risk of partner homicide,[22] and increase the chances of attempted and completed suicide.[47] At the same time, the chronic nature of battering—coupled with battered women's fear, shame, loss of self-esteem and personal power, isolation, lack of social support, and development of other health problems (e.g., chronic pain, depression)—may make it harder for them to break free of drug or alcohol dependency.[9,40,48–50] For some women, chronic violence and substance abuse become enmeshed. Substance abuse among battered women also is thought to increase the likelihood that these women will be held inappropriately responsible for their victimization by those in a position to help them, such as the police, judges, social service workers, and health care workers.[44,51–53]

Among men who are batterers and are also substance abusers, there are good reasons to believe that their substance abuse is an impediment to getting them to stop using violence against their partners. In the next section, we discuss the ways that drinking might be a factor in the etiology of men's violence (e.g., cognitive impairment, drinking associated with male power needs, alcohol as an excuse for violence). Although there is not a clear consensus about the nature and magnitude of alcohol's relationship to battering, there is little disagreement that it is contributory in some way. Moreover, there appears to be a growing disagreement that it is contributory in some way. Moreover, there appears to be a growing consensus that it is necessary to address alcohol and drug problems to achieve the best results with respect to the battering problem.[54,55] However, batterers' programs may not wish to deal with the substance abuse problems of their clients within their own programs. Nevertheless, many such programs recognize the need for substance abuse treatment to maximize long-term violence-free outcomes for violent men. It also seems likely that family conflict may be a risk factor for relapse to substance abuse among those batterers in treatment.[27] Substance abuse, battering, and family conflict are probably related to each other in complex ways.

3. Explanation of the Alcohol–Domestic Violence Relationship

Despite the high correlation of drinking and drinking problems to domestic violence, there is considerable controversy about alcohol's role in connection with the violence. Psychosocial interpretations of the alcohol–domestic violence relationship include the following:

1. Alcohol-induced cognitive impairment may result in misinterpretation of spouses' verbal–behavioral cues and intentions and increase the likelihood of violent interactions[56,57]; a similar interpretation suggests

that alcohol causes a "myopia" that can have dangerous behavioral effects.[58]

2. Alcohol interacts with the male's need to exert personal power and control in marital relationships[55,59–61]; the relevance of power and control is also thought to be a major factor in family violence independent of alcohol.[62–64]

3. Socially learned alcohol expectancy effects lead individuals to think that alcohol induces violence and that it may be an acceptable excuse for family violence[24,65–67]; an expectancy effect for alcohol-induced aggression has been demonstrated in controlled laboratory experiments.[68–70] These expectancy effects have sociocultural roots.[71]

4. Using a complex explanatory framework that combines multiple causal views, Leonard,[72] in a National Institute on Alcohol Abuse and Alcoholism (NIAAA) monograph, suggested that multiple distal factors (background influences, drinking patterns, marital discord) combine with proximal influences, such as situational cues and acute alcohol effects, in the context of aversive interpersonal interactions to produce physical aggression between spouses (p. 256).

A common feature of these psychosocial interpretations appears to be that alcohol use in and of itself is not sufficient for a man to commit acts of domestic violence. In particular, interpretations that focus on issues of male power and control, or on socially learned expectancies related to alcohol, suggest that underlying social or attitudinal problems must be dealt with if a male batterer is to stop his behavior.[73] Under these theoretical interpretations, should a batterer stop drinking but nothing be done about these other issues, the battering is likely to continue, or the batterer may resume drinking to provide an excuse to resume the pattern of abuse (i.e., the socially learned expectancy explanation). Not surprisingly, then, programs for batterers consider the violence to be a behavioral choice on the part of the batterer.[55,74] Further, both the Minnesota Coalition for Battered Women[38] and Levy and Brekke[74] recommended that programs for batterers place a strong emphasis on the batterers assuming responsibility for their behaviors and that the programs challenge excuses for battering (e.g., "I was drunk").

In contrast to programs for batterers that focus on psychosocial issues and behavioral responsibility, the "disease concept" of alcoholism and the Minnesota (or Hazelden) model of treatment are popular with many alcohol treatment programs.[75–77] Specifically, Roman and Blum[77] stated that alcoholism is characterized as a progressive disease (p. 758), marked by the inability to control one's drinking, and in later stages by physical tolerance and withdrawal symptoms.[78,79] As summarized by Chiauzzi and Liljegren[75] (p. 305), the Minnesota model of treatment is characterized by (1) psychological counseling and educational approaches to build awareness of the consequences of addiction; (2) involvement of recovering personnel in therapeutic roles; (3) acceptance of the disease concept of alcoholism; (4) emphasis on attending

Alcoholics Anonymous (AA) meetings and doing what the Institute of Medicine[76] referred to as "stepwork" (p. 56); and (6) use of group counseling to confront denial. An important underlying feature of this model is that alcoholism is viewed as a primary problem requiring treatment in its own right.[76]

By definition, alcohol treatment programs will focus primarily on a client's use of alcohol, the consequences of this use, and development of a way of living that involves abstinence from alcohol. However, the primary focus on recovery from alcohol abuse or dependence can mean that perpetrators of domestic violence who are in alcohol treatment may go undetected, allowing the domestic violence to continue. If issues of domestic violence are detected in the course of alcohol treatment, the emphasis on the disease concept of alcoholism can lead domestic violence to be viewed as a problem secondary to the abuse of alcohol, as opposed to a problem requiring special intervention in its own right.[80] Consequently, programs, counselors, and clients adhering to an alcoholism treatment approach that emphasizes the disease concept of alcoholism may assume that behavior change (i.e., cessation of battering) will occur once a client stops drinking and begins to achieve some measure of sobriety.[80,81]

A different set of issues is raised if the female victim of battering has a substance abuse problem. Good evidence on the relationship between the female domestic violence victim and substance abuse is sparse, but it seems most likely that the woman's substance abuse problem is usually either independent of the battering problem or is a response to battering. Regardless of the etiology of battering and substance abuse for the battering victim, it is advisable to treat both problems. If a woman has an active alcohol or drug problem, she will be less likely to have the cognitive, emotional, and other resources needed to take constructive actions to protect herself and her children, leave the violent relationship, or do both.

4. Examples of Current Linkage

Bennett and Lawson[54] surveyed substance abuse programs and domestic violence programs in Illinois to learn more about the types of service linkages between both types of programs, as well as barriers to cooperation. Their sample consisted of all 45 domestic violence programs in Illinois and a random sample of 150 licensed substance abuse treatment programs in the state. A total of 388 staff from 74 programs participated in the study (249 staff from 53 substance abuse treatment programs and 139 staff from 21 domestic violence programs), for agency response rates of 47% for the domestic violence programs and 35% for the substance abuse treatment programs.

Although response rates were low and the focus of the study was on service linkages within a single state, the study represents an attempt to use survey research methods to document the extent and types of service linkages between substance abuse treatment and domestic violence programs, as well as to indicate the relative importance of possible barriers to linkage. Key findings from their study regarding the extent and types of service linkages include the following:

1. Formal screening for cross-problems (e.g., screening for domestic violence among substance abuse treatment clients) was relatively rare, done possibly by about 10% of programs. However, "screening" tended to consist of one or two questions and tended not to be very systematic. Among substance abuse treatment clients, for example, histories of domestic violence tended to be identified only if a client reported incidents in the course of counseling.

2. One exception to the general pattern of haphazard screening was that screening for substance abuse tended to be more systematic and structured in programs for male batterers. Many of these programs used the Michigan Alcoholism Screening Test (MAST).[82]

3. Although sizable percentages of substance abuse treatment and domestic violence programs indicated that they had an in-house "specialist" on staff (35% of the treatment programs and 24% of the domestic violence programs), such expertise was not often based on formal training. For example, substance abuse specialists in domestic violence programs often consisted of staff who were recovering from their own chemical dependency.

4. Approximately 70% of substance abuse treatment and domestic programs indicated some form of formal linkage agreement with the complementary program. However, only about 20% of directors of substance abuse treatment programs indicated that they met sometimes or frequently with staff from domestic violence programs, compared with nearly 70% of domestic violence program directors who indicated that they met with staff from substance abuse treatment programs.

5. Nearly one in four (23%) of substance abuse treatment staff indicated that they never referred clients to domestic violence programs, compared with only 5% of domestic violence staff who did not refer clients to substance abuse treatment.

We have also had conversations about service linkage with approximately 25 individuals who do research or deliver services in the domestic violence and substance abuse fields. These conversations confirm that linkage to address both domestic violence and substance abuse is infrequent. And although our conversations cannot be said to have been with a representative sample of researchers and service providers, two observations can be made: Programmatic linkage attempts are more common for batterer programs than for victim programs, and programs that do try to deal with the coexistent domestic violence and substance abuse problems typically do so by referral. In other words, the most common pattern we have seen is for batterers' programs to refer their clients who have alcohol or drug problems to substance abuse treatment. This is probably not surprising given the impediments to linkage we have already discussed (e.g., differing treatment philosophies, organizational boundaries).

We have identified a few batterer treatment programs operating at several locations that incorporate both substance abuse and domestic violence treatment as part of a single programmatic entity.[55,80,83] The Amend Program, for example, operating at several locations in Colorado, has counselors trained as both substance abuse and domestic violence counselors.[80] The Amend Program attempts to deal with both substance abuse and violent behavior problems among batterers' problems in spite of the difficulties of integrating the two treatments already discussed. It is not clear whether it is feasible to adopt this approach widely, or whether it requires special circumstances, such as a strong commitment, to deal explicitly with both problems.

5. Linking Services

Given the strong evidence of the relationship between alcohol abuse and domestic violence, a number of researchers and service providers have suggested the need for greater integration of treatment services for alcohol and domestic violence problems, such that both problems can be addressed.[38,54,74,80,84] The situation with substance abuse and domestic violence may be analogous to other dually occurring problems, such as psychiatric comorbidities. Although the problems are interrelated, the systems that have been designed to intervene in the problems operate essentially independent of one another. Stated more generally, the dilemma is that although research evidence continues to mount, showing that many psychosocial problems are highly interrelated (i.e., people with one problem tend to have many other problems as well), our systems of care tend to be narrowly focused on a specific problem, and the systems operate independently.

The set of problems existing around the alcohol–domestic violence relationship may be a particularly complex situation for integrating services. The configuration of problems includes the following:

1. The needs of the victim and her children related to injury, housing, subsistence, safety, and so on, and whether to continue the existing family unit.
2. Possible substance abuse treatment needs of the victim.
3. Intervention to deal with the violent behavior of the offender.
4. Possible substance abuse treatment needs of the offender.

It is unlikely that the full set of needs for families with the dual problems of violence and substance abuse can be dealt with by a single program.

Attempting to link services provided by multiple programs raises several issues that may make linkage problematic:

1. The philosophies and goals of treatment for programs may not be compatible.
2. Mechanisms and logistics for linking services may not exist.
3. Funding and other resources to support linkage may be limited.

Domestic violence programs usually have a strong advocacy component that focuses on protecting and promoting the safety and interests of women victims. A corollary of this perspective emphasizes personal accountability for men who batter. As discussed previously, substance abuse programs often operate under the view that addiction is a disease, implicitly deemphasizing personal accountability for actions that took place during the active disease state. Moreover, most domestic violence programs view the violence that is perpetrated against women to have its roots in men's desire to exercise power and control over their partners. Substance abuse programs often view addiction as a pervasive condition that has broad negative physiological, psychological, and behavioral effects that can include violence. The logical implications of the views of domestic violence and substance abuse treatment programs for dealing with the problems they try to ameliorate are at odds with each other. This is an impediment to linking substance abuse and domestic violence services. Indeed, Bennett and Lawson[54] found that having conflicting beliefs about the issue of personal responsibility for behavior was the leading factor cited as a possible reason for noncooperation between substance abuse treatment and domestic violence programs; this factor was endorsed by 55% of all respondents as a possible reason for noncooperation, as well as by 65% of respondents in domestic violence programs and 45% of staff in substance abuse treatment programs.

The problem of conflicting perspectives that underlie programmatic interventions is further complicated for female domestic violence victims with alcohol or drug problems who may find themselves in substance abuse treatment programs, operating under the disease concept. In such programs, there may be an implicit tendency to see the domestic violence they suffer as associated with their own alcohol or drug problem (i.e., that their substance abuse contributed to their victimization). Under this view, the substance abuse problem receives primary attention. Sobriety first is likely to be the goal of substance abuse programs; safety first will usually be the first priority for domestic violence programs.[38,73] Fundamental differences of perspective make it difficult for collegial cooperation between domestic violence and substance abuse treatment programs.

The problem of different treatment paradigms also impedes dealing effectively with the multiple problems of substance abuse and domestic violence, even within single program types. Because domestic violence programs view some of the traditional substance abuse treatment approaches with skepticism or hostility, and because they may not have an alternative treatment paradigm that is effective, successful responses to alcohol and drug problems for their clients may be absent. Substance abuse programs may ignore the violence that their clients engage in, assuming that if the substance abuse treatment is successful, the violence problem will be solved. There is evidence that battering does not cease unless the problem is explicitly addressed.[74,80] And substance abuse treatment programs do not typically focus on the violence problem, particularly for the male batterer.

Resource scarcity or the absence of appropriate resources is a common problem in domestic violence and substance abuse treatment programs. Domestic violence programs may not have the expertise to recognize the presence of an alcohol or drug problem. Even if a problem is recognized, the resources or programmatic expertise to deal with it may not be available. In fact, some domestic violence programs will not accept women with active substance abuse problems because it may interfere with their care of women and children in their programs who are not substance abusers. Similarly, substance abuse treatment programs do not usually have programmatic components that address either battering problems or problems associated with being a victim of domestic violence.

The linkage of alcohol and domestic violence services is also impeded by organizational boundaries and financial limitations. Domestic violence and alcohol treatment programs are usually independent of one another. They are organized separately, have intervention philosophies and program approaches shaped to their unique perspectives and goals, and may have resource limitations that prevent integration of services. Financial support for both alcohol and domestic violence programs is usually modest and limits the scope of programming. Financial impediments to integration of services may also be formal. For example, during our interviews at both types of programs, we were told of an alcohol treatment program that was prevented from dealing with domestic violence because hours could not be billed for these services.

The organizational placement and method of funding domestic violence and substance abuse treatment services make service linkage difficult. Domestic violence and substance abuse treatment programs tend to be located in different parts of the social service and health bureaucracies. The domestic violence and substance abuse treatment functions are often independent entities in state, county, or municipal governments. Or, the two program types are located in different parts of the governmental structure (e.g., health, mental health). These formal boundaries make it more difficult to embark on joint ventures, such as attempting to deal with the related aspects of domestic violence and substance abuse problems. The collaboration problem is difficult enough when the two kinds of services are organized separately but in the same departmental unit, such as when domestic violence and substance abuse programs come under a Department of Mental Health. When different departments are involved, a consensus to do something collaborative is even more complicated.

In recent years, the courts have begun to mandate that domestic violence offenders participate in batterers' programs as a condition of their sentences. This approach, however appropriate for protecting women victims, may introduce another layer of complexity for linkage, given the involvement of the criminal justice system.

6. Models for Service Linkage

Recognition that many individual and family problems are multifaceted has led to a movement toward services integration, which has been defined by Agranoff[85] as "the quest for the development of systems that are responsive to the multiple needs of persons at risk" (p. 533). Born largely out of the War on Poverty that was launched by the Johnson Administration in the mid-1960s, efforts at improving services integration have flourished, but they also have encountered substantial barriers.[86]

Although many services integration efforts have been broad-based, it is clear that there are potential benefits to integration on a more limited scale. For example, experiences of programs attempting to establish integrated substance abuse treatment and primary care have demonstrated that it is feasible to improve the integration of these services and beneficial to do so.[87] On a somewhat broader scale, evaluation of the National Institute of Mental Health's Child and Adolescent Service System Program demonstration showed that integration of services for severely emotionally disturbed children and adolescents could be improved at the state and local levels, and that doing so could result in more effective service delivery.[88]

Examples of attempts to integrate alcohol abuse and domestic violence interventions include programs in the Amend Program at several Colorado locations,[80] the Intercede Program of Longford Health Sources in Massillon, Ohio,[83] and Pittsburgh Veterans Affairs Medical Center.[55] Beyond these examples, however, little information has been documented about the extent of integration of alcohol-related and domestic violence services and mechanisms for integrating both services when integration is attempted. An exception is a study of domestic violence and chemical dependency program linkages in Illinois. Bennett and Lawson[54] surveyed statewide samples of these programs and found that programs thought linkage would benefit clients; however, the authors noted that "in-house expertise in the cross-problem was minimal for both chemical dependency and domestic violence agencies" (p. 281).

A recent study of linking drug abuse treatment to primary medical by Schlenger et al.[87,89] provides some guidance for the linkage of domestic violence and substance abuse programming. The study developed an a priori taxonomy of basic linkage approaches that were being implemented. This taxonomy was based on the perspective of the service user, and it identified four different models: (1) centralized, where drug treatment and primary care services are offered at a single location ("one-stop shopping"); (2) decentralized, where different services are offered at different locations, with clients being referred to different locations, depending on their service needs; (3) mixed, where a limited number of primary care and drug treatment services are offered at a single location,but most services are delivered at separate locations; and (4) transitional, in which the location of services changes over the user's treatment history.

It was observed, however, that the a priori conceptualization of models of linkage was probably more complicated than what existed in reality. Based on observations of linkage demonstration projects, it was hypothesized that specific linkage efforts may be best understood as lying along a continuum that ranges from decentralized through centralized. At one extreme, virtually all drug treatment and primary care services are delivered at separate locations, and linkage occurs by referral; in these highly decentralized systems, case management appears to be a key ingredient for ensuring that referrals are kept and for providing some continuity of care. At the other extreme of the linkage continuum, a full range of both primary care and drug treatment services is located in a single location (i.e., the one-stop shopping approach), with linkage occurring through the physical proximity of services.[90] It would not be surprising to find a similar decentralized to centralized continuum of domestic violence and substance abuse treatment integration among the linkages observed in this area although too few examples exist to be sure.

In addition, findings from the national linkage evaluation suggested some important benefits of having services in a single location. In particular, having services in a single location appeared to make services more accessible to clients and facilitated client enrollment and retention in treatment. In addition, having services in a single location almost always increased both formal and informal interaction among providers, contributing to a more holistic approach to treatment.

Furthermore, the linkage demonstration study revealed that attempts to bring together two service systems that have historically been separate can often expose philosophical differences in approaches to treatment that need to be addressed and overcome if linkage is to occur. Specifically, it was learned through contacts with some grantees that primary care providers sometimes viewed the structure and rules of some drug treatment programs as being overly rigid, while drug treatment providers sometimes viewed primary care providers as "rescuing" or "enabling" a substance abuser. Similarly, then, we might expect philosophical differences between alcohol treatment and domestic violence providers to be an important reason why these services remain separate, as well as a potential barrier to integration when programs attempt to establish linkages.

It may also be difficult to sustain the linkage of services across different agencies over time. A research demonstration project to link substance abuse, health, employment, and housing services for homeless drug-using adults illustrates the problem. In a recent discussion on service linkages, Erickson *et al.*[90] noted that the Amity Settlement Services for Education and Transition Program found that the networking needed to sustain service linkage "wilted away" over time (p. 343).

Some domestic violence service providers and advocates downplay the role of alcohol in incidents of domestic violence. Many domestic violence service providers consider drinking as an excuse for acting violently or think it is offered as an excuse after the fact to avoid accountability. Moreover, a commonly held view is that the principal causes of domestic violence are sociocultural factors that support the use of violence against women and reinforce the social and economic advantages of men. From this perspective, a focus on alcohol as an important contributory factor in domestic violence may detract from a focus on what are viewed as the more important cultural, social, and economic causes. For example, Cayouette[91] cited the concern that men in a batterers' program who subsequently enter a recovery program for alcoholism can have their focus diverted from attention to their battering problem. Cayouette also expressed the concern that some men can use their involvement in a recovery program (e.g., frequent attendance at AA meetings) as a way of continuing to avoid family responsibilities. Furthermore, application of terms from the self-help movement, such as "codependent" or "enabler," to female victims of domestic violence has been cited as a new form of victim-blaming, in which the woman is made to feel partly responsible for the alcoholic batterer's problem.[80,91] It is the view of some domestic violence advocates and service providers that empowerment for women victims and behavioral accountability and attitudinal change for batterers are the major goals to be sought.

Based on anecdotal evidence regarding the substance abuse–domestic violence service linkage and on general findings about linking multiple kinds of services, some tentative inferences can be drawn. Our conversations with individuals in both the domestic violence and substance abuse treatment fields suggest that linkage is rare or at least infrequent. (The Bennett and Lawson[54] study in Illinois is consistent with this conclusion.) This is true for each program type and for both domestic violence victims and offenders. Domestic violence programs for victims often will not accept women with substance abuse problems. Programs for male batterers usually do not deal with alcohol and drug problems; if they recognize that a substance abuse problem exists, they will usually refer the individual to a substance abuse treatment program. Substance abuse treatment programs do not usually recognize or deal with the violent experiences or violent behavior of their clients. One implication of the scarcity of existing linkages is that well-developed models for accomplishing linkage do not exist. This means that significant programmatic development and evaluation are needed. It would be premature to recommend implementation of widespread attempts at linking substance abuse and domestic violence services in the absence of well-developed and effective models for doing so.

Based on anecdotal evidence from domestic violence treatment providers, linkage is sometimes not possible until the victim's or offender's substance abuse problem is dealt with, particularly for male batterers. The substance abuse problem can be a serious impediment to meaningful cognitive and psychological engagement in programming to address problems related to domestic violence. The anecdotal evidence we have gathered indicates that domestic violence treatment providers usually refer victims and batterers who have serious alcohol or drug problems to a substance abuse program to deal with this problem. In our experience, it is rare that victim or offender domestic violence programs deal simultaneously with the domestic violence programming.

The domestic violence program services provided to victims and offenders differ. Programming for victims emphasizes safety, shelter, child care services, legal advocacy, and so on. Programming for male batterers emphasizes anger and conflict management, acceptance of responsibility for violent behavior, meeting family responsibilities, and so on. Due to the different program foci, the optimal approaches to linking substance abuse and domestic violence services may differ for victims and offenders. For example, the simultaneous treatment of both substance abuse and problems related to domestic violence victimization may work well, whereas a serial approach in which the substance abuse problem is dealt with first for batterers may be better in the case of offenders.

At the current state of development of domestic violence and substance abuse treatment linkage, the linkage mechanism that seems most appropriate is a brokering or case management approach. A case manager approach to delivery of therapeutic services involves assessing individual's needs and arranging for services to address those needs. So, in the case of linking domestic violence and substance abuse services, for example, a case manager would evaluate whether a victim or offender has a substance abuse problem, assess its severity, identify available treatment resources, make a referral to treatment, and monitor treatment progress. Because so little is currently known about dealing with the domestic violence and substance abuse problems within a single programmatic context, the case management model seems appropriate. When more is learned about how to integrate programming for the two kinds of problems, dealing with both in a single program might be effective. What does seem clear though is that domestic violence and substance abuse are highly correlated. Regardless of the exact nature of their causal relationship (or the absence thereof), dealing with both problems may be beneficial. It remains to be demonstrated whether synergistic benefits result from linking domestic violence and substance abuse services, but there is every reason to expect that dealing with both problems when they coexist will pay high individual and social dividends.

7. Next Steps

Based on the strong empirical association between alcohol and domestic violence and on evidence from practitioners, it is reasonable to infer that services for the two kinds of problems should be linked. But linkage is both problematic and uncertain. There are philosophical, structural, and practical impediments to linkage, as we have discussed. Moreover, no existing scientific evaluation evidence indicates that linkage is successful. Two needs are certain: (1) study of the feasibility of linkage and identification of promising approaches to linkage, and (2) evaluation of the effects of linkage.

One focus of feasibility work should be the study of attitudes and beliefs toward the alcohol–domestic violence relationship among service providers and the implications of these beliefs for service linkage.[54] If the attitudes and beliefs among a range of service providers in both the domestic violence and chemical dependency fields were documented, it likely would be possible to develop plans for linkage that have a high probability of succeeding. Another line of linkage inquiry should focus on structural factors likely to affect efforts to link services. The bureaucratic placement and organization of the two kinds of services, as well as the method and level of financing of the services, are likely to influence both the feasibility and implementation of linkage.

Ultimately, evaluation of the domestic violence–chemical dependency service linkage will be the arbiter of its long-term use. At the present time, this presents a real challenge, given the infrequency of linkage in the real world. The first set of steps should probably involve conducting process and implementation evaluation work with the few existing examples of programmatic service linkage. Subsequently, outcome evaluation work using experimental or quasi-experimental designs could address questions of effectiveness.

The evaluation of linkage will be a complex undertaking, given the need to consider three major outcomes (success of victim services, batterer violence cessation, and chemical dependency recovery) and the involvement of multiple program types. Even when the technical evaluation methodology challenges are dealt with successfully, the findings are likely to be ambiguous. For example, some aspects of linkage such as batterer violence cessation may succeed, but others such as chemical dependency recovery may fail.

Given the high coincidence and seriousness of the domestic violence and chemical dependency problems, it is reasonable to begin linkage activities before evaluation results are in. Bennett and Lawson[54] argued that chemical dependency and domestic violence programs ought at least to assess for the cross-problems, making an argument that not to do so is at best programmatically unsatisfactory and at worst irresponsible. Given the very high personal and societal costs involved, we agree with their conclusion.

It is not premature to document the existence of chemical dependency problems among domestic violence victims and offenders and to attempt to determine whether violent victimization or violent behavior co-occur with a chemical dependency problem. Uncovering the problems can be the first step toward amelioration, and establishing the magnitude of the coexistent problems among clients may itself create an impetus toward service linkage.

ACKNOWLEDGMENT. The authors appreciate the editorial support of Richard S. Straw and the word-processing support of Catherine A. Boykin during the preparation of this chapter.

References

1. Straus MA, Gelles RJ, Steinmetz SK: *Behind Closed Doors: Violence in the American Family.* New York, Anchor Doubleday, 1980.
2. US Department of Health and Human Services: *Healthy People 2000: National Health Promotion and Disease Prevention Objectives* (DHHS publication PHS 91-50212). Washington, DC, US Government Printing Office, 1991.

3. Louis Harris and Associates Inc: *The Commonwealth Fund Survey of Women's Health*. New York, The Commonwealth Fund, 1993.

4. National Committee for Injury Prevention and Control: *Injury Prevention: Meeting the Challenge*. New York, Oxford Press, 1989.

5. Kurz D, Stark E: Not-so-benign neglect: The medical response to battering, in Yllo K, Bograd M (eds): *Feminist Perspectives in Wife Abuse*. Newbury Park, CA, Sage, 1988, pp 249–266.

6. McLeer S, Anwar R: Education is not enough: A systems failure in protecting battered women. *Ann Emerg Med* 18:651–653, 1989.

7. McLeer S, Anwar R: A study of battered women presenting in an emergency room. *Am J Public Health* 79:65–66, 1989.

8. Stark E, Flitcraft A, Frazier: Medicine and patriarchal violence: The social construction of a private event. *Int J Health Serv* 9:461–493, 1979.

9. Stark E, Flitcraft A: Spouse abuse, in Rosenberg ML, Fenley MA (eds): *Violence in America: A Public Health Approach*. New York, Oxford University Press, 1991, pp 123–157.

10. Harlow CW: *Female Victims of Violent Crime* (NCJ-126826). Washington, DC, US Department of Justice, Office of Justice Programs, Bureau of Justice Statistics, 1991.

11. Domino JV, Haber JD: Prior physical and sexual abuse in women with chronic headache: Clinical correlates. *Headache* 26:310–314, 1987.

12. Haber JE, Roos C: Effects of spouse abuse and/or sexual abuse in the development and maintenance of chronic pain in women. *Adv Pain Res Ther* 9:889–895, 1985.

13. Larsson G, Anderson M: Violence in the family: Morbidity and mortality consumption. *Scand J Soc Med:* 161–166, 1989.

14. Helton A: *Protocol of Care for the Battered Women: Prevention of Battering during Pregnancy* (prepared June 1986 at Texas Women's University through grant from Metropolitan Houston Chapter of March of Dimes Birth Defects Foundation). White Plains, NY, March of Dimes Birth Defect Foundation, 1987.

15. McFarlane J: Battering during pregnancy: Tip of an iceberg revealed. *Women Health* 15:69–84, 1989.

16. Drossman DA, Leserman J, Nachman G: Sexual and physical abuse in women with functional or organic gastrointestinal disorders. *Ann Intern Med* 113:828–833, 1990.

17. Koss MP: The women's mental health research agenda: Violence against women. *Am Psychol* 45:374–380, 1990.

18. Post R, Willett AB, Franks RD, et al: A preliminary report on the prevalence of domestic violence among psychiatric inpatients. *Am J Psychiatry* 137:974–975, 1987.

19. Rosewater LB: Battered or schizophrenic? Psychological tests can't tell, in Yllo K, Bograd M (eds): *Feminist Perspectives on Wife Abuse*. Newbury Park, CA, Sage, 1988, pp 200–216.

20. Walker LE: *The Battered Women Syndrome* (Springer Series: Focus on Women, vol 6). New York, Springer, 1984.

21. Amaro H, Fried LE, Cabral H, Zuckerman B: Violence during pregnancy and substance use. *Am J Public Health* 80:575–579, 1990.

22. Browne A: *When Battered Women Kill*. New York, Free Press, 1987.

23. Mercy IA, Saltzman IE: Violence among spouses in the United States, 1976–85. *Am J Public Health* 79:595–599, 1989.

24. Coleman DH, Straus MA: Alcohol abuse and family violence, in Gottheil E, Druley KA, Skoloda TE, Waxman HM (eds): *Alcohol, Drug Abuse, and Aggression*. Springfield, IL, Charles C. Thomas, 1983, pp 104–124.

25. Kantor GK, Straus MA: The "drunken bum" theory of wife beating. *Soc Probl* 34:213–231, 1987.

26. Kantor GK, Straus MA: Substance abuse as a precipitant of wife abuse victimizations. *Am J Drug Alcohol Abuse* 15:173–189, 1989.

27. Gondolf EW, Foster RA: Wife assault among VA alcohol rehabilitation patients. *Hosp Community Psychiatry* 42:74–79, 1991.

28. Hamilton CJ, Collins JJ: The role of alcohol in wife beating and child abuse, in Collins JJ Jr

(ed): *Drinking and Crime: Perspectives on the Relationships between Alcohol Consumption and Criminal Behavior*. New York, Guilford Press, 1981, pp 253–287.

29. Hotaling G, Sugarman D: An analysis of risk markers in husband to wife violence: The current state of knowledge. *Violence Vict* 1:101–124, 1986.

30. Leonard KE, Bromet EJ, Parkinson DK, *et al*: Patterns of alcohol use and physically aggressive behavior in men. *J Stud Alcohol* 46:279–282, 1985.

31. National Woman Abuse Prevention Project: *Alcohol Abuse and Domestic Violence* (Domestic Violence Fact Sheet). Springfield, IL, Illinois Department of Public Aid, n.d.

32. Rounsaville BJ: Theories in marital violence: Evidence from a study of battered women. *Victimology* 3:11–31, 1978.

33. Gayford JJ: Wife battering: A preliminary survey of 100 cases. *Br Med J* 1:194–197, 1975.

34. Carlson BE: Battered women and their assailants. *Soc Work* 22:455–460, 1977.

35. Roy M: A current survey of 150 cases, in Roy M (ed): *Battered Women: A Psychosociological Study of Domestic Violence*. New York, Van Nostrand Reinhold, 1977, pp 24–44.

36. Lehmann N, Krupp S: Alcohol-related domestic violence: Clinical implications and intervention strategies. *Alcohol Treat Q* 1(4):111–115, 1984.

37. Jones A, Schechter S: *When Love Goes Wrong: What to Do When You Can't Do Anything Right*. New York, HarperCollins, 1992.

38. Minnesota Coalition for Battered Women: *Safety First: Battered Women Surviving Violence When Alcohol and Drugs Are Involved*. Saint Paul, MN, Minnesota Coalition for Battered Women, 1992.

39. Barnett OW, Fagan RW: Alcohol use in male spouse abusers and their female partners. *J Fam Violence* 8(1):1–25, 1993.

40. Berenson AB, Stiglich NJ, Wilkinson GS, Anderson GD: Drug abuse and other risk factors for physical abuse in pregnancy among white non-Hispanic, black and Hispanic women. *Am J Obstet Gynecol* 164:1491–1499, 1991.

41. Erble PA: Alcohol abusers and non-users: A discriminant analysis of differences between two subgroups of batterers. *J Health Soc Behav* 23:260–271, 1982.

42. Frieze I, Knoble J: The effects of alcohol on marital violence. Paper presented at annual meeting of American Psychological Association, Montreal, Quebec, Canada, 1980.

43. Van Hasselt VB, Morrison RL, Bellack AS: Alcohol use in wife abusers and their spouses. *Addict Behav* 10:127–135, 1985.

44. Smith PH, Chescheir N: *Services Integration for Substance-Abusing Battered Women: Final Report*. Raleigh, NC, North Carolina's Governor's Institute for Alcohol and Substance Abuse, 1994.

45. Center for Substance Abuse Treatment: *Practical Approaches in the Treatment of Women Who Abuse Alcohol and Other Drugs* (DHHS publication SMA 94-3006). Rockville, MD, US Department of Health and Human Services, Public Health Service, Substance Abuse and Mental Health Services Administration, 1994.

46. Hankin J, Ortay IS: *Mental Disorder and Primary Medical Care: An Analytical Review of the Literature* (publication ADM 78-661, series D, no 5). Washington, DC, US Department of Health and Human Services, 1979.

47. Gomberg ESL: Suicide risk among women with alcohol problems. *Am J Public Health* 79:1363–1366, 1989.

48. Haver B: Female alcoholics: IV. The relationship between family violence and outcome 3–10 years after treatment. *Acta Psychiatr Scand* 77:449–455, 1987.

49. Korlath MJ: Alcoholism in battered women: A report of advocacy services to clients in a detoxification facility. *Victimology Int J* 292–299, 1979.

50. Smith PH, Gittelman DF: Psychological consequences of battering: Implications for women's health and medical practice. *NC Med J* 55(9):2–7, 1994.

51. Aramburu B, Leigh BC: For better or worse: Attributions about drunken aggression toward male and female victims. *Violence Vict* 6:31–41, 1991.

52. Corenblum B: Reactions to alcohol-related marital violence: Effects of one's own abuse experience and alcohol problems on causal attributions. *J Stud Alcohol* 11:665–674, 1983.

53. Richardson DC, Campbell JL: Alcohol and wife abuse: The effect of alcohol on attributions of blame for wife abuse. *Pers Soc Psychol Bull* 6:51–56, 1980.

54. Bennett L, Lawson M: Barriers to cooperation between domestic-violence and substance-abuse programs. *Fam Soc J Contemp Human Services* 75:277–286, 1994.

55. Gondolf EW: Alcohol abuse, wife assault, and power needs. Manuscript submitted for publication, Indiana, PA, Mid-Atlantic Abduction Training Institute, Indiana University of Pennsylvania, 1993.

56. Pernanen K: Alcohol and crimes of violence, in Kissin B, Begleiter H (eds): *The Biology of Alcoholism*, vol 4: *Social Aspects of Alcoholism*. New York, Plenum Press, 1976, pp 351–444.

57. Pernanen K: Theoretical aspects of the relationship between alcohol use and crime, in Collins J (ed): *Drinking and Crime: Perspectives on the Relationship between Alcohol Consumption and Criminal Behavior*. New York, Guilford Press, 1981, pp 1–69.

58. Steele CM, Josephs RA: Alcohol myopia: Its prized and dangerous effects. *Am Psychol* 45:921–933, 1990.

59. Frieze IH, Browne A: Violence in marriage, in Ohlin L, Tonry M (eds): *Family Violence*. Chicago, University of Chicago press, 1989, pp 163–218.

60. McClelland D: *Power: The Inner Experience*. New York, Wiley, 1975.

61. McClelland DC, Davis WN: The influence of unrestrained power concerns on drinking in working-class men, in McClelland DC, Davis WN, Kalin R, Wanner E (eds): *The Drinking Man*. New York, Free Press, 1972, pp 142–161.

62. Bowker L: *Beating Wife-Beating*. Lexington, MA, Heath, 1983.

63. Dobash RE, Dobash RP: *Violence Against Wives*. New York, Free Press, 1979.

64. Dobash RE, Dobash RP: *Women, Violence, and Social Change*. New York, Routledge, 1992.

65. Collins JJ: Alcohol and crime aetiology, in Russell J (ed): *Alcohol and Crime: Proceedings of a Mental Health Foundation Conference*. London, England, Mental Health Foundation, 1993, pp 22–32.

66. Fagan J: Intoxication and aggression, in Tonry M, Wilson JQ (eds): *Drugs and Crime*. Chicago, University of Chicago Press, 1990, pp 241–320.

67. Spieker G: What is the linkage between alcohol abuse and violence? In Gottheil E, Druley KA, Skiloda TE, Waxman HM (eds): *Alcohol, Drug Abuse and Aggression*. Springfield, IL, Charles C. Thomas, 1983, pp 125–136.

68. Bushman BJ, Cooper HM: Effects of alcohol on human aggression: An integrative research review. *Psychol Bull* 107:341–354, 1990.

69. Lang AR, Goeckner DJ, Adesso VJ, Marlatt GA: Effects of alcohol on aggression in male social drinkers. *J Abnorm Psychol* 84:508–518, 1975.

70. Taylor SP, Gammon CB: Effects of type and dose of alcohol on human physical aggression. *J Pers Soc Psychol* 32:169–175, 1975.

71. MacAndrew C, Edgerton RB: *Drunken Comportment: A Social Explanation*. Chicago, Aldine, 1969.

72. Leonard KE: Drinking patterns and intoxication in marital violence: Review, critique, and future directions for research, in Martin SE (ed): *Alcohol and Interpersonal Violence: Fostering Multidisciplinary Perspectives* (research monograph 24, NIH publication 93-3496). Rockville, MD, National Institute on Alcohol Abuse and Alcoholism, 1993, pp 253–280.

73. New York State Office for the Prevention of Domestic Violence: *Adult Domestic Violence: The Alcohol Connection*. Rensselaer, NY, New York State Office for the Prevention of Domestic Violence, 1993.

74. Levy AJ, Brekke JS: Spouse battering and chemical dependency: Dynamics, treatment, and service delivery, in Potter-Efron RT, Potter-Effron PS (eds): *Aggression, Family Violence and Chemical Dependency*. New York, Haworth Press, 1990, pp 81–97.

75. Chiauzzi EJ, Liljegren S: Taboo topics in addiction treatment: An empirical review of clinical folklore. *J Subst Abuse Treat* 10:303–316, 1993.

76. Institute of Medicine: *Broadening the Base of Treatment for Alcohol Problems*. Washington, DC, National Academy Press, 1990.

77. Roman PM, Blum TC: The medicalized conception of alcohol-related problems: Some social

sources and some social consequences of murkiness and confusion, in Pittman DJ, White HR (eds): *Society, Culture, and Drinking Patterns Reexamined.* New Brunswick, NJ, Rutgers Center of Alcohol Studies, Publications Division. 1991, pp 753–774.

78. Jellinek EM: *The Disease Concept of Alcoholism.* New Haven, CT, College and University Press, 1960.

79. Jellinek EM: Phases of alcohol addiction,in Pittman DJ, White HR (eds): *Society, Culture, and Drinking Patterns Reexamined.* New Brunswick, NJ, Rutgers Center of Alcohol Studies, Publications Division, 1991, pp 403–416.

80. Rogan A: Domestic violence and alcohol: Barriers to cooperation. *Alcohol Health Res World* 10:22–27, 1985/86.

81. Harner IC: The alcoholism treatment client and domestic violence. *Alcohol Health Res World* 12:150–152, 160, 1987/88.

82. Selzer M: The Michigan Alcoholism Screening Test: The quest for a new diagnostic instrument. *Am J Psychiatry* 127:1653–1658, 1971.

83. Burkins M: *Informational Packet on Individualized Care.* Massillon, OH, Longford Health Sources at Massillon Community Hospital, 1995.

84. Lindquist CU: Battered women as coalcoholics: Treatment implications and case study. *Psychotherapy* 23:622–628, 1986.

85. Agranoff R: Human services integration: Past and present challenges in public administration. *Public Admin Rev* 51:533–542, 1991.

86. US Department of Health and Human Services: *Services Integration: A Twenty-Year Retrospective.* Washington, DC, Office of the Inspector General, 1991.

87. Schlenger WE, Kroutil LA, Roland EJ, et al: *National Evaluation of Models for Linking Drug Abuse Treatment and Primary Care: Linking Drug Treatment and Primary Care: A Casebook* (report prepared for Clinical Medicine Branch, Division of Clinical Research, National Institute on Drug Abuse, contract 283-90-0001). Research Triangle Park, NC, Research Triangle Institute, 1992.

88. Schlenger WE, Etheridge RM, Hansen DJ, et al: Evaluation of state efforts to improve systems of care for children and adolescents with severe emotional disturbances: The CASSP initial cohort study. *J Ment Health Admin* 19:131–142, 1992.

89. Schlenger WE, Kroutil LA, Roland EJ, Dennis ML: *National Evaluation of Models for Linking Drug Abuse Treatment and Primary Care: Descriptive Report of Phase 1 Findings* (report prepared for Clinical Medicine Branch, Division of Clinical Research, National Institute on Drug Abuse contract 283-90-0001). Research Triangle Park, NC, Research Triangle Institute, 1992.

90. Erickson JR, Chong J, Anderson C, Stevens S: Service linkages: Understanding what fosters and what deters from service coordination for homeless adult drug users. *Contemp Drug Probl* 22:343–362, 1995.

91. Cayouette S: *The Addicted or Alcoholic Batterer.* Boston, EMERGE, 1990.

Contents of Previous Volumes

Index

ISBN 0-306-45358-4

90000